Lecture Notes in Computer Science 13079

More information about this subseries at http://www.springer.com/series/7409

Siuly Siuly · Hua Wang ·
Lu Chen · Yanhui Guo ·
Chunxiao Xing (Eds.)

Health
Information Science

10th International Conference, HIS 2021
Melbourne, VIC, Australia, October 25–28, 2021
Proceedings

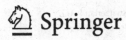

Editors
Siuly Siuly (iD)
Victoria University
Footscray, VIC, Australia

Lu Chen (iD)
Swinburne University of Technology
Melbourne, VIC, Australia

Chunxiao Xing (iD)
Tsinghua University
Beijing, China

Hua Wang (iD)
Victoria University
Footscray, VIC, Australia

Yanhui Guo (iD)
University of Illinois at Springfield
Springfield, NY, USA

ISSN 0302-9743   ISSN 1611-3349   (electronic)
Lecture Notes in Computer Science
ISBN 978-3-030-90884-3   ISBN 978-3-030-90885-0   (eBook)
https://doi.org/10.1007/978-3-030-90885-0

LNCS Sublibrary: SL3 – Information Systems and Applications, incl. Internet/Web, and HCI

This Springer imprint is published by the registered company Springer Nature Switzerland AG
The registered company address is: Gewerbestrasse 11, 6330 Cham, Switzerland

Preface

The International Conference Series on Health Information Science (HIS) provides a forum for disseminating and exchanging multidisciplinary research results in computer science/information technology and health science and services. It covers all aspects of health information sciences and systems that support health information management and health service delivery.

The 10th International Conference on Health Information Science (HIS 2021) was held in Melbourne, Australia, during October 25–28, 2021. Founded in April 2012 as the International Conference on Health Information Science and Their Applications, the conference continues to grow to include an ever broader scope of activities. The main goal of these events is to provide international scientific forums for researchers to exchange new ideas in a number of fields that interact in-depth through discussions with their peers from around the world. The scope of the conference includes the following: (1) medical/health/biomedicine information resources, such as patient medical records, devices and equipment, and software and tools to capture, store, retrieve, process, analyze, and optimize the use of information in the health domain; (2) data management, data mining, and knowledge discovery, all of which play a key role in decision-making, management of public health, examination of standards, and privacy and security issues; (3) computer visualization and artificial intelligence for computer-aided diagnosis; and (4) development of new architectures and applications for health information systems.

The conference solicited and gathered technical research submissions related to all aspects of the conference scope. All the submitted papers were peer-reviewed by at least three international experts drawn from the Program Committee. After the rigorous peer-review process, a total of 16 full papers and seven short papers among 56 submissions were selected on the basis of originality, significance, and clarity and were accepted for publication in the proceedings. The authors were from Australia, Bangladesh, China, the Czech Republic, India, Iran, the Netherlands, Pakistan, Serbia, Spain, and the USA.

The high quality of the program – guaranteed by the presence of an unparalleled number of internationally recognized top experts – is reflected in the content of the proceedings. The conference was therefore a unique event, where attendees were able to appreciate the latest results in their field of expertise and acquire additional knowledge in other fields. The program was structured to favour interactions among attendees coming from many different areas, scientifically and geographically, from academia and from industry.

Finally, we acknowledge all those who contributed to the success of HIS 2021 but whose names are not listed here.

October 2021

Siuly Siuly
Hua Wang
Lu Chen
Yanhui Guo
Chunxiao Xing

Organization

General Co-chairs

Fernando Martin-Sanchez   Institute of Health Carlos III, Spain
Hua Wang   Victoria University, Australia

Program Co-chairs

Siuly Siuly   Victoria University, Australia
Yanhui Guo   University of Illinois at Springfield, USA
Chunxiao Xing   Tsinghua University, China

Publicity Co-chairs

Enamul Kabir   University of Southern Queensland, Australia
Varun Bajaj   IIITDM Jabalpur, India
Abdulkadir Sengur   Firat University, Turkey
Yong Zhang   Tsinghua University, China

Publication Co-chairs

Rui Zhou   Swinburne University of Technology, Australia
Lu Chen   Swinburne University of Technology, Australia

Local Arrangement Co-chairs

Jiaying Kou   Victoria University, Australia
Supriya Supriya   Victorian Institute of Technology, Australia

Workshop Chair

Manik Sharma   DAV University, India

Website Chair

Yong-Feng Ge   La Trobe University, Australia

Finance Chair

Sudha Subramani   Victoria University, Australia

HIS Steering Committee Representative

Yanchun Zhang   Victoria University, Australia

Program Committee

Venkat Achalam   Christ University, India
Nahida Afroz   Comilla University, Bangladesh
Ashik Mostafa Alvi   Victoria University, Australia
Alaleh Aminzadeh   University of Melbourne, Australia
Varun Bajaj   IIITDM Jabalpur, India
Genlang Chen   Zhejiang University, China
Lu Chen   Swinburne University of Technology, Australia
Soon Chun   City University of New York, USA
Yong-Feng Ge   La Trobe University, Australia
Yanhui Guo   University of Illinois at Springfield, USA
Zakir Hossain   University of Dhaka, Bangladesh
Zhisheng Huang   Vrije Universiteit Amsterdam, The Netherlands
Md Rafiqul Islam   University of Technology Sydney, Australia
Samsad Jahan   Ahsanullah University of Science and Technology,
                                   Bangladesh
Enamul Kabir   University of Southern Queensland, Australia
Smith Khare   Shri Ramdeobaba College of Engineering and
                                   Management, India
Humayun Kiser   Comilla University, Bangladesh
Jiaying Kou   Victoria University, Australia
Shaofu Lin   Beijing University of Technology, China
Gang Luo   University of Washington, USA
Jiangang Ma   Federation University Australia, Australia
Fernando Martin-Sanchez   Instituto de Salud Carlos III, Spain
Mehdi Naseriparsa   Federation University Australia, Australia
Fatemeh Noroozi   University of Tartu, Estonia
Khushbu Patel   The Children's Hospital of Philadelphia, USA
Yongrui Qin   University of Huddersfield, UK
Atikur Rahman   Jahangirnagar University, Bangladesh
Muhammad Tariq Sadiq   University of Lahore, Pakistan
Joy Shao   Northumbria University, UK
Ravinder Singh   Victoria University, Australia
Siuly Siuly   Victoria University, Australia
Sudha Subramani   Victoria University, Australia
Weiqing Sun   University of Toledo, Spain
Supriya Supriya   Victoria University, Australia
Sachin Taran   IIITDM Jabalpur, India
Md. Nurul Ahad Tawhid   Victoria University, Australia
Hua Wang   Victoria University, Australia
Kate Wang   RMIT University, Australia

Fangxiang Wu	University of Saskatchewan, Canada
Da Zhang	Harvard Medical School, USA
Guo-Qiang Zhang	Case Western Reserve University, USA
Yong Zhang	Tsinghua University, China
Xiaolong Zheng	Chinese Academy of Sciences, China
Youwen Zhu	Nanjing University of Aeronautics and Astronautics, China

Additional Reviewers

Akbari, Hesam
Kamble, Ashwin
Kamble, Kranti
Malik, Shahida

Neupane, Ashish
Pujari, Medha
Singh, Ravinder
Subramani, Sudha

Contents

Medical Data Analysis

Medical Record Mining (I)

Medical Data Mining (II)

Medical Data Processing

COVID-19

Research on the Fluctuation Characteristics of Social Media Message Sentiment with Time Before and During the COVID-19 Epidemic

Chaohui Guo[1], Shaofu Lin[1,2(✉)], Zhisheng Huang[3], Chengyu Shi[1], and Yahong Yao[1]

[1] Faculty of Information Technology, Beijing University of Technology, Beijing 100124, China
linshaofu@bjut.edu.cn
[2] Beijing Institute of Smart City, Faculty of Information Technology, Beijing University of Technology, Beijing, China
[3] Department of Computer Science, Vrije University Amsterdam, Amsterdam, The Netherlands

Abstract. "Tree hole" refers to a social media formed after the death of a social media user, in which other users continue to leave messages due to emotional resonance. This paper focuses on exploring the fluctuation of emotions with time in a "tree hole" of social media such as Microblog, and provides ideas and support for suicide warning, rescue, and user portraits of patients with depression in the "tree hole". In this paper, the dataset of 2,356,066 messages captured from the "tree hole" Microblog with the "tree hole" agent (i.e., an AI program) and pre-processed. Subsequently, the effective dataset was labeled by a text sentiment analysis model based on BERT and BiLSTM, and accordingly the sentiment was scored. Then the scored data was visualized and analyzed in the time dimension. Finally, it was found that the sentiment of the "tree hole" messages reached a trough at 4:00 am and a peak around 8:00 am. In addition, the overall trend of "tree hole" sentiment has fluctuated downwards from Monday to Sunday. We have concluded that the sentiment of patients with depression fluctuates regularly at some special time points, and special events such as the outbreak of COVID-19 and so on, have a great impact on the emotions of patients with depression. Therefore, it is necessary to strengthen warning and intervention for those who has expressed thoughts of suicide at special points to prevent the spread and fermentation of suicidal emotions in the "tree hole" in time. In addition, the rescue volunteers for patients with depression as Tree Hole Rescue Team should make corresponding adjustments to the rescue strategy when special events occur. This research is of great significance for the emergency response of "tree hole" depressed users in major events such as COVID-19 epidemic.

Keywords: Microblog tree hole · Message sentiment · COVID-19 epidemic · Scrapy-Redis · BERT-BiLSTM

This research is partially funded by the high-level foreign talent fund program of Beijing (No. C202004).

S. Siuly et al. (Eds.): HIS 2021, LNCS 13079, pp. 3–14, 2021.
https://doi.org/10.1007/978-3-030-90885-0_1

1 Introduction

Depression has become a common disorder. More than 300 million people are living with depression all around the world. It can happen to anybody and begin at any time [1]. According to the 2019 China Mental Health Survey, major depressive disorder was the most prevalent sentiment disorder [2]. Depression brings huge burdens and sufferings to individuals and their friends, leading to an extremely high suicide rate among depressed patients [3]. Close to 800,000 people die due to suicide every year [4]. According to the United Nations report, suicide has become the second leading cause of unnatural death among young people [5]. In addition, more and more young people are addicted to the Internet. As of December 2020, the number of Chinese Internet users has reached 989 million, and the Internet penetration rate has reached 70.4% [6]. With the increasing number of users in the virtual world, online social media has gradually become the main way of socializing for people [7]. The freedom of expression and the instant delivery feature of Microblog [8] have allowed many young patients with depression to express their suicidal feelings and wishes through this platform.

The term "tree hole" comes from a fairy tale. The barber knew that the emperor had a pair of donkey ears, but was afraid to tell others the secret. So, he told the secret to a hole in a big tree on the mountain [9]. With the popularity of the Internet, more and more people are inclined to tell their secrets through online social media platforms. Many patients with depression often express their real thoughts through social media platforms (such as Microblog) when they have suicidal thoughts, and thus the social media platforms turn to be "tree holes" in the virtual world. On March 17, 2012, the depressed patient with a nickname "Zou Fan" committed suicide after posting the last message on her Microblog account. Since then the message area of the Microblog account of "Zou Fan" has become a "tree hole" for many patients with depression in the virtual world. From 2012 to 2020, "Zou Fan Tree Hole" has more than 2.3 million messages, and it has become the largest "tree hole" in Microblog. Professor Zhisheng Huang has developed a "tree hole" agent (i.e., an AI program) that patrols large "tree holes" in social media and automatically screens people with obvious suicidal tendencies [10].

In different time periods, the sentiments of Microblog "tree hole" users are various, especially when a special event occurs during a specific time period, the overall sentiment of the Microblog "tree hole" will fluctuate, such as the outbreak of COVID-19 epidemic. Most previous analysis of "tree hole" message data was only aimed at the time characteristics of the number of messages [11, 12], whereas the time characteristics of the sentiment of the "tree hole" messages were less analyzed. In this research, we mainly scored the emotional characteristics of the messages from the largest "tree hole" on Microblog, the "Zou Fan Tree Hole", and analyzed the fluctuation of the emotion of the messages in the "tree hole" in time dimension. Furthermore, we analyzed the reasons for "tree hole" emotion fluctuations with time, and provided ideas and data support for suicide warning and intervention.

2   Methods

2.1   Models

Model Selection
There are two main models of sentiment classification. One is based on deep learning, and the other is based on dictionary [13]. The characteristics of the "tree hole" message include short text, large number of messages, and complex thoughts expressed.

The sentiment classification model based on dictionary needs to expand a large number of labelled vocabularies, meanwhile the analysis effect of short text is poor. In addition, the sentiment classification model based on dictionary cannot analyze the relationship between vocabularies and context in the message text. The sentiment classification model based on deep learning have strong generalization ability and outstanding effect on short text analysis. And it also takes into account the order and semantic characteristics of words. Therefore, the sentiment classification model based on deep learning is more suitable for analyzing the emotion of "tree hole" messages.

BERT (Bidirectional Encoder Representations from Transformers)
Since the Microblog comment texts are short texts, the text vectorization layer of this sentiment polarity analysis model does not use the commonly used word2vec [14] text vector representation. And word2vec takes words as processing unit, which needs to go through text preprocessing, feature extraction, feature vector representation, vector stitching, and finally to generate a vector representation of the text. However, BERT offers an advantage over the traditional models such as word2vec. BERT model uses the characters as the processing unit and maps each word into the form of an n-dimensional word vector.

BiLSTM (Bi-directional Long Short-Term Memory)
BiLSTM layer [14] is composed of two parts: forward LSTM and backward LSTM. If only the LSTM model is used to determine the polarity of message sentiment, there will be an inability to encode the message from backward to forward. The structure of LSTM and BiLSTM are shown in Figs. 1 and 2:

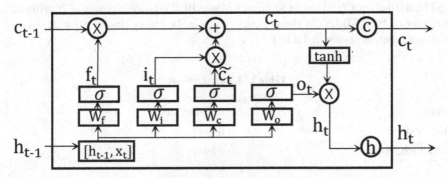

Fig. 1. Structure of LSTM

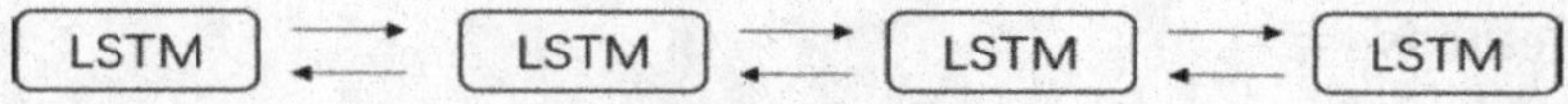

Fig. 2. Structure of BiLSTM

Compared with other neural networks, BiLSTM can extract text sequence information more effectively, so it has a much better performance in solving the problem of text sentiment classification. The gates in Fig. 1 are expressed in the equations as the following.

Equation (1) is Forget gate:

$$f_t = \sigma(U_f \cdot c_{t-1} + W_f x_t + b_f) \tag{1}$$

Equation (2) is Input gate:

$$i_t = \sigma(U_f \cdot h_{t-1} + W_f x_t + b_i) \tag{2}$$

Equation (3) is Output gate:

$$O_t = \sigma(U_o \cdot h_{t-1} + W_o x_t + b_o) \tag{3}$$

Equation (4) is Memory cell gate:

$$\tilde{c}_t = tanh(U_c \cdot h_{t-1} + W_c x_t + b_c) \tag{4}$$

Equation (5) is Memory cell gate:

$$c_t = f_t \circ c_{t-1} + i_t \circ \tilde{c}_o \tag{5}$$

Equation (6) is Final gate:

$$h_t = O_t \circ tanh(c_t) \tag{6}$$

Model Evaluation

This research uses the BERT-BiLSTM to predict the sentiment of the Treehole message. The accuracy of the BiLSTM model used in text analysis tasks is higher than that of the LSTM and the TextCNN [15]. In addition, because BERT utilizes a powerful Transformer mechanism, BERT-BiLSTM shows better results in the binary classification analysis of text sentiment, as shown in Table 1.

Table 1. Labeled dataset

Models	AccuracyMetric
BiLSTM	0.7548
BERT-BiLSTM	0.8941

2.2 Emotion Scoring Algorithm

This paper uses the mathematical expectation of calculating message sentiment to score each message. The higher the score, the more positive of the message, as shown in Eq. (7).

$$S = P \times \hat{P} + N \times \hat{N} \tag{7}$$

In this paper, for the convenience of calculation, the weight of P (Positive) is set to 1, and the weight of N (Negative) is set to 0. $\hat{P}$ and $\hat{N}$ refer to the positive and negative probabilities of the message sentiment calculated by the sentiment analysis model, respectively. S represents the total score of the message sentiment, the value range is [0,1]. And the closer S is to 1, the more positive the sentiment is.

Emotion Scoring Algorithm Based on Every Hour in a Day

$$y = \frac{\sum_{i=1}^{max} S(Hour = x)_i}{max} x \in [0, 23] \tag{8}$$

Where i, max and $Hour$ is the serial number, the largest serial number, and the Hour value of each data item in the dataset, respectively. And S is the Eq. (7) under the condition of $Hour = x$. Therefore, the value of y is the average of the sentiment scores of all messages in the dataset, where $Hour$ is equal to x. The value range of y is [0,1], and the sentiment at $y = 0.5$ is neutral.

Emotion Scoring Algorithm Based on Every Day in a Week

$$y = \frac{\sum_{i=1}^{max} S(Week = x)_i}{max} x \in [1, 7] \tag{9}$$

Where i, max and $Week$ is the serial number, the largest serial number, and the Week value of each data item in the dataset, respectively. And S is the Eq. (7) under the condition of $Week = x$. Therefore, the value of y is the average of the sentiment scores of all messages in the dataset, where $Week$ is equal to x. The value range of y is [0,1]. And the larger the value of y, the more positive the sentiment, and the sentiment at $y = 0.5$ is neutral.

3 Data Pre-processing and Sentiment Prediction

3.1 Data Source

The data source of this paper is the Microblog message of "Zou Fan". The "tree hole" agent is used to capture messages sent by Microblog users through the "tree hole". And the Scrapy-Redis distributed crawler [17] was written to complete and correct the missing and incorrect fields of the message data. The 2,356,066 messages from March 18, 2012 to August 31, 2020 finally constituted "Raw dataset 1.0", as shown in Table 2.

Table 2. Raw dataset 1.0

Date	Time	Message-ID	User-ID	User-Name	Message	Other
2012-03-18	10:54	Null	123	Alan	Come back soon	Null
...	...	...	...	...	...	...
2020/08/31	21:29	123456	456	Bob	I will live	Chen XX

3.2 Data Preprocessing

In this experiment, we chose the Scrapy crawler framework to fix the errors and missing fields in the "Raw dataset 1.0". Since the Scrapy crawler framework does not have distributed characteristics, this experiment used the Redis in-memory database with distributed characteristics to improve the Scrapy crawler framework. Finally, a distributed crawler framework with Scrapy-Redis is formed.

It can be observed that "Raw dataset 1.0" has many problems, such as inconsistent data format and invalid information in the message. In order to solve these problem, we wrote a program to process the "Raw dataset 1.0" as follows: (1) Normalize the time information of each data item in the data set. (2) Calculate the day of the week by year, month, and day. (3) Sort the message data in chronological order to form a "Preprocessed data set", as shown in Table 3.

Table 3. Preprocessed dataset

Year	Month	Day	Hour	Minute	Week	User-ID	User-Name	Message
2012	03	18	10	54	7	123	Alan	Come back soon
...	...	...	...	...	...	...	...	...
2020	08	31	23	59	1	456	Bob	I will live

3.3 Sentiment Prediction

Training Dataset

This paper used the deep learning method to determine the sentiment polarity of the "tree hole" message, so a tremendous amount of labelled data is needed as the training set of the deep learning model. In this experiment, we randomly selected 100,000 pieces of data from the "Preprocessed dataset" as the "Labelled dataset". The sentiment polarity of the messages in the "Labelled dataset" was automatically determined by a publicly available generic sentiment analysis tool [18], where the label "0" represents negative sentiment and the label "1" represents positive sentiment. However, public sentiment analysis tools are not effective in specific scenarios. This experiment used a combination of public sentiment analysis tools and manual screening. After labelling the "Labelled dataset" by sentiment analysis tool, we wrote rules to further filter the "Labelled dataset". The main rules are as follows: (1) Delete messages where the emotions represented by the emoji and the emotion represented by the labels are different; (2) Delete non-Chinese messages; (3) Delete messages composed of symbols; (4) Delete redundant messages, and only keep emotion labels and message texts. Finally, the "Labelled dataset" consisting of 40,000 messages with positive emotions and 40,000 messages with negative emotions was retained after screening, as shown in Table 4.

Table 4. Labelled dataset

Target	Message
1	Thanks for the hug. I'm much better. Good night
...	...
0	Suddenly want to die

Model Training and Output

The experiment chose a deep learning model based on BERT-BiLSTM for the sentiment polarity analysis. The vector dimension output after the BiLSTM layer is the specified units, which is different from the vector dimension of the label. Therefore, this experiment adds a fully connected layer after the BiLSTM model. Finally, the model outputs the results to the sentiment prediction output layer [19].

The sentiment prediction output layer of this model is the SoftMax function, which maps the input to real numbers between 0 and 1 and ensures that the sum of the probabilities of classification is exactly 1. In this experiment, the output of the SoftMax function is $(\hat{x}, \hat{y})$, where $\hat{x}$ is the probability of the message sentiment being negative, and $\hat{y}$ is the probability of the message sentiment being positive, and the sum of both is exactly 1.

Dataset Sentiment Prediction

In the experiment, the "Labelled dataset" was divided into training set, validation set and test set according to the ratio of 9:0.5:0.5.

This paper selected the BERT-BiLSTM as the training model to judge the sentiment polarity of all messages in the "Preprocessed dataset". And the "Sentiment prediction dataset" is obtained, as shown in Table 5. The value of Emotion represents the sentiment polarity of the message, which is divided into positive emotion (1) and negative emotion (0), $\hat{P}$ and $\hat{N}$ represent the probability of positive emotion and negative emotion of the message, respectively. The prediction results of the BERT-BiLSTM model are shown in Table 5.

Table 5. Sentiment prediction dataset

Year	Month	Day	Hour	Minute	Week	Message	Emotion	$\hat{P}$	$\hat{N}$
2012	03	18	10	54	7	Come back soon	1	0.272	0.728
...	...	...	...	...	...	...	...	...	...
2020	08	31	23	59	1	I will live	1	0.273	0.727

4   Experimental Results and Analysis

4.1   Analysis of "Tree Hole" Message Sentiment in a Day

In order to study the impact of the COVID-19 epidemic on the sentiment of the "tree hole", the "Sentiment prediction dataset" was divided into two parts, that is, the data from 2012 to 2019 and the data formed after the outbreak of the COVID-19 in 2020.

This paper uses Eq. (8) to score the information sentiment of every one hour period of a day and plot the results. The result is shown in Fig. 3.

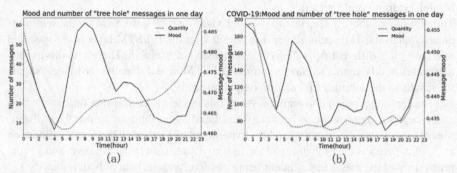

Fig. 3. The number and the fluctuation of sentiment of "tree hole" messages during 24 h a day before the COVID-19 epidemic (a) and during the epidemic (b)

It can be seen that there is obvious difference between the sentiment of the "tree hole" on Microblog before the COVID-19 epidemic and during the epidemic.

1. In daily life before the COVID-19 epidemic, the lowest point of "tree hole" sentiment in a day appeared around 4 am. The highest point of "tree hole" sentiment appeared in the early morning from 7 am to 9 am. After that the sentiment in the "tree hole" gradually declined until 12 at noon when there was a rebound, and reached the peak around 1 pm. After 1pm, the sentiment in the "tree hole" gradually declined, and reached the second low point of sentiment around 6 pm. Then the sentiment in the "tree hole" started to rise rapidly and reached to the peak at about 1 am.
2. From the above curves, it can be found that negative emotions dominate in the "tree hole". And the emotions in the "tree hole" during the epidemic were much lower than those in the "tree hole" before the epidemic. The peak point of "tree hole" emotion

in a day during the epidemic became around 0:00 a.m., while the lowest point was around 10 am.

3. The number of messages was correlated with the sentiment in the "tree hole". The sentiment of the messages was also relatively positive during the time period when the number of messages was high, and conversely the sentiment of the messages was relatively low. However, there was an anomaly in the early morning from 7am to 8 am. The sentiment turned to be relatively positive in that time period, but the number of messages was low.

4.2 Analysis of "Tree Hole" Message Sentiment in a Week

After analyzing the sentiment fluctuations of the "tree hole" within a day, we continued to draw and analyze the weekly sentiment fluctuations of the "tree hole" before and during COVID-19 epidemic.

This paper uses Eq. (9) to score the information sentiment of each time period of the day and plot the results. The result is shown in Fig. 4. The x-axis represents Monday to Sunday, and the y-axis represents the "tree hole" sentiment score.

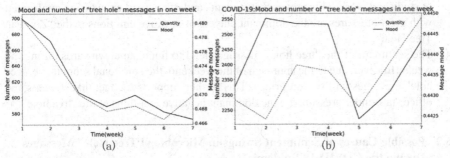

(a)   (b)

Fig. 4. The number and the fluctuation of sentiment of "tree hole" messages during a week before the COVID-19 epidemic (a) and during the epidemic (b)

As can be seen from Fig. 4, the situation of messages and sentiment swings within a week during the epidemic differed significantly from that during the epidemic.

1. In general, the sentiment in the "tree hole" of Microblog fluctuates and decreases throughout the week. The highest point of the "tree hole" sentiment usually appeared on Monday, and this sentiment gradually declined day by day until a brief rebound on Friday and then continued to go down on weekend.
2. The highest point of "tree hole" sentiment during the epidemic was also much lower than the lowest point of "tree hole" sentiment before the epidemic. The sentiments of "tree hole" users during the epidemic reached its lowest point on Friday, the opposite of the daily situation.
3. Under normal circumstances, the number of "tree hole" messages in a week showed a downward trend in daily situations. During the epidemic, the number of "tree hole" messages showed big fluctuations in a week. The number of "tree hole" messages during the epidemic was less on Tuesday and Friday, and more on weekends.

5 Discussion and Suggestions

5.1 Possible Causes of Sentiment Swings of Microblog "Tree Hole" Messages in General

As shown in Figs. 3a and 4a, we can infer that the possible reasons for forming the sentiment fluctuation pattern of the "tree hole" messages in daily situation are as follows.

1. The sentiment in the "tree hole" fluctuates regularly over time. But the negative sentiment always dominates in the "tree hole" messages.
2. In the tree hole, users are most negative at 4 am, and most active at around 8 am. This shows that "tree hole" users who stay up late and have insomnia will have a lot of negative sentiment. On the contrary, after a moderate amount of sleep, the sentiment of "tree hole" users will be relieved, leading to a rise in emotions of the "tree hole". This shows that sleep condition has a direct impact on the sentiment of the "tree hole" users.
3. Around 6 pm is also the time when there are more negative emotions in the "tree hole" message, because people need to vent their negative emotions during a day of study and work. This proves that students and office workers who are confronted with great pressures are the dominant players of negative emotions in the "Zou Fan Tree Hole".
4. The sentiment of the "tree hole" messages tend to fluctuate downwards during the week. However, due to the approach of the weekend, the emotional score in the "tree hole" messages will rise on Friday. This further supports the fact that students and office staff under pressure are the dominant negative emotions in the "tree hole".

5.2 Possible Causes of Sentiment Swings in Microblog "Tree Hole" Messages During the COVID-19 Epidemic

As shown in Figs. 3b and 4b, we can infer the sentiment fluctuation pattern and possible causes of the "tree hole" messages during the COVID-19 epidemic are as follows.

1. After the outbreak of the COVID-19 epidemic, the sentiments of the "tree hole" has changed significantly, showing a trend different from previous fluctuations.
2. During the epidemic, the daily sentiment swing in the "tree hole" became more dramatic. This led to four troughs in the sentiment of the messages every day. These four troughs appeared at 4 a.m., 10 a.m., 3 p.m., and 6 p.m.
3. During the epidemic, "tree hole" sentiment was lower than normal throughout the week.

5.3 Suggestions

Based on the above analysis, the following suggestions are made for suicide warning and rescue of "tree hole" users.

1. It is suggested that the Tree Hole Rescue Team should enhance suicide prevention and control mechanisms based on monitoring and warning suicide information. Mainly aimed at the "double low" period when mood is extremely low and the number of people is small, and passive early warning is transformed into active intervention.
2. The sensitivity of suicide warning in "tree hole" is adjusted dynamically according to the changing law of message mood. It is recommended to allocate more rescue resources at the lowest emotional point of the "tree hole" within a certain period.
3. Increase the attention on the "tree-hole" users who send messages early in the morning, maybe staying up late and suffering from insomnia. Actively discover "tree hole" crowds with irregular work and rest, and accordingly increase the alert sensitivity to such crowds.
4. The Tree Hole Rescue Team should stay vigilant persistently in the event of the COVID-19 epidemic or other special event. The intensity of suicide warning and suicide intervention should be adjusted according to the changing law of the sentiments of "tree hole" users. For example, during the COVID-19 epidemic, the Tree Hole Rescue Team should improve the intensity and sensitivity of suicide warning, especially on Fridays at 4 am, 10am and 6 pm. If necessary, we should take the initiative to post positive messages in the "tree hole" to stop the spread of negative emotions. This can be used to intervene in advance of suicide. By intervening in suicidal tendencies in advance, our research results can be helpful to the Tree Hole Rescue Team to better carry out rescue work.

6   Conclusion and Outlook

In this paper, we analyze the sentiment and quantity of messages in the "tree hole" of Microblog in time dimension, and we can conclude that the overall sentiment of the messages in the "tree hole" fluctuates regularly with time. And the fluctuation pattern will change when certain big events occur. In addition, few messages and low sentiment of the "double bottom" time period, should be appropriate to increase the sensitivity of suicide warning. If necessary, sending positive messages to the "tree hole" through the rescue team during the "double bottom" period turns passive rescue into active early intervention. This can assist the rescue team to carry out better work.

This paper has completed the analysis of the temporal characteristics of the sentiment of the Microblog "tree hole" messages in terms of hours in a day and days in a week, and compared the changes of sentiment fluctuations before and during the COVID-19 epidemic. However, we haven't analyzed the temporal characteristics of the sentiment of "tree hole" messages in terms of months and years. Since the data is only available until August 2020, we haven't analyzed the temporal characteristics of the sentiment of the "tree hole" messages in the context of regular epidemic prevention and control. Therefore, we will continue to complete the dataset and expand to more social media. And we plan to use more sentiment analysis methods to analyze the sentiment of the "tree hole" messages in a month, a year and other temporal dimensions.

References

1. Losekam, S., Konrad, C.: Depression. In: Kircher, T. (ed.) Kompendium der Psychotherapie, pp. 101–143. Springer, Heidelberg (2019). https://doi.org/10.1007/978-3-662-57287-0_7

2. Huang, Y., et al.: Prevalence of mental disorders in China: a cross-sectional epidemiological study. Lancet Psychiatry **6**(3), 211–224 (2019)
3. Zhu, W.: The formation, harm and response of depression. J. Polit. Sci. Eng. **2021**(03), 70–71 (2021)
4. WHO TEAM: Suicide in the world. World Health Organization, pp. 1–32 (2019)
5. Rozanov, V.A., Rakhimkulova, A.S.: Suicidal ideation in adolescents—a transcultural analysis. In: Kumar, U. (ed.) Handbook of Suicidal Behaviour. Springer, Singapore (2017). https://doi.org/10.1007/978-981-10-4816-6_15
6. CNNIC: The 47th China Statistical Report on Internet Development. The 47th China Statistical Report on Internet Development, pp. 1–118 (2021)
7. Li, C.: Research on group loneliness in online social media environment. Huazhong Normal University (2019)
8. Yang, F., Huang, Z., Yang, B., Ruan, J., Nie, W., Fang, S.: Analysis of suicidal ideation of Microblog "tree hole" users based on artificial intelligence technology. J. Nurs. **34**(24), 42–45 (2019)
9. Lv, S.: On the anonymity effect of tree hole communication. Literary Educ. **2021**(12), 33–34 (2021)
10. Feng, X.-H., Huang, Z.: Using AI to brighten the lives of depressed patients. China Sci. Technol. Ind. **2019**(10), 65–66 (2019)
11. Gong, J., Lin, S., Huang, Z.: Study on the spatial characteristics of depression patients' data on Microblog "tree holes." China Digit. Med. **15**(04), 70–74 (2020)
12. Jing, X., Lin, S., Huang, Z.: Research on the behavior pattern of microblog "tree hole" users with their temporal characteristics. In: Huang, Z., Siuly, S., Wang, H., Zhou, R., Zhang, Y. (eds.) Health Information Science. HIS 2020. LNCS, vol. 12435, pp. 25-34. Springer, Cham (2020). https://doi.org/10.1007/978-3-030-61951-0_3
13. Zhang, J.: A combination of Lexicon-based and classified-based methods for sentiment classification based on Bert. J. Phys.: Conf. Ser. 1802(3), 032113 (2021)
14. Mikolov, T., Chen, K., Corrado, G.S., et al.: Efficient estimation of word representations in vector space. In: International Conference on Learning Representations (2013)
15. Liu, W., Li, Y., Luo, J., Li, W., Fu, S.: Chinese short text sentiment analysis based on BERT and BiLSTM. J. Taiyuan Normal Univ. (Nat. Sci. Edn.) **19**(04), 52–58 (2020)
16. Fu, Y., Liao, J., Li, Y., Wang, S., Li, D., Li, X.: Multiple perspective attention based on double BiLSTM for aspect and sentiment pair extraction. Neurocomputing **438**, 302–311 (2021)
17. Yin, F., He, X., Liu, Z.: Research on scrapy-based distributed crawler system for crawling semi-structure information at high speed. In: 2018 IEEE 4th International Conference on Computer and Communications (ICCC), pp. 1–6 (2018)
18. Baidu.Sentiment_Classify[EB/OL]   (2019).   https://ai.baidu.com/tech/nlp/sentiment/_classify
19. Yan, Y.: Research on text sentiment analysis of microblog hot topics based on deep learning. Nanchang University (2020)

Advancing Health Information System with System Thinking: Learning Challenges of E-Health in Bangladesh During COVID-19

Samsad Jahan[1] and Forkan Ali[2(✉)]

[1] Ahsanullah University of Science and Engineering, Dhaka, Bangladesh
[2] School of Humanities and Social Sciences, UNSW Canberra, Canberra, Australia

Abstract. *Background*: Public health system is connected to a complex dynamic of overall systematic processes of socio-political structure. Therefore, ensuring a high-quality digital healthcare system has inter-connected impacts on the war of COVID-19 prevention and beneficial for the health and welfare of people. Adopting an electronic vaccination registration system in Bangladesh has already made a huge impact in bringing the huge population under the vaccine scheme in a responsive manner. However, the country still has been struggling to achieve a systematic and technical strength due to a range of issues such as technical knowledge of healthcare professionals in providing services (for instance, e-healthcare services), use of tech tools and their application, developing and managing data, data visualization, and data availability.

Objective: The advancement of the health information system (HIS) develops the entire healthcare service in a country. This paper aims to explore how a developing country like Bangladesh has been fighting the COVID-19 pandemic and how the adoption of a robust digital health information system can impact the overall health and living conditions of the large population at stake.

Method: Based on system thinking and modeling, this study provided and described information based on existing data obtained from different inter-connecting sources with contributions to the systematic approach indicating a brief statistical data analysis.

Results: This study finds out that adopting a rigorous digital health information system during COVID-19 helped Bangladesh immensely to fight the ongoing pandemic and minimized the overall risks, but she still has a lot of scope to improve.

Keywords: Digital health information system · E-health in Bangladesh · Systematic analysis

1 Introduction

Unexpectedly, Coronavirus (COVID-19) disease emerged in December 2019 in China and spread all over the world exponentially. The COVID-19 is still rising continuously, and thus the healthcare systems require more healthcare facilities and clinical services.

© Springer Nature Switzerland AG 2021
S. Siuly et al. (Eds.): HIS 2021, LNCS 13079, pp. 15–23, 2021.
https://doi.org/10.1007/978-3-030-90885-0_2

To support the management of COVID-19 cases, modern medicine needs faster, efficient, and effective digital health technologies. Calton et al. provided several tips to applying telemedicine as one of the measures to decline the transmission of COVID-19 [1]. Keesara et al. conducted a study on the capabilities and potential of digital health to fight against COVID-19 [2]. Fagherazzi et al. has concentrated on the great potentiality of digital technology for COVID-19 control and prevention [3]. Scholars emphasized that COVID-19 should be considered as a high priority crisis of the healthcare system during this overwhelming time. Alwashmi has explored the potentiality of digital health technologies implementation in different stages of COVID-19 outbreak such as disease surveillance, screening, triage, detection, etc. [4]. Over the pandemic period, digital health tools and technology can support the organization and societies with more competency. These tools are beneficial for the distribution of information widely, transmission tracking time, virtual meetings and daily official activities including visits of the patients through telemedicine. These practices are discussed by several public health experts [5].

Developing countries have started adopting digital technology as a means of fighting COVID-19, too. Bangladesh as a developing nation has also made a notable advancement in digital health system in recent years. Through one of the world's largest deployments of the open-source District Health Information Software 2 (DHIS2), the country now has a national public sector health data warehouse [6].

In this paper, we examined contemporary literature on health information system (HIS) while connecting some major areas of e-health—"the intersection of medical informatics, public health and business, referring to health services and information delivered or enhanced through the internet and related technologies" [7]—during COVID-19 pandemic. Therefore, the questions that we attempt to answer are: (i) how a developing country like Bangladesh has been fighting the COVID-19 pandemic, and (ii) how the adoption of a robust digital health information system can impact the overall health and living conditions of the large population at stake. We find that there are less studies conducted on how high-quality digital health care system has a positive impact in the war of COVID-19 prevention and overall beneficial for health and welfare of common people, particularly for developing country like Bangladesh [7–9]. Relying on system science application in public health informatics, we offer an analysis of existing (statistical) data and present a systematic analysis of how to address this existing gap in an intellectual manner to provide the ways forward. Moreover, few studies discuss how to tackle the newer challenges derived from emerging health crisis like COVID-19 pandemic in Bangladesh [7–9]. We have addressed this with system science [8, 9] to bring the diverse developments of data in one plate to study the overall e-healthcare system, management, and challenges for Bangladesh with an overview of the current COVID-19 situation.

2   Method

This study relies on system thinking and modeling, "relating different types of structures that shape our lives, including the biological systems of our bodies, the organizational systems in which we work, and the political systems with which we govern public affairs"

[9]. In this study, first, we brought current scenarios of COVID-19 in Bangladesh and consider this scenario as a part of whole social-political, health and technical system. According to Midgley, "the whole concept of public health is founded on the insight that health and illness have causes or conditions that go beyond the biology and behavior of the individual human being" [8]. Then, systematically, we have described information based on existing data obtained from different sources (COVID-19 data, digital healthcare policy, recent developments of digital health information system including e-health developments in Bangladesh) with contributions of the systematic approaches indicating a brief statistical analysis, based on healthcare systems hierarchy as shown in Fig. 1 below where (digital) systems adopted by the government reaches to the people of the community as a form of service through healthcare institutions.

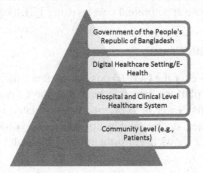

Fig. 1. Healthcare systems hierarchy in Bangladesh

3 Description, Interpretation and Discussion of Digital Healthcare System in Bangladesh

3.1 The Roadmap of E-Health in Bangladesh

Bangladesh government announced a 5-year roadmap of health information system (HIS) and e-healthcare plan for 2011–2016 [10]. The objective of this roadmap was to improve the health information system and develop infrastructure and create the necessary environment for effective HIS, e-health, and medical biotechnology. Their specific purpose was to advance the health information system through- (a) development and operation of population-based HIS, (b) strengthen the institution-based HIS, (c) Strengthening program based HIS, (d) to develop and strengthening logistic tracking, and inventory management and procurement system, (e) developing financial management system, (f) expansion of GIS health service, (g) improve the infrastructure and human resource capacity necessary for HIS, and finally (h) sustaining the HIS initiatives and encourage public–private partnership. Another specific purpose is to improve e-health through several ways including Mobile phone health services, video conferencing and public–private partnership.

3.2   Telemedicine Service

High-quality Telemedicine Services are available in different levels of the hospital all over the country. There are two specialized hospitals—for example, Bangabandhu Sheikh Mujib Medical University and National Institute of Cardiovascular Diseases—and some district-level hospitals and subdistrict level hospitals that are included in this program. Through this service patients from district and sub-district level hospitals can get the suggestions without the necessity of visiting the higher-level hospitals. Webcams and Skype are being used to give telemedicine services in these hospitals. Telemedicine service through community clinics is also available in a rural area in Bangladesh. A total of 18,000 community clinics will provide healthcare services to rural citizens. Moreover, The Access to Information (A2I) program under the Prime Minister's Office runs Union Information and Service Centers (UISCs) in 4,536 unions in Bangladesh to give various services to the local people at a nominal cost by using ICT tools.

3.3   Covid-19 Telehealth Center

To ensure the e-healthcare for the COVID positive patients, the Bangladesh government has developed a digital platform which is known as the COVID-19 telehealth Center. The main purpose of this center is to provide health-related information, advice, and counseling through medical doctors and health information officers over mobile phones (Audio/video). The Fig. 2 shows the information[1] on telehealth services provided by the telehealth center.

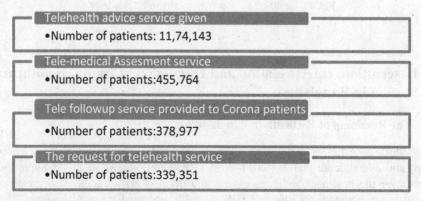

Fig. 2.   The information on telehealth services provided by the telehealth center

One can have an overall information of tele health center service from Fig. 2. It is seen that about 455,764 got telemedicine health care assessment services and 1,174,143 telehealth advice services were provided till 7th July 2021 by this center.

---

[1] Source: COVID-19 Telehealth Center Daily Report, dated 8th July 2021 Website: http://103. 247.238.92/webportal/pages/; Data: DGIS website: http://103.247.238.92/webportal/pages/.

3.4 Current Covid Situations in Bangladesh

From COVID-19 Dynamic Dashboard for Bangladesh, one can easily get day-to-day information on the COVID situation. We have observed and analyzed the COVID situation during the period of May 15 to July 15 here. Number of daily deaths and the death rate is shown through Fig. 3.

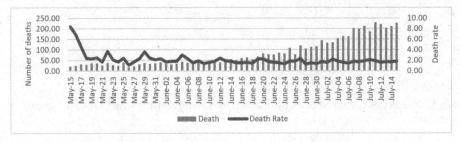

Fig. 3. Daily deaths and death rate from May-15 to July 14, 2021

Due to the second wave of Corona, the number of death cases has been increased significantly. In Fig. 4, it is seen that number of death cases on July 15, 2021, was 226 which was the highest during the period May 15 to July 14. In brief, the death rate was reduced from 8.40% on May 15, 2021, to 1.80% on July 15, 2021. It is clear that death rate was reduced due to the increased number of COVID-19 affected patients. The number of confirmed cases and case rate[2] during the above period is also represented.

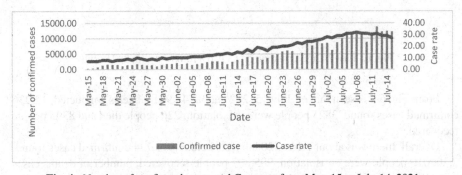

Fig. 4. Number of confirmed cases and Case rate from May-15 to July 14, 2021

From Fig. 5 it is visible that, Dhaka division reports the maximum number of confirmed cases which is about 4,95,695 affected cases and the Mymensingh division is in the last position with 19,950 cases. The case rate was highest in Khulna division (21%). Whereas in Sylhet and Chittagong division it was least (11%) among all division. We can get a clear picture of the COVID situations of Bangladesh which reflects

---

[2] website: http://103.247.238.92/webportal/pages/covid19.php.

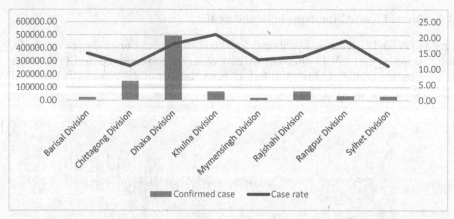

Fig. 5. Number of confirmed cases by division: the overall division wise COVID-19 spreading scenario[3]

that Dhaka and Khulna is mostly affected and in a danger zone. This information is essential for the government and related organizations to take the further decision to fight against COVID-19. People can also get the last 24-h COVID situation information from COVID-19 Dynamic Dashboard for Bangladesh.

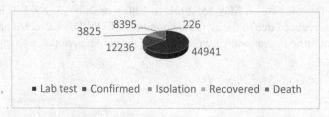

Fig. 6. Last 24 h information on COVID-19 on July 15, 2021 (ibid)

From Fig. 6 it is seen that on July 15, 2021 about 44,941 lab tests conducted, 12,236 confirmed cases found, 3825 people were in isolation, 226 people died and 8395 people recovered.

Overall, there was about 7,144,420 lab tests held, 1,071,774 confirmed cases found, 2,36, 010 people were on isolation, 905,807 people recovered, number of deaths cases were 17,278. Finally, the number of people who administered second dose vaccination were 4,284,959.

3.5 Vaccination Registration Through Online

Bangladeshi citizens can register for vaccination through digital services through a website (https://surokkha.gov.bd) which is a government-run online service and hence this website is playing a vital role in ensuring COVID vaccination to all. People complete their

---

[3] Source: DGIS website: http://103.247.238.92/webportal/pages/).

registration process for covid vaccination simply through their national ID card. This website has made the registration process easier by providing the facility of online registration. Now people do not need to go in person to register for vaccination. According to the information from Dynamic Dashboard for Bangladesh, about 4,284,959 people have already been administered the second dose. Gradually all people will be fully vaccinated through this e-registration system.

4   Challenges to Implement the E-healthcare System

Although Bangladesh has achieved great advancement in e-healthcare and digital health information system, there are some challenges too. These challenges are interconnected to the various socio-technical and political issues and part of the complex system where a smooth hierarchical responsibility and flow of transparency is required.

4.1   Insufficient ICT Infrastructure

There is a shortage in ICT infrastructure support like computers, internet connectivity, printers, webcam, electricity for e-health. Moreover, only a small proportion of people get computer access [11]. Bangladesh Telecommunication Commission (BTRC) reports 2014 show that only 4.5% of people use the internet among the total population [12]. Today, this amount has increased due to availability of the 3G/4G mobile network system. Internet cost, slow internet bandwidth, and insufficient power supply is another barrier for implementation of e-health.

4.2   Insufficient Finance

The establishment, implementation, and use of e-health systems are quite expensive [13]. According to WHO, lack of finance is one of the key barriers to adopt e-health in developing countries [14]. Bangladesh is not out of this. Most of the time government needs to depend on foreign investment, the world bank, and other developed countries for the implementation of a large project.

4.3   Lack of Motivation for Learning New

Old and experienced staff in the hospital sectors in Bangladesh are used to the manual system and less interested to implement new technology in their known setup. This lack of motivation is typically regarded as resistance to change [11]. Administrative staff, policymakers, Doctors, Nurses might think that a computerized healthcare system could make some people redundant. Some are resistant to a new change in their familiar environment [15]. Usability and user acceptance, lack of policy and regulation, Interoperability of Systems are also reasons for the development of e-health in Bangladesh [16].

5   Conclusion

The health sector in Bangladesh is quite undeveloped but the advancement is seen during COVID-19 period, providing daily basis information, telehealth service, online immunization registration service. But this is not enough. To augment the likelihood of success requires understanding of how "different types of structures that shape our lives [during COVID-19], including the biological systems of our bodies [overall human health], the organizational systems in which we work [care providers and institutions], and the political systems [governmental body] with which we govern public affairs" [8] are interconnected. For growing IT literacy, robust finance, and human motivation, a strong inter-institutional cooperation, communication, and socio-technical support building is the key to way forward. We also recognize that "systems-oriented inquiry may point the way toward a promising new frontier" for advancing health information system and "for public health action in response to the critical challenges" [9] like COVID-19 Pandemic.

References

1. Fagherazzi, G., Goetzinger, C., Rashid, M., Aguayo, G., Huiart, L.: Digital health strategies to fight COVID-19 worldwide: challenges, recommendations, and a call for papers. J. Med. Internet Res. **22**(6), 9284 (2020)
2. Alwashmi, M.F.: The use of digital health in the detection and management of COVID-19. Int. J. Environ. Res. Public Health **17**(8), 2906 (2020)
3. Joshi, A.U., et al.: Impact of emergency department tele-intake on left without being seen and throughput metrics. Acad. Emerg. Med. **27**(2), 139–147 (2020)
4. Langabeer, J., et al.: Telehealth-enabled emergency medical services program reduces ambulance transport to urban emergency departments. West J. Emerg. Med. **17**(6), 713–720 (2016)
5. Torous, J., Jän Myrick, K., Rauseo-Ricupero, N., Firth, J.: Digital mental health and COVID-19: using technology today to accelerate the curve on access and quality tomorrow. JMIR Ment. Health **7**(3), 18848 (2020)
6. Khan, M.A.H., Oliveira Cruz, V., Azad, A.K.: Bangladesh's digital health journey: reflections on a decade of quiet revolution. WHO South-East Asia J. Public Health **8**(2), 71–76 (2020)
7. Eysenbach, G.: What is e-health? J. Med. Internet Res. **3**(2), 20 (2001)
8. Midgley, G.: Systemic intervention for public health. Am. J. Public Health **96**, 466–472 (2006)
9. Leischow, S.J., Milstein, B.: Systems thinking and modeling for public health practice. Am. J. Public Health **96**(3), 403–405 (2006)
10. Alam, J.: E-Governance in Bangladesh: present problems and possible suggestions for future development. Int. J. Appl. Inf. Syst. (IJAIS) **4**(8), 21–25 (2012)
11. Uddin, G.: E-governance of Bangladesh: present scenario, expectation, ultimate target and recommendation. Int. J. Sci. Eng. Res. **3**(11), 1–20 (2012)
12. BTRC: Internet Subscribers in Bangladesh, Bangladesh Telecommunication Regulatory Commission Report (2014)
13. Khan, S.Z., Shahid, Z., Hedstrom, K., Andersson, A.: Hopes and fears in implementation of electronic health records in Bangladesh. Electron. J. Inf. Syst. Dev. Count. **54**, 1–18 (2012)
14. WHO: Program and Project: Global Observatory for e-Health. World Health Organization (2013). http://whqlibdoc.who.int/publications/2011/9789241564168_eng.pdf. Accessed 17 Aug 2013

15. Khalifehsoltani, S.N. Gerami, M.R.: E-Health challenges, opportunities and experiences of developing countries. In: International Conference on e-Education, eBusiness, e-Management, and e-Learning, Sanya, China (2010)

16. Hoque, M.M., Fahami. B.Y: e-Health in Bangladesh: current status, challenges, and future direction. Int. Technol. Manag. Rev. 4(2), 87–96 (2014)

17. Calton, B., Abedini, N., Fratkin, M.: Telemedicine in the time of coronavirus. J. Pain Symptom Manage. **60**(1), 12–14 (2020)

18. Keesara, S., Jonas, A., Schulman, K.: Covid-19 and health care's digital revolution. N Engl. J. Med. **382**(23), 82 (2020)

Developing Telerehabilitation in Low-Income Countries During COVID-19: Commencement and Acceptability of Telerehabilitation in Rohingya and Host Community People

Rasel Ahmed[1] and Forkan Ali[2(✉)]

[1] Centre For Disability in Development (CDD), Dhaka, Bangladesh
[2] School of Humanities and Social Sciences, UNSW Canberra, Canberra, Australia

Abstract. *Background.* The world has witnessed a major change in providing and viewing the treatment continuum for medical and rehabilitation services because of the COVID-19 epidemic. Demand for digital health services like telemedicine and telerehabilitation has been increasing rapidly due to the COVID-19 factors (e.g., isolation, lockdown) in play. Though telemedicine in lower-income countries like Bangladesh has a little history, telerehabilitation is quite new and the first of its kind addressed through this study.

Objective. This study aims to explore the present status of digital health services like telemedicine and telerehabilitation in Bangladesh and examines the commencement and acceptability of telerehabilitation services during COVID-19 to offer the outcomes of it.

Method. Relying on the phenomenological qualitative method of analyzing collected data, this research paper recognizes Rohingya and host community members' perspectives on the Tele-rehabilitation service during the COVID-19 pandemic.

Results. Results of the conducted study show commencement of telerehabilitation in Bangladesh has positive outcomes and can be adopted widely in various related sectors, expanding options and possibilities for people with disabilities and the Rohingya population. This study has opened new doors for many people to lift their life, ensuring their safety as well as ensuring therapeutic outcomes by utilizing telerehabilitation services daily.

Keywords: Telerehabilitation · Telemedicine · Digital health system

1 Introduction

During this unforeseen and ongoing COVID-19 pandemic, healthcare providers and experts across the world dramatically converted their face-to-face mode of health care services into online, providing services through telehealth technology [1]. As the number of cases of Coronavirus disease rises across the country, the healthcare systems of Bangladesh struggle to balance the need to reduce provider exposure and personal protective equipment use while maintaining high-quality patient care. Medical service

S. Siuly et al. (Eds.): HIS 2021, LNCS 13079, pp. 24–32, 2021.
https://doi.org/10.1007/978-3-030-90885-0_3

and rehabilitation services needed to consider new approaches to providing home and community-based rehabilitation care, particularly, to the huge number of Rohingya and host community people in Cox's Bazar district [2]. As practitioners in community-based settings, hospitals, nursing homes, outpatient clinics, disability service centers, and schools transitioned into utilizing telehealth techniques to serve their clients [3].

The epidemic has hastened the global adoption of telehealth services, providing healthcare from distance often using telecommunication or virtual technology. Telerehabilitation has become effective in treating several chronic illnesses including persons with disabilities and diversities [4]. Telehealth incorporates all remote health services, while telerehabilitation refers to the use of information and communication technology (ICT) to provide rehabilitation treatments to individuals in their homes or other settings. Tele rehabilitation aims to increase client access to care by enabling them to get therapy beyond the confines of a conventional rehabilitation facility. As a result, the rehabilitation care becomes consistent. Rehabilitation professionals employ a wide range of technology, from basic day-to-day applications, such as phone calls, emails, pictures, and videos to more advanced technologies, such as encrypted video conferencing, sensor-based monitoring, and virtual gaming. This way of providing services can be used to make things more accessible and cost-effective for rehabilitation [5]. The World Health Organization (WHO) created a worldwide observatory for e-health in 2005 to track the advancement of ICT for health care, including telemedicine, and to offer accurate information and recommendations on best practices, regulations, and standards. According to a recent analysis, telemedicine has progressed slowly in lower-income countries both in terms of the number of nations with services delivered and the number of countries that are piloting telemedicine services [6]. Nonetheless, numerous telemedicine networks across the world provide humanitarian aid regularly, with many of these services going to low-income nations. Moreover, there are fewer studies conducted around the inception, development, and progresses of telemedicine in developing countries like Bangladesh and hardly any research was found on telerehabilitation commenced in this country [5, 6].

This study, therefore, not only addresses this wide gap informing the status of telemedicine in lower-income countries but also creates an intellectual bridge between global public health intervention and telerehabilitation services in developing countries like Bangladesh. This study attempts to answer the following questions: (a) what is the present status of digital health services (for instance, telemedicine and telerehabilitation) in Bangladesh? and (b) how can we examine the commencement and acceptability of telerehabilitation services during COVID-19 to offer the outcomes of it? Relying on the phenomenological qualitative method of analyzing collected data, this research paper recognizes Rohingya and host community members' perspectives on the Tele-rehabilitation service during the COVID-19 pandemic.

2 Brief Review of Telehealth and the Commencement of Telerehabilitation in Bangladesh

According to Leochico, Austria, and Espiritu, "telerehabilitation, a subset of telehealth and telemedicine, refers explicitly to the remote provision of rehabilitation services" particularly in countries with inadequate health facilities and lack of healthcare providers in comparison to the total population [17, 18]. Rehana stated that in Bangladesh, numerous organizations assist individuals with disabilities, however, they are insufficient [7]. Some of the organizations working sensitively for the disabled include the Centre for the Rehabilitation of the Paralyzed (CRP), Handicap International, Center for Disability in Development (CDD), BRAC, Action Aid Bangladesh, Bangladesh Protibondhi Kollyan Somity (BPKS), and ADD International. To provide medical treatments, such as physiotherapy and occupational therapy, and speech and language therapy to persons with disabilities in Bangladesh's rural and remote locations like Cox's Bazar's world largest Rohingya crisis, the Centre for Disability in Development (CDD) runs a tremendous project on "Inclusive Humanitarian Response for Rohingya Crisis: Access to Rehabilitation & Disability Mainstreaming" (see CDD: https://cdd.org.bd/). In which CDD provides wide-ranging rehabilitation services to Rohingya and host community people at Cox's Bazar. When the world was driven to lockdown due to the COVID-19 epidemic, the medium of disability service supply changed. Then, instead of providing door-to-door service in the community, CDD designed a telerehabilitation protocol so that practitioners can still reach out and give rehabilitation services while maintaining appropriate communication and keeping COVID-19 safeguards in mind. As part of their tremendous obligation to provide ongoing rehabilitation services to Rohingya and host community members, they employed telehealth in rehabilitation also known as telerehabilitation, as a medium of digital disability service.

3   Description of Research Method

Chowdhury and Ashrafuzzaman et al. 2015 reviewed that in the Bangladeshi situation, telemedicine is a quite effective approach to spread health services to rural Bangladesh while using the country's limited resources [8]. In mid-1999, Bangladesh began to engage in telemedicine operations. The availability of high bandwidth is critical to the productivity and usability of telemedicine data. Bangladesh's information and communication infrastructure have seen massive growth in recent years. Moreover, Bangladesh is expanding its operations to the country's most remote districts. Internet access is virtually universal in many districts of Bangladesh. With government and business sectors initiatives where the necessary measures are taken, patients in rural areas can contact doctors over the internet. The graph below shows the rapid growth of the use of telemedicine during the COVID-19 Pandemic while the figure is replicating the trend of COVID-19 cases by Outcome, 08 March-23 November 2020, Bangladesh (Fig. 1).

When the international community pressured Bangladesh to lock down, CDD (https://cdd.org.bd/) launched a telerehabilitation program for its beneficiaries mostly persons with disabilities (PWD) in Cox's Bazaar and other districts where they had ongoing initiatives. The recipients of the Cox's Bazaar host community and Rohingya people had never heard of telehealth or telerehabilitation services before. Some of them cannot even operate the mobile phone smoothly and other technological devices. Hussain and Heeks stated that the bulk of these Rohingyas have limited or no access to technology, including almost no access to the Internet [10]. Despite this, innovation in the form of digital content production and sharing has blossomed in mobile phone repair/recharge establishments. With a total of three mechanisms, this article presents a

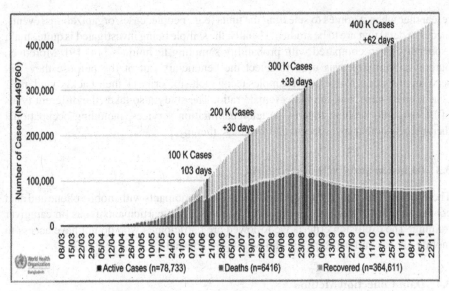

Fig. 1. Use of Telemedicine in Bangladesh during the COVID-19 pandemic [9]

mechanism-based explanation of this form of device innovation. The following factors are taken into consideration: (1) the communications and technological infrastructure built around mobile phone shops; (2) the motivation and social, cultural, and political belief structures of Rohingyas; and (3) the legal and technical infrastructure that applies to Rohingyas in Bangladeshi refugee camps.

We have used the phenomenological qualitative method, which is descriptive, exploratory, and contextual to determine the acceptability and understanding of people regarding the telerehabilitation services [11]. This method aims to describe the life experience of people in a particular setting to understand their perspectives [12]. The most prominent criterion is the participants' experience with the phenomenon under the study [13], as we investigate the phenomenon which is described and interpreted by the participants about their attitude towards acceptance and practice of telerehabilitation.

3.1 Study Setting/Data Collecting Setting

Qualitative method design focuses on ordinary events in natural settings. According to the literature we observed and interacted with the individual in the participant's context. The study focused on the participant who primarily received rehabilitation and continuingly receiving rehabilitation service from CDD projects.

3.2 Sampling and Recruitment

Participants were selected by purposive sampling where purposive sampling represents a group of different non-probability sampling techniques. Also known as judgmental, selective, or subjective sampling, purposive sampling relies on the judgment of the researcher when it comes to selecting the units (e.g., people, cases/organizations, events, pieces of data) that are to be studied. Usually, the sample being investigated is quite small, especially when compared with probability sampling techniques [14, 19]. Moreover, purposive sampling was used to select the beneficiary out of the purpose they will serve in this study. We selected samples using inclusion criteria, their background, their educational status, and the male–female ratio. The study also takes the different types of therapy into account to provide telerehabilitation services, including occupational therapy, physiotherapy, speech, and language therapy.

3.3 Inclusion and Exclusion Criteria

The inclusion criteria we followed are as follows: participants with mobile phone and data connection, both male and female, adult patients, child participants focus on caregiver training. The exclusion criteria we followed are participants who do not have access to mobile phones and participants who won't give consent.

3.4 Data Collection Method

After getting permission from the authority of CDD and the campsite coordinator, we started the data collection process. Semi-structured interviews were conducted by a self-developed question, including basic demographic questions and about their perspective and willingness to take telerehabilitation services and know about the COVID-19 pandemic. In this case, most of the questions were open-ended so that we can find out the objectives of the study. During interviews, we have taken permission from all candidates in the consent form, and we used a voice call recorder to record the exact answer of the candidates.

3.5 Interview Guide/Data Collection Instrument

During interview time, we used self-developed questionnaire forms, mobile phone, voice call recorder to collect the conversation or interview with all the participants, pen, pencil, paper (white), clipboard, consent form, laptop, internet data.

3.6 Data Analysis

Thematic approach was taken. The thematic analysis in this research used is a kind of descriptive approach focused on lived experience, which referred to participants' experiences of the world. The philosophy of phenomenology is the study of a phenomenon, for example, something as it is experienced (or lived) by a human being that means how things appear in our experiences.[21] we did the same in considering the Rohingya participants. Tuddin and Mamun reviewed that maintenance of critical rehabilitative services over the continuum of care is considered a core component of high-value care [15]. This study described the perspectives of Rohingya and host community members who have been influenced by COVID-19 in the medical rehabilitation sector. Recommendations are made for adjusting rehabilitative services during lockdown limitations, progressive relaxation of restrictions, and in the post-lockdown period, particularly after phases of working with rehabilitation doctors and other trained professions, such as therapists that specialize in rehabilitation. Wootten and Geissbuhler stated that more and better evidence is needed to guarantee successful and appropriate use of telehealth in resource-constrained settings [6]. We provided better evidence within the limited resources used.

Moreover, information and communication technologies (ICTs) have advanced in recent years, allowing society to swiftly access services that support economic and social growth. Telehealth/Telemedicine/E-health is an ICT blessing and perhaps the most notable e-business service that may have a significant visible impact on society's growth [16]. Thus, we selected the population based on the uses of mobile phones with data connectivity and provided telerehabilitation services through telehealth medium, and received consent for uses of information regarding the perspective of telerehabilitation services.

4 Results

We have selected 50 participants from the entire population including 20 Rohingya beneficiaries and 30 host community beneficiaries who met the inclusion criteria. Most participants were members of the host community who had benefited from the CDD Rohingya emergency response project "Inclusive Humanitarian Response for Rohingya Crisis "Access to Rehabilitation & Disability Mainstreaming." We have selected the number of samplings following the type of beneficiaries: their background and how many therapies they are receiving. Tele-rehabilitation services were provided via cell phone, 45-min sessions were held three times a week, with a 15-day follow-up. In Cox's Bazar, Bangladesh, the chosen participants exhibited a significant increase in their understanding and acceptance of telerehabilitation services.

During the implementation of the telerehabilitation service, most of the beneficiaries responded well to receiving telerehabilitation service from CDD staff. When we conducted key person interview, we found that the acceptance of the telerehabilitation service among both host communities and Rohingya community beneficiaries was fruitful, whereas, preliminary, female participants showed less interest as some female beneficiaries didn't feel comfortable sharing information with a male therapist. Though there were some cultural barriers, aged male participants' confidence was boosted up as they were using the tech tools in the treatment procedure.

While interviewing, we also found that there was a huge need for telemedicine and telehealth in telerehabilitation services in both communities. We also found the gap in their need and tried to meet the need by reaching out for external and medical referrals for the beneficiaries who needed basic medical services.

Furthermore, those who got telerehabilitation services improved more quickly and had a better therapeutic outcome than those who did not. During the COVID-19 epidemic, some of them learned to use the telerehabilitation medium to overcome a variety of physical, emotional, and financial obstacles in their everyday lives.

5 Discussion

Like Cox and Scrivener's study [4], this research describes a short intervention to aid telerehabilitation deployment in community rehabilitation. The implementation approach addressed important behaviors such as knowledge, resources, social support, and ideas about consequences, which were identified as obstacles to telerehabilitation. The intervention was highly accepted, and it resulted in some practice changes, but it had only a little impact on perceived barriers and obstacles and enablers to telerehabilitation implementation. Changes in workload, availability of equipment and technical assistance, and time restrictions have all been highlighted as hurdles to adopting telerehabilitation in clinical practice. Our study finds that clinician education is also essential for telehealth adoption to be successful. Although telerehabilitation implementation does not happen in a vacuum. Moreover, we found that more than a third of chronically sick people have never used the internet, and 30 percent to 40 percent have little interest in using telehealth to receive rehabilitative treatments. The ability or experience of the patient with telerehabilitation was not considered in this study, but it might have had a direct impact on clinician perceptions of the appropriateness of telerehabilitation.

Nessa and Ameen followed that the development of the information and telecommunications infrastructure is critical to the effective spread of Teleconsultation [16]. Due to a lack of communications infrastructure in the past, telehealth deployment was difficult. Currently, the scenario favors telemedicine. In recent years, Bangladesh's telecommunications sector has seen tremendous growth. Several commercial and public telecommunications companies are expanding their reach into the most remote locations, as well as focusing on improving network performance and introducing new technologies to the public [9].

The goal of this short study was to commence a telerehabilitation service with the most vulnerable group of Rohingya refugees in Cox's Bazar's hill track region, where their fundamental needs were still unfulfilled. We focused on the viewpoints of these populations on the treatment continuum that was required at the time for their improvement. We have observed that the implementation of telerehabilitation in Bangladesh has positive outcomes and can be carried out for better impacts.

6 Limitations

This study encountered several obstacles, including a lack of time to educate the recipients about the benefits of telehealth and telerehabilitation. The absence of communication gadgets and internet connectivity was a disaster. The information was gathered during telerehabilitation therapy sessions. There were some cultural barriers and, also, some female beneficiaries didn't feel comfortable sharing information with a male therapist.

7 Recommendations

This discovery helps future researchers initiate telerehabilitation services in Bangladesh's rural areas, as well as anywhere else in the globe. The study suggests that participants and telerehabilitation service professionals be prepared in advance for more accurate results and fewer difficult scenarios.

8 Conclusion

To conclude, because of the COVID-19 epidemic, immense changes have occurred in providing and viewing the treatment continuum for rehabilitation services. Therefore, the demand for digital health services like telemedicine and telerehabilitation have been increasing rapidly. This study has shown that the launch of a telerehabilitation services in Cox's Bazar, Bangladesh, has expanded options and possibilities for people with disabilities and the Rohingya population. It has opened new doors for many people of lower-income countries to lift their life, ensuring their safety as well as ensuring therapeutic outcomes by utilizing telerehabilitation services daily.

References

1. Dahl-Popolizio, S., Carpenter, H., Coronado, M., Popolizio, N.J., Swanson, C.: Telehealth for the provision of occupational therapy: reflections on experiences during the COVID-19 pandemic. Int. J. Telerehabil. **12**(2), 77–92 (2020)
2. Humphreys, J., et al.: Rapid implementation of inpatient telepalliative medicine consultations during COVID-19 pandemic. J. Pain Sympt. Manag. **60**, 54–59 (2020)
3. Little, L.M., Pickett, K.A., Proffitt, R., Cason, J.: Keeping PACE with 21st century healthcare: a framework for telehealth research, practice, and program evaluation in occupational therapy. Int. J. Telerehabil. **13**(1) (2021)
4. Cox, N.S., et al.: A brief intervention to support implementation of telerehabilitation by community rehabilitation services during COVID-19: a feasibility study. Arch. Phys. Med. Rehabil. **102**, 789–795 (2021)
5. Gefen, N., Steinhart, S., Beeri, M., Weiss, P.L.: Lessons learned during a naturalistic study of online treatment for pediatric rehabilitation. Int. J. Environ. Res. Public Health **18**(12), 6659 (2021)
6. Wootton, R., et al.: Long-running telemedicine networks delivering humanitarian services: experience, performance and scientific output. Bull. World Health Org. **90**, 341–3477 (2012)
7. Parvin R.: Perception of the patients and providers regarding telehealth service of disabled people's organization (DPO) through centre for the rehabilitation of the paralysed (CRP). Thesis, Bangladesh Health Professions Institute, Faculty of Medicine (2018)
8. Chowdhury, S.M., Kabir, M.H., Ashrafuzzaman, K., Kwak, K.-S.: A telecommunication network architecture for telemedicine in Bangladesh and its applicability. Int. J. Digit. Content Technol. Appl. **3**, 4 (2009)
9. Khan, M.M., Rahman, S.T., AnjumIslam, S.T.: The use of telemedicine in Bangladesh during COVID-19 pandemic. E-Health Telecommun. Syst. Netw. **10**, 1 (2021)
10. Hussain, F., Wall, P.J., Heeks, R.: Digital innovation by displaced populations: a critical realist study of Rohingya refugees in Bangladesh. In: Bass, J.M., Wall, P.J. (eds.) International Conference on Social Implications of Computers in Developing Countries. IFIP Advances in Information and Communication Technology, vol. 587, pp. 54–65. Springer, Cham (2020). https://doi.org/10.1007/978-3-030-65828-1_5
11. Kvale, S., Brinkmann, S.: Interviews: Learning the Craft of Qualitative Research Interviewing. Sage (2009)
12. Alanko, T., Karhula, M., Kröger, T., Piirainen, A., Nikander, R.: Rehabilitees perspective on goal setting in rehabilitation–a phenomenological approach. Disabil. Rehabil. **41**, 2280–2288 (2019)
13. Sundler, A., Lindberg, E., Nilsson, C., Palmér, L.: Qualitative thematic analysis based on descriptive phenomenology. Nurs. Open **6**, 733–739 (2018)

14. Campbell, S., et al.: Purposive sampling: complex or simple? Research case examples. J. Res. Nurs. **25**(8), 652–661 (2020)
15. Uddin, T., et al.: Rehabilitation perspectives of COVID-19 pandemic in Bangladesh. J. Bangladesh Coll. Physicians Surg. **38**, 76–81 (2020)
16. Nessa, A., Ameen, M., Ullah, S., Kwak, K.S.: Applicability of telemedicine in Bangladesh: current status and future prospects. In: 2008 Third International Conference on Convergence and Hybrid Information Technology. IEEE (2008)
17. Sarfo, F.S., Adamu, S., Awuah, D., Sarfo-Kantanka, O., Ovbiagele, B.: Potential role of tele-rehabilitation to address barriers to implementation of physical therapy among West African stroke survivors: a cross-sectional survey. J. Neurol. Sci. **381**, 203–208 (2017)
18. Leochico, C.F.D., Austria, E.M.V., Espiritu, A.I.: Global online interest in telehealth, telemedicine, telerehabilitation, and related search terms amid the COVID-19 pandemic: an infodemiological study. Acta Medica Philippina **10** (2020)
19. Rai, N., Thapa, B.: A study on purposive sampling method in research. Academia. Kathmandu School of Law, Kathmandu (2015)

Towards a User-Level Self-management of COVID-19 Using Mobile Devices Supported by Artificial Intelligence, 5G and the Cloud

Sajjad Ahmed(✉) ⓘ, Anup Shrestha ⓘ, and Jianming Yong ⓘ

School of Business, University of Southern Queensland, Toowoomba, Australia
{Sajjad.ahmad,anup.shrestha,jianming.yong}@usq.edu.au

Abstract. The fatal outbreak of COVID-19 has placed its fear around the globe since it was first reported in Wuhan, China, in November 2019. COVID-19 has placed all countries and governments across the world in an unstable position. Most countries underwent partial or full lock down due to the dearth of resources to fight the COVID-19 outbreak, primarily due to the challenges of overloaded healthcare systems. The tally of confirmed COVID-19 cases via laboratory continues to increase around the globe, with reportedly 60.5 million confirmed cases as of November 2020. Evidently, innovation has an imperative function to empower the omnipresent health technologies in order to counter the impacts of COVID-19 in a post-pandemic period. More specifically, the Fifth Generation (5G) cellular network and 5G-empowered e-health and Artificial Intelligence (AI) based arrangements are of on the spotlight. This research explores the use of AI and 5G technologies to help alleviate the effects of COVID-19 spread. The novel approach is based on the premises that the COVID-19 vaccine may take years to rollout effectively, whereas the AI and 5G technologies offer effective solutions to reduce the Covid-19 spread within weeks. Currently, the approaches such as contact tracing and virus testing are not secure and reliable; and the cost of testing is high for end users. The proposed solution offers a self-diagnostic mechanism without any security risk of the users' data with very low cost using cloud-based data analytics using mobile handsets.

Keywords: COVID-19 · Pandemic · AI · 5G · e-Health

1 Introduction

The COVID-19 is a contagious virus family named *Corona viridae*. It is a family of positive-sense RNA, single-stranded viruses. This virus causes the ailments of fever, fatigue, cough and difficulty in breathing by attacking the respiratory system of its victim. The actual source of this virus is still undefined but, the scientists have mapped the sequence of its genome and identified the virus as the member of COVID-19 family with genera of β-CoV and originates its foundation of genes from rodents and bats [1]. The first reported case of this virus to affect the human life was reported in December

© Springer Nature Switzerland AG 2021
S. Siuly et al. (Eds.): HIS 2021, LNCS 13079, pp. 33–43, 2021.
https://doi.org/10.1007/978-3-030-90885-0_4

2019 from the city of Wuhan in China's province of Hubei. Since then, the COVID-19 virus is spreading like a wildfire throughout the globe and has affected 213 countries and independent territories, and caused 3.5 billion people to stay in some form of self-isolation or restrictions. Around the globe, as of in the second week of November 2020, there have been over 60.5 million confirmed cases of COVID-19, including over 566,355 deaths, reported by the World Health Organization (WHO) [2]. Figure 1 depicts the statistics of the worst affected countries, the total number of cases and tally of fatalities in those countries, respectively. This exponential rise in the number of cases of COVID-19 has stimulated the necessity for instantaneous countermeasures to curtail the cataclysmic effect of the spread. This paper evaluates the role of Artificial Intelligence (AI) and Fifth Generation (5G) telecommunication essential in mitigation of the opposing effects of this outbreak and aid in the recovery phase.

As per the report of W.H.O, the infections due to the different types of Corona viruses are continuously emerging and posing severe community health issues [1].

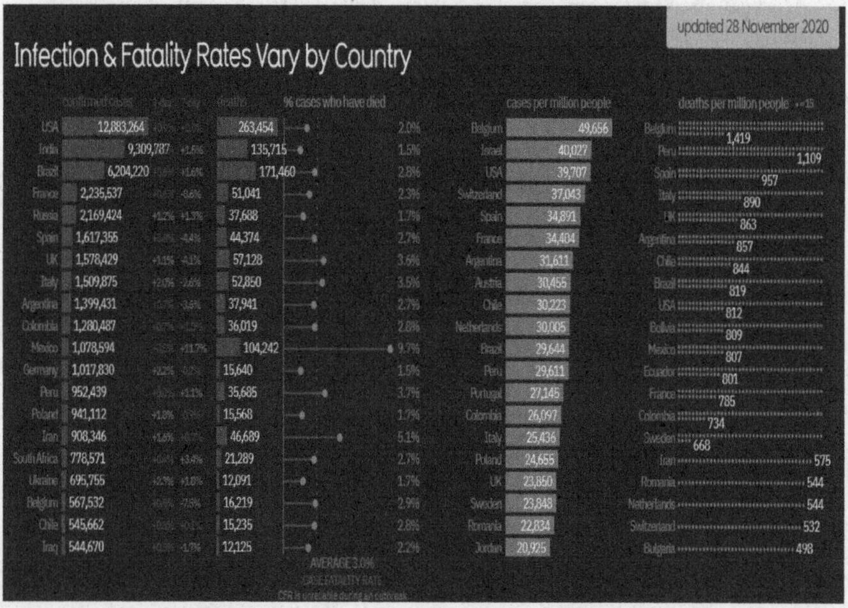

Fig. 1. Statistics of worst affected countries

The rest of the paper is arranged like this. In Sect. 2, we discuss existing status of ongoing activities by researchers on the COVID-19 epidemic. In the following sections, we provide an all-inclusive overview of the use of AI and 5G technologies as a way to effectively manage COVID-19 pandemic. The last section will conclude the paper with the presentation of smartphone-based framework for self-diagnosis which can help in and reducing the COVID-19 spread.

2 Related Works

After the outbreak of COVID-19, different laboratories, researchers, scientists and organizations worldwide were being prompted to conduct the wide-scale research to aid the development of vaccines, drugs and other treatment methodologies. However, there is very less literature available that attempt to provide the role of 5G and AI technologies on the management of COVID-19 pandemic. This presents the need for research which provides every possible view of the COVID-19 in terms of clinical aspects, prevention methodologies, diagnosis and possible treatments to determine the role of technologies to assuage the impact of its outbreak.

3 Incipient Technologies for Extenuating the Influence of the Covid-19 Pandemic

As the spread of novel COVID-19 continues around the world, the nations are staggering under the weight of struggling economies and other socio-economic setbacks. Sadly, billions of individuals are as yet under a consistent danger of the virus, with the situation not showing any signs of improvement in the immediate forthcoming future. Notwithstanding, an entire host of innovative ideas has been proposed to manage the challenges of the COVID-19 pandemic. Among them, advanced technologies such as AI and 5G have been considered [3]. As per the WHO and the Centers of Disease Control & Prevention (CDC) in the US, advanced technologies can support general public health based on the positive response to the COVID-19 pandemic. In the accompanying segments, we present the previously discussed technology advances in mitigating the COVID-19 pandemic.

3.1 Artificial Intelligence

Since the advent of AI, it has proved to be a milestone in technological advancement. AI can be standing as an extremely effective instrument against the COVID-19 pandemic if used properly. Early detection with AI can reduce the spread of COVID-19 by 40% [4]. Surveillance of ailment, prediction of COVID-19 spread risk, clinical diagnosis and screening, identification of the source hosts, and enforcement of the lockdown measures are some of the genuine measures by which AI can help the government and relevant administrations towards combating COVID-19 challenges.

Contact Tracing. Containing the COVID-19 virus has proven successful with aggressive contact tracing and isolation of suspected or confirmed cases. Published literature have suggested that digital rather than manual contact tracing might be more effective in containing the pandemic.

Contact tracing is a significant process to help decrease the frequency of new instances of virus. Contact tracing applications are being created to help fighting COVID-19 in public and with worldwide scope, such as CovidSafe App in Australia, TraceTogether App in Singapore, StopCovid App in France, and the Application Programming Interface (API) offered by Google and Apple. In all the applications referenced above, the government control the clusters data and have access to the information's. The data accumulated by Apple and Google, which permits information exchange between mobile phones on iOS and Android frameworks, has incredibly supported contact tracing and determining people who are tested positive with COVID-19. In Canada, the COVI application was created which uses AI towards contact tracing to help the administration of general health strategies. With AI trend of COVID-19 spread can be generated, the infected person data can be used for back tracking for the source and potential outbreak from the infected person while tracing all his contacts.

Monitoring of Ailment. The appropriate forecast and monitoring of the virus is essential. Blue Dot (B-Dot), a health surveillance company based in Toronto was successful to report and impend the outbreak of COVID-19 on December 2019, 9 days prior to W.H.O. announcement. Computer based intelligence model of B-Dot use different AI devices to recognize developing aliments. This AI model of B-Dot had the option to follow the spread of the COVID-19 and figure its episode a long time before the other human associations.

Risk Prediction. One of the possible boulevards of application of AI against COVID-19 is prediction of risk. The AI model for risk prediction of getting infected by disease would be very complex due to the fact that, this model will depend on various functions such as age, medical history of person and his/her family, recent health status, diet habits, hygiene and existing medical history etc. Prolific outcomes cannot be expected from this model if we model it directly using mathematical models of these aforementioned functions. However, more reliable and precise risk prediction profile can be generated as more all-inclusive analysis of all the functions with AI techniques are incorporated.

Diagnosis and Screening of Patients. Swift identification of the COVID-19 patients can permit governments to acquire effectual reaction procedures to stop the diseases from further spread. The global scarcity of testing kits has made it difficult for the establishments to bear out across-the-board diagnostic testing. Numerous available AI gear are being repurposed, while some new ones are being worked to address this problem. For example, 93% of the Shanghai population was tested with AI based quick scan. In this subsection, we inspect how AI is changing the cycle of COVID-19 infection screening and diagnosis.

Face Scanners. Since Various hospitals, medical centers and heavily crowded areas such as malls, airports etc., are using cameras with AI based scanning technology to decrease the exposure of COVID-19 victims to front line personnel [5]. These AI based cameras not only can monitor the temperature of individuals in crowded areas but can also enable authorities to analyze their movement with face tracking.

Medical Imaging. Various efforts have already been made to deploy AI based medical imaging and screening of COVID-19. For example, a collaboration of an Ontario-based AI start up with the academic researchers of University of Waterloo has come up with a Convolutional Neural Network (CNN) to identify COVID-19 using chest X-Rays. They named their AI model as COVID-Net and calculation for the framework is made open source by the makers to encourage the improvement of AI instrument over their model.

Enforcing the Lockdown Measures. Several nations and states around the globe, including USA, India, China, and the UK, are using AI-based technologies to enforce social segregation and lockdown processes. One of the largest AI-based companies in China has infrared cameras operated by computers that monitor public spaces. These cameras can not only detect people with high body temperature, but through their facial recognition system, they can also distinguish citizens who do not follow lockdown procedures. The first launch of AI in the USA - Landing AI, given to one of the world's top AI connectors - Andrew Ng developed a public awareness tool similar to contact tracing tool used in Australia and Singapore [6].

3.2 Fifth Generation Cellular Technologies

Fifth Generation Cellular Network, which is commonly known as 5G, is wireless cellular technology [7]. 5G is able to support mobile communication worldwide. 5G has a potential of revolutionizing the healthcare sector like its concomitant technologies such as the Internet of Medical Things (IoMT), AI and Blockchain. The response mechanism of COVID-19 pandemic in China is already transformed by the commercialization of 5G technology. 5G is capable of providing better assistance to the frontline medical staff and government authorities for contact tracing as well as able to facilitate the virus tracking, patient screening, data analysis and data collection. With Network slicing emergency services can be prioritized with 5G, high throughput, low latency, more connections, network efficiency and spectral efficiency will help to deal with COVID-19 type of pandemic with help of 5G. In this subsection we will discuss the different ways, in which 5G technologies has assisted countries impacted by COVID-19 pandemic. 5G with help of other digital technologies like IOT, Big Data, AI and blockchain can be used for monitoring, detection, protection, surveillance and mitigating of COVID-19 [8].

5GC Telemedicine. The practice of keeping distance from patients of disease while monitoring them is supported by telemedicine. While the use of drones, smart phone accessories, and mobile apps can provide telemedicine functionality, 5G network technology can enable that functionality. Different emergency clinics in China have introduced 5G telemedicine screens for COVID-19 patients. For instance:

- West China Hospital has propelled the Corona infection 5G-C broadcast communications stage with the help from China Telecom.
- An emergency health facility partnered with Kunming Medical University has propelled an online 5G-based demonstrative stage and free COVID-19 management therapy [9].

5G Medical Imaging. Recent medical imaging processes such as Photo Archive and Communication Systems (PACS) have been identified as an important part of testing and management. Cloud based CT scan were used as an alternate of RT-PCR tests and smartphone surveillance was a key method used for contract tracing. At a particular emergency clinic at the Wuhan Center, Leishenshan Hospital, 5G-empowered clinical stages take into consideration ongoing conclusion of COVID-19 patients, and in doing as such, diminish the workload on clinical staff [10].

5G Thermal Imaging. Thermal imaging technology, originally designed to protect anti-aircraft equipment, is now in full swing in the health care sector, where it has been shown to be particularly helpful in COVID-19 management. The development of 5G networks has facilitated the development of 5G enabled user systems that can have multiple health protection and care systems. The 5GC IR progressed checking framework can empower continuous temperature of moving bodies with more prominent exactness and accuracy. The information gathered by the projects can be moved to the focal test framework through Ultra-low inactivity utilizing 5G systems. With the coming of COVID-19, this activity could mean checking the clock's open temperature. In China, 5G warm hopeful frameworks have been incorporated into robots and Unmaned Arial Vehicles (UAV), which are appropriated in open regions of a few urban areas to lessen the spread of COVID-19 [10].

5GC Robots. Following the spread of COVID-19, a few endeavors have been made worldwide to create and convey robots to lessen the workload of first-line health authorities. This segment centers chiefly around ground-breaking 5G robots. Notwithstanding having extra usefulness, 5G-empowered robots are commonly more proficient at performing errands allotted to them as robot will be working with low latency and high bandwidth which is only possible with 5G technology. Robot can be used for disinfection of surfaces, temperature testing, food delivery and medicine delivery to infected peoples to reduce the direct contact of medical staff.

Thailand's Deployed 5G Robots. In Thailand, Advanced Info Services (AIS), the world's biggest versatile administrator, has introduced 5G innovation in different approaches to battle the COVID-19 flare-up. AIS has introduced 5G systems in 20 medical clinics and conveyed a few 5G robots to assist medical clinics with extending their broadcast communications offices. Apart from acting as a connection with medical staff and patients, these robots can perform autonomous health examinations [11].

Wuhan's Cloudminds' 5G Robots. A field clinical facility, with various 5G-engaged robots, opened in Wuhan, China. These robots, given by a Beijing-based association called Cloud Minds, can clean and disinfect the zone, pass taking drugs to patients, and measure their temperature. The workplace, for the most part known as Smart Field Hospital, has used the use of other IoT devices to lessen the workload on the center staff. Patients at the center wore wristbands and arm groups agreed with the Cloud Minds 'man-made insight stage so medical specialists could continue watching their patients' basic signs, including temperature, heartbeat, and blood oxygen levels, without requiring steady physical contact with them [12].

Patrolling Robots in Several Cities of China. A robot organization situated in Guangzhou, China deployed robots with 5G connections along with AI, IoT, and distributed computing. These robots have five infrared thermometers and high-end cameras that permit them to gauge internal heat levels of up to ten individuals concurrently. Furthermore, using characteristic sensors, these robots can decide if an individual is wearing a mask or not. At whatever point a robot experiences an individual who isn't wearing a mask or has a high fever is quickly alerted to the nearby specialists. These robots have been circulated in open territories of numerous Chinese urban communities, including Shanghai, Guangzhou, and Guiyang [13].

Challenges. Since the spread of COVID-19, various technological arrangements have been proposed to decrease its effect. Among them, IoT, drone innovation, and AI are at the bleeding edge. To understand the groundbreaking capacities of this innovation, there is a requirement for a portable system that can beat transfer speed, idleness, and adaptability issues related with current system innovation. The capacity of this lays on the up and coming age of portable systems. The combination of devices, for example, UAVs, robots, and 5G-with zero contact. Currently, however, the use of 5G networks faces a number of challenges, some of which are discussed below:

- With the launch of 5G is still in its early stages, one of its difficulties is the absence of foundation to help its tasks. Furthermore, the significant expenses related with the establishment and upkeep of 5G systems have made worldwide transportation hard for governments and telecom administrators.
- 5G systems cannot impact the health sector by itself. They can just appear to work, when utilized pair with other accessible advancements, for example, Internet of medical things (IoMT), AI, and distributed computing.
- Currently, there are no agreed rules overseeing the utilization of gathered patient protection utilizing 5G social insurance frameworks. Apart from information classification, a couple of other security issues identified with utilization of 5G are yet to be settled. While the far and wide applications of 5G systems in the social insurance industry may take few years, a developing number of clinical establishments are thinking about 5G-empowered wellbeing frameworks to improve clinical assistance quality and patient experience, diminish clinical consideration costs, and lessen trouble on human services [14].

5GC Internet of Things. With Internet of things, there will be millions of connected devices and sensors in smart cities which is not possible with 4G network as per GSMA. Mobile IOT is considered the trusted IOT and sensor data can be transmitted to cloud solutions with help of 5G networks. With IOT contact tracing, robotic interviews, crowd temperature sensing with cameras, use of drones for surveillance and IOMT for medical Internet of things are few examples to help and reduce the COVID-19 spread [15]. This kind of technology advancements bring up astonishing possibilities outside the pandemic scenario. Some examples are IoT based electrocardiograms that can be used to detect early arrhythmias [16] and other systems with the goal to improve the accessibility to health records [17, 20] and even predict web page accesses, which can benefit the health industry [18, 19].

3.3 A Proposed Framework for Covid-19 Management Using AI & 5G

Future management of the COVID-19 and similar virus can be done with the help of mobile device. End user can have full access to their own assessment and tracking without going to medical centers and hospital for testing. Accessing and storing personal data on cloud can help to combat spread of COVID-19. Similar to patient fall detection technologies implemented by Apple and researched almost a decade ago, the individuals' mobile handset data will be easily available which can be used for diagnosis of COVID-19 virus. The current diagnostic process is expensive and not available for everyone especially in remote areas of third world countries. Likewise, in advance economies like Australia and Singapore, the end users were reluctant to use the tools like contact tracing. Therefore, this proposed solution is more cost effective and easily available to everyone. Comparison of voice and photos with AI based apps can help the patient to monitor and diagnose the symptoms of COVID-19 virus. A high-level framework and journey of COVID-19 control is presented in Fig. 2.

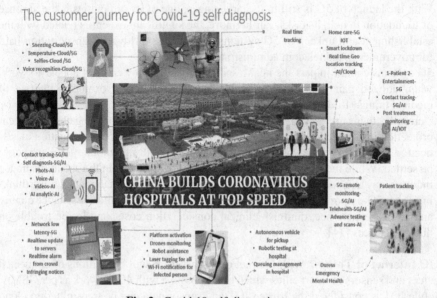

Fig. 2. Covid-19 self-diagnosis system

The framework explains the process from the initial symptoms to the post treatment. Each setup in the framework is linked with use of Cloud, AI, 5G with smartphones. The tracking, monitoring, diagnosis, robot control, patient tracking, in room entertainment, homecare the contact tracing etc. are all dependent on use of smartphones with cloud computing platforms.

The proposed framework consists of Smartphones, 5G network, Cloud computing storage, AI analytic using the data collected from the smartphones and finally linking it to the government databases like census data, demographic of people living in a geographic area and then pushing the data through mobiles apps to the users again for self-diagnosis.

The smartphones will have the capabilities to run the analytic from cloud in real time using the high speed 5G networks. The cloud storage will have enough storage for photos, voice recording, and health data uploaded by the end users. The data analytic part is the most critical one as mobile phones will be used for uploading the data to cloud and retrieving the data from cloud but the AI analytic will be done using the cloud computing.

A high-level data flow is given in Fig. 3 below.

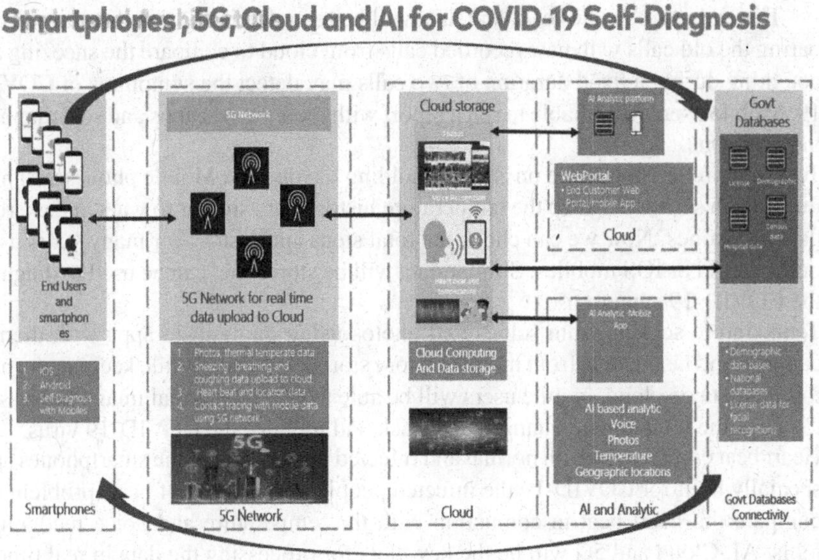

Smartphones , 5G, Cloud and AI for COVID-19 Self-Diagnosis

Fig. 3. Data flow for self-Diagnosis using smartphones

1. Image processing with comparison of selfies: similar to crowd monitoring with high-definition fever detection thermal imaging system, in the future this can be done by mobile phones with help of AI, old selfies and new ones can be compared to identify infected people and end mobile users will be able to compare old photos from google cloud, this will allow mobile user to self-identify and diagnose the COVID-19 symptoms. Just like Google photos are uploaded and kept on google drive by end users, the selfies and AI based algorithm can be used to run a comparison of the photos and generate the reports. Similar to Thermal imaging cameras by Remark Holdings, Feevr, FLiR, UniView, Hikvision, Chubb Fire & Security, Bytronic Automation, Athena Security have launched thermal security cameras for fever detection for crowd monitoring but deployment of these at a high scale is impossible. Smartphones specially IOS and Android with AI, thermal cameras and combining the contact tracing, voice recognition with AI, facial recognition and apps like Therm-App and FlirOne can be used to upload the real time data to cloud with high speed 5G network and AI based computing on edge of the 5G for fast analysis and results.

2. Voice recognition and comparison for breathing difficulties, sneezing and coughing. The banking sector in Australia is already using voice recognition for customers verification and same technology can be used to store the personal data to cloud and run the AI based analysis for COVID-19 symptoms detection. The smartphone users can manage the recoded data and compare it with old calls for self-detection. The sampling of infected people can be used to optimize the AI based tool for better prediction and further research in this area can be focused by government similar to contact tracing apps. The focus is on smartphones, real time data transmission with 5G network and AI based application on public cloud for storage and analysis purpose of voice recoded.

The end users' voices call, and data will be recorded in the cloud storage. Comparing the old calls with new recorded calls from cloud to compare the sneezing and coughing during a fixed duration of two calls may detect the symptoms of COVID-19. Mobile users will be able to run a report with their phones apps and self-diagnose the problems.

3. Temperature sensing while on call and holding the phones. Mobile phones will have the built-in sensors to keep the temperature history data similar to walk and exercise data on phones. Now we can check the total steps and history for many years using our Android or IOS mobiles. Similar data will be stored and can be used to diagnose the COVID-19 symptoms.

4. Temperature sensing from selfies and photos using the built-in apps with thermal cameras and health data from mobile history stored on cloud. While keeping the photos and data on cloud, mobile users will be able to use the thermal image processing to check the temperature changes and track and monitor the COVID-19 virus.

5. Heart beat comparison with normal and infected person. Using the smartphones apps specially built for COVID-19 the infected people with history of heart problem can compare the heart beat in conjuction with the temperature and voice recognition tools. AI, Cloud and 5G will be the key tools for processing the data in real time.

6. Social distancing alarms with mobiles and keeping track of full day report using Wi-Fi and cellular technologies for connecting to nearby devices.

7. People counting, location tracking, geographical movement, international traveling and all other kinds of travelling history can be available from telecom operator's big data, and end user will have full control of managing their own data.

4   Conclusion

As the individuals around the world keeps on understanding the effect of COVID-19 pandemic, blending endeavors of an assortment of cutting-edge advancements, for example, AI and 5G, are trying to minimize its adverse impact. Recognition of that as the supporting of this exertion, we present the absolute most up to date approaching on the COVID-19 pandemic. This paper begins with a comprehensive appraisal of the COVID-19 itself, in which we see the sights of its clinical highlights, transmission system, and diagnosis techniques. Following this, we list the different treatment endeavors being made to stop the pandemic and the preventive measures to be followed till the time that is conceivable. Finally, we propose the use of cutting-edge advancements in AI and 5G to self-manage COVID-19 using mobile handsets. Until a formidable solution for COVID-19 is presented, the responsibility to self-regulate and manage this pandemic may be undertaken with the use of our smartphones on a very basic level using the benefits of Cloud, AI and 5G.

Acknowledgment. The statements made here are the sole responsibility of the authors.

References

1. Cascella, M., Rajnik, M., Cuomo, A., Dulebohn, S.C., Di Napoli, R.: Features, Evaluation, and Treatment of Coronavirus. StatPearls Publishing, Statpearls (2020)

2. WHO: Coronavirus disease (COVID-19) pandemic (2021). https://www.who.int/emerge ncies/diseases/novel-coronavirus-2019. Accessed 25 July 2021

3. Bakshi, S.K., Ho, A.C., Chodosh, J., Fung, A.T., Chan, R.V.P., Ting, D.S.W.: Training in the year of the eye: The impact of the COVID-19 pandemic on ophthalmic education. Br. J. Ophthalmol. **104**, 1181–1183 (2020). https://doi.org/10.1136/bjophthalmol-2020-316991

4. Zhong, L., Mu, L., Li, J., Wang, J., Yin, Z., Liu, D.: Early prediction of the 2019 novel coronavirus outbreak in the Mainland China based on simple mathematical model. IEEE Access **8**, 51761–51769 (2020). https://doi.org/10.1109/ACCESS.2020.2979599

5. Obeidat, S.: How artificial intelligence is helping fight the COVID-19 pandemic. Entrep. Middle East 19–21 (2020)

6. Naudé, W.: Artificial intelligence against COVID-19: an early review. IZA Discuss. Pap. (2020)

7. Qualcomm: Everything you need to know about 5G. Q : What is 5G ? (2021). https://www. qualcomm.com/5g/what-is-5g. Accessed 25 July 2021

8. Ting, D.S.W., Carin, L., Dzau, V., Wong, T.Y.: Digital technology and COVID-19. Nat. Med. **26**, 459–461 (2020). https://doi.org/10.1038/s41591-020-0824-5

9. Chunming, Z., He, G.: 5G applications help China fight against COVID-19. China Acad. Inf. Commun. Technol. 1–4 (2020)

10. Deloitte Consulting: Combating COVID-19 with 5G opportunities to improve public health systems (2020)

11. Tortermvasana, K.: AIS uses 5G, robots in pandemic war (2020)

12. Charles, A., Ruan, S.: In China, robot delivery vehicles deployed to help with COVID-19 emergency—UNIDO (2020)

13. Happich, J.: 5G edge patrol robots deployed in China to detect Covid-19 cases (2020)

14. Li, D.: 5G and intelligence medicine—how the next generation of wireless technology will reconstruct healthcare? Precis. Clin. Med. **2**, 205–208 (2019). https://doi.org/10.1093/pcm edi/pbz020

15. Vaishya, R., Haleem, A., Vaish, A., Javaid, M.: Emerging technologies to combat the COVID-19 pandemic. J. Clin. Exp. Hepatol. **10**, 409–411 (2020). https://doi.org/10.1016/j.jceh.2020. 04.019

16. He, J., Rong, J., Sun, L., Wang, H., Zhang, Y., Ma, J.: A framekwork for cardiac arrythmia detection from IoT-based ECGs. World Wide Web **23**(5), 2835–2850 (2020)

17. Khalil, F., Wang, H., Li, J.: Integrating Markov model with clustering for predicting web page accesses. In: Proceeding of the 13th Australasian World Wide Web Conference (AusWeb 2007), pp. 63–74 (2007)

18. Vimalachandran, P., Liu, H., Lin, Y., Ji, K., Wang, H., Zhang, Y.: Improving accessibility of the Australian my health records while preserving privacy and security of the system. Health Inf. Sci. Syst. **8**(1), 1–9 (2020)

19. Supriya, S., Siuly, S., Wang, H., Zhang, Y.: Automated epilepsy detection techniques from electroencephalogram signals: a review study. Health Inf. Sci. Syst. **8**(1), 1–15 (2020). https:// doi.org/10.1007/s13755-020-00129-1

20. Sarki, R., Ahmed, K., Wang, H., Zhang, Y.: Automated detection of mild and multi-class diabetic eye diseases using deep learning. Health Inf. Sci. Syst. **8**(1), 1–9 (2020). https://doi. org/10.1007/s13755-020-00125-5

EEG Data Processing

Auto-correlation Based Feature Extraction Approach for EEG Alcoholism Identification

Muhammad Tariq Sadiq[1,2(✉)] [iD], Siuly Siuly[3], Ateeq Ur Rehman[4],
and Hua Wang[3]

[1] School of Automation, Northwestern Polytechnical University, Xi'an, China
tariq.sadiq@mail.nwpu.edu.cn
[2] Department of Electrical Engineering, The University of Lahore, Lahore, Pakistan
muhammad.sadiq1@ee.uol.edu.pk
[3] Victoria University, Melbourne, VIC 3011, Australia
{siuly.siuly,hua.wang}@vu.edu.au
[4] Government College University, Lahore 54500, Pakistan

Abstract. Alcoholism severely affects brain functions. Most doctors and researchers utilized Electroencephalogram (EEG) signals to measure and record brain activities. The recorded EEG signals have non-linear and nonstationary attributes with very low amplitude. Consequently, it is very difficult and time-consuming for humans to interpret such signals. Therefore, with the significance of computerized approaches, the identification of normal and alcohol EEG signals has become very useful in the medical field. In the present work, a computer-aided diagnosis (CAD) system is recommended for characterization of normal vs alcoholic EEG signals with following tasks. First, dataset is segmented into several EEG signals. Second, the autocorrelation of each signal is computed to enhance the strength of EEG signals. Third, coefficients of autocorrelation with several lags are considered as features and verified statistically. At last, significant features are tested on twenty machine learning classifiers available in the WEKA platform by employing a 10-fold cross-validation strategy for the classification of normal vs alcoholic signals. The obtained results are effective and support the usefulness of autocorrelation coefficients as features.

Keywords: Electroencephalography · Computer-aided diagnosis · Alcoholism · Autocorrelation · Classification

1 Introduction

Alcohol addiction is perhaps the most widely recognized mental problem related to extensive horribleness and mortality [1]. As per the World Health Organization (WHO) report in 2014, practically 3.3 million individuals (5.9%) of overall

Supported by organization x.

deaths are because of alcohol utilization [2], which is the fifth driving reason for passings [3] and is the principal risk factor for early demise and handicap [4]. There is a wide scope of health impacts in wellbeing due to alcohol dependency, for example, liver and heart diseases, mental deficiency, certain malignant growths, and so forth. Likewise, alcohol consumption is a critical reason for different vandalization, like street crimes, road collisions, social issues, and adds to family breakdown [5,20]. Alcoholics go through various intellectual insufficiencies, for example, learning and memory deficiencies, issues with motor abilities, and enduring conduct changes that incorporate nervousness and melancholy [6,7].

The electroencephalogram (EEG) is one of most significant medical procedure for considering brain occasions, capacities, and problems. EEG signals measure recorded electrical movement produce by the firing of neurons around different brain regions [8,22,39,42]. These recorded EEG signals are extremely intricate in nature and add to a lot of information to be taking into account. Usually, visual assessment is adopted to distinguish dissimilarities in EEG signals by talented clinicians whether the signs come from normal or alcoholic subjects. Indeed, even experienced clinicians can fail to identify the differences in signals because of the presence of noises [9,40,41,43]. Subsequently, the inspiration of this study is to foster a programmed examination framework for the determination of alcoholism with worthy exactness, because of the expanded requirement for appropriate analysis and instruction of neurological anomalies. It will assist us to early admonitions about the approaching sicknesses [21].

For automated identification of alcoholic and normal EEG signals, in literature time-dependent, frequency-dependent, non-linear features based, Autoregressive and time-frequency approaches are available. Either time or frequency domain methods are not suitable for non-stationary signals analysis because these signals have dynamic characteristics thus, time-frequency analysis is obligatory. In study [13], AR and fast Fourier transform (FFT) methods were utilized to estimate power circulation of EEG signals for classification purpose. In [14], a computerize method is proposed by integrating AR model, fuzzy-based adaptive approach and principal component analysis (PCA).

Several non-linear features such as approximate entropy (ApEn), largest Lyapunov exponent (LLE), sample entropy (SampEn), correlation dimension (CD), Hurst exponent (H), along with higher order spectral features are employed in studies [10–12] to classify normal and alcoholic EEG signals. In studies [15], time-frequency approaches are suggested for discrimination of normal vs alcoholic EEG signals. A spectral entropy based approach is proposed in research [16] indicating the suitability of gamma band to extract useful information related to alcoholism. Recently a graph based approach along with non-linear features is presented for identification of alcoholic subjects signals. Despite the extensive work in alcoholism EEG field, there is still gap to develop a stable automated system with few features in a way to provide high classification results with several performance measures.

Subject to the aforementioned issues, the proposed study presents a stable computer-aided diagnosis framework, which utilizes only one feature to obtain high classification outcomes for different performance evaluation parameters. In the alcoholism EEG field, most of the work focus only on classification accuracy and utilized several distinct features for the classification of EEG signals [29, 30]. In the proposed computerized system, we first divide each category's EEG data into several segments with an optimal time interval, and artifacts are removed from each segment. We consider each segment as one signal. Secondly, we executed the auto-correlation of each EEG signal to enhance its quality and avoid its dependency on noises. Thirdly, we consider coefficients of autocorrelation as features, and these features are concatenated for decision making. At last, the statistically significant features are provided as an input to bayesnet, naïve Bayes, support vector machine with the linear and sigmoid kernel, logistic regression, multi-layer perceptron, simple logistic, sequential minimum optimization, voted perceptron, k-nearest neighbor, k star, locally weighted learning, AdaBoost, bagging, logit boost, rotation forest, decision stump, Hoeffding tree, J48, logistic model tree, random forest, and random tree. The results from these classifiers are verified with several performance measures named accuracy, sensitivity, specificity, precision, F-measure, area under the receiver operating curve (AUC), and Matthews correlation coefficient (MCC).

2   Materials

The EEG alcoholism dataset is acquired from human brains of alcoholic and control subjects. This dataset is publically available at (https://archive.ics.uci.edu/ml/datasets/EEG+Database). for research purposes. This dataset provides the 64 electrodes recoding on the scalps of the subjects. The places of the electrodes were situated with standard sites (American Electroencephalographic Association 1990). The examining frequency of recorded EEG signal 256 Hz. There are two categories of subjects: normal vs alcoholic EEG. In the two categories, there are 122 subjects and each subject finished 120 preliminaries. They give 32s EEG information division. There are three forms of the EEG datasets collections: the small collection, the large informational collection, and the full dataset. In this investigation, the small dataset collection is utilized for experimental purposes [17, 18].

Figure 1 shows the visual representation of alcoholic and control EEG signal.

3   Methods

In this investigation, an auto-correlation based approach is presented for categorization of normal and alcoholic EEG signals. The whole cycle of proposed framework is partitioned into following modules: pre-processing, auto-correlation as feature extraction, and classification as displayed in Fig. 2. The beforehand mentioned modules are examined underneath.

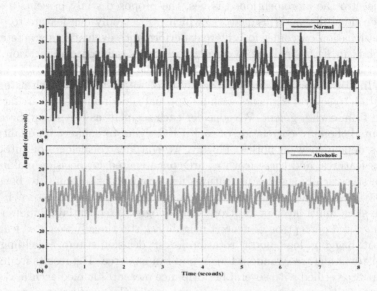

Fig. 1. Graphical representation of normal and alcoholic EEG signals

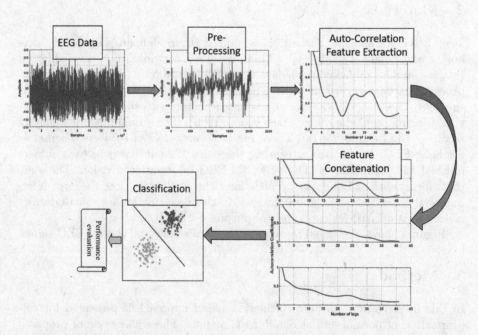

Fig. 2. Block diagram of the proposed auto-correlation framework for classification of normal and alcoholic EEG signals

3.1   Module 1: Pre-processing

The dataset includes the recorded EEG signals 256 Hz sampling rate and 12-bit resolution for 32 s (about 16400 samples). In this study investigations are done utilizing smaller data sets where the baseline filter effectively removes artefacts such as blinking and muscle movements ($>73.3\,\mu v$). The huge EEG recordings are divided into an eight-second window comprising 4 equal sections of 2048 samples for further investigation.

3.2   Module 2: Auto-correlation as Feature Extraction

A signal can also be correlated with its own other segments. The technique is known as autocorrelation by executing a cross correlation of same signal. The Autocorrelation function essentially measures how strongly a signal is correlated with shifting variants. Autocorrelation is helpful in identifying portions of a repeated signal and provide information how the signal corresponds to its neighbours. Determining how the next segments of a signal relate to each other gives some insight into the way in which intervening processes have created or changed the signal. For instance, a signal that remains exceptionally corresponded with itself throughout some duration more likely than not been delivered, or altered, by some interaction that considered past values of the signal. Such a process can be depicted as having memory, since it should recollect past values of the signal and utilize this data to shape the signal present qualities. The more drawn out the memory, the more the signal remaining parts somewhat connected with moved adaptations of itself. The mathematical formulation of autocorrelation function is given as follows [19],

$$A_{aa}[k] = \frac{1}{M} \sum_{m=1}^{M} a[m]a[m+k] \quad k = 0, 1, 2, \ldots K \qquad (1)$$

where M denotes the data points, k is a displacement and varies from 0 to K, and K changes dependent on the treatment of endpoints. Specifically, this approach involves matching the signal to K periods in which K might be fairly large. This shifting k is also named as lag and specify the amount of samples shifted for a specific correlation. If the autocorelation signals included time functions originally, lags may be translated into time shifts in seconds. Feature extraction chooses and/or incorporates elements into functions to efficiently reduce the quantity of data to be processed whilst also representing the actual range of data properly and thoroughly [25, 26]. In the EEG-based alcoholism field, several feature extraction approaches such as time domain, frequency domain, time-frequency domain, linear or non-linear approaches, however, each method inherent a deficiencys. Despite the intensive work, there is still a need to present effective features for the classification of normal and alcoholic EEG signals. In the present work, we employed autocorrelation coefficients as features. We executed autocorrelation functions for different lag values to obtain autocorrelation coefficients. After empirical evaluation, the lag value is set to 40 for each trial. Figure 3 represents the autocorrelation coefficients for trial 1 of normal and alcoholic class EEG signal. It is noted that there is significant difference among different class coefficients, representing the potential of features for better discrimination.

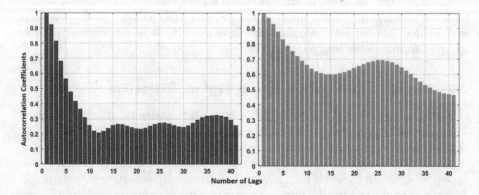

Fig. 3. Autocorrelation coefficients for alcoholic (blue color) and normal (red color) EEG signal (Color figure online)

3.3   Module 3: Classification

To segregate normal and alcoholic EEG signal features, we employed bayesnet (C1), naïve Bayes (C2), support vector machine with the radial basis function, linear and sigmoid kernels (C3, C4 and C5), logistic regression (C6), multi-layer perceptron (C7), simple logistic (C8), sequential minimum optimization (C9), voted perceptron (C10), k-nearest neighbor (C11), k star (C12), locally weighted learning (C13), adaBoost (C14), bagging (15), logit boost (C16), rotation forest (C17), decision stump (C18), Hoeffding tree (C19), J48 (C20), logistic model tree (C21), random forest (C22), and random tree classifiers (C23) [23,24].

4   Results and Discussions

The statistical significance of features extracted from all trials is tabulated in Table 1, where, T represents the trial. It is clearly shown that there is significant difference among mean and standard deviation (STD) of both categories. The probability (P) values for all features are also very small, indicating the statistical significance of features.

The performance of the proposed framework is measure by following performance measures [27,28]:

- Accuracy: Ratio of estimated labels to total labels.
- True Positive Rate (TPR): The potential to recognize alcohol EEG signals accurately.

Table 1. Statistical analysis of features

TN	P value	TN	P value	TN	P value	TN	P value
T1	1.87E−10	T31	0.307658736	T61	1.40E−09	T91	0.003809647
T2	0.067701185	T32	4.76E−07	T62	1.47E−10	T92	0.985201584
T3	0.187866423	T33	1.71E−08	T63	4.95E−08	T93	0.015897659
T4	2.45E−05	T34	0.023643606	T64	1.62E−08	T94	0.032168645
T5	7.05E−11	T35	0.334793983	T65	2.21E−12	T95	2.65E−07
T6	5.18E−10	T36	0.095051701	T66	7.82E−06	T96	0.831090268
T7	0.504304297	T37	0.008676098	T67	0.030706396	T97	0.081242124
T8	0.398703039	T38	5.55E−12	T68	0.015106959	T98	3.29E−12
T9	7.82E−06	T39	0.024221499	T69	9.02E−11	T99	0.896695472
T10	4.86E−05	T40	0.181724138	T70	0.028620174	T100	3.23E−06
T11	0.642860408	T41	0.559041346	T71	1.36E−05	T101	1.35E−06
T12	0.696898409	T42	0.004040789	T72	1.18E−06	T102	1.96E−07
T13	0.000331869	T43	0.00695999	T73	0.992600474	T103	0.00735772
T14	0.155918907	T44	0.061018565	T74	9.29E−06	T104	4.56E−11
T15	4.95E−08	T45	0.022523622	T75	2.77E−05	T105	0.089667607
T16	0.008915276	T46	0.005246546	T76	4.57E−12	T106	5.24E−07
T17	0.001515339	T47	8.10E−05	T77	5.43E−09	T107	7.21E−05
T18	3.39E−05	T48	0.388419066	T78	1.48E−12	T108	2.78E−07
T19	5.93E−05	T49	0.181724138	T79	1.08E−10	T109	3.38E−06
T20	1.29E−11	T50	0.000814155	T80	5.38E−13	T110	0.000471719
T21	0.001564445	T51	0.918745005	T81	7.07E−13	T111	0.002350955
T22	4.87E−12	T52	0.007775722	T82	6.78E−09	T112	1.71E−06
T23	1.18E−13	T53	0.015497872	T83	2.94E−11	T113	1.46E−08
T24	3.92E−07	T54	0.773732579	T84	0.00023159	T114	1.77E−11
T25	0.000621327	T55	5.20E−12	T85	0.079636674	T115	6.75E−12
T26	0.067701185	T56	0.294652789	T86	5.83E−10	T116	3.51E−12
T27	0.344171785	T57	0.041321047	T87	0.001564445	T117	1.21E−12
T28	2.25E−06	T58	0.050367755	T88	2.77E−08	T118	0.334793983
T29	2.94E−11	T59	0.963015093	T89	0.200608161	T119	0.000993741
T30	0.001775879	T60	2.88E−05	T90	0.911387363	T120	7.33E−07

- True Negative Rate (TNR): The capability to recognize normal EEG signals accurately.
- Precision: The closeness between alcoholic and normal EEG signals.
- F-measure: A single numeric value measure to explore balance between sensitivity and precision.

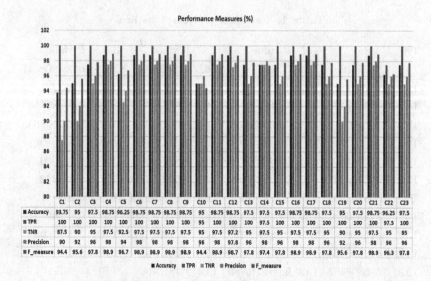

Fig. 4. Classification results for proposed framework

	C1	C2	C3	C4	C5	C6	C7	C8	C9	C10	C11	C12	C13	C14	C15	C16	C17	C18	C19	C20	C21	C22	C23
▪ Accuracy	93.75	95	97.5	98.75	96.25	98.75	98.75	98.75	98.75	95	98.75	98.75	97.5	97.5	97.5	98.75	98.75	97.5	95	97.5	98.75	96.25	97.5
▪ TPR	100	100	100	100	100	100	100	100	100	95	100	100	100	97.5	100	100	100	100	100	100	100	97.5	100
▪ TNR	87.5	90	95	97.5	92.5	97.5	97.5	97.5	97.5	95	97.5	97.2	95	97.5	95	97.5	97.5	95	90	95	97.5	95	95
▪ Precision	90	92	96	98	94	98	98	98	98	96	98	97.8	96	98	96	98	98	96	92	96	98	96	96
▪ F_measure	94.4	95.6	97.8	98.9	96.7	98.9	98.9	98.9	98.9	94.4	98.9	98.7	97.8	97.4	97.8	98.9	98.9	97.8	95.6	97.8	98.9	96.3	97.8

- Matthews correlation coefficient (MCC): It consider true positive, true negative, false positive and false negative to measure the quality of alcoholic and normal EEG classification.
- Area Under the Receiver Operating Curve (AUC): AUC measures a value between 0 and 1, the value near to 1 indicating the authenticity of a classifier for classification of alcoholic and normal EEG signals.

Figure 4 shows the accuracy, TPR, TNR and F-measure classification performance measures (in %). In term of classification accuracy the proposed framework deliver 98.75% classification accuracy results for 10 classifiers, which indicate the effectiveness and flexibility of framework. The minimum classification accuracy of 93.75% is achieved by bayesnet (C1), which is only 5% less than the highest results. The TPR i.e. detection capability of classifiers for alcoholism EEG class is 100% for most of the cases, whereas, TNR i.e. detection ability of classifiers for normal EEG signals is 97.5%. It is worth noting that the difference between TPR and TNR is only 3.5% indicating that the proposed framework is fairly stable in recognition of alcoholic and normal EEG signals. Additionally, precision and F-measure best results are 98% and 98.9% accordingly. Figure 5 indicates the MCC and AUC results deliver by all classifiers. It is seen in Fig. 5 that C7, C8, C15, C17, C21 and C22 obtained 1 value which indicate that these classifiers provide accurate results. In addition, 0.95 value is achieved by C1 and the difference among different classifier results is very small as seen in Fig. 5. On the other hand, C4, C6, C7, C8, C9, C11, C16, C17, and C21 deliver 0.98 value which is also very closed to 1. These results clearly indicate that proposed framework is effective and stable and can be utilized for classification of alcoholic and normal EEG signal identification.

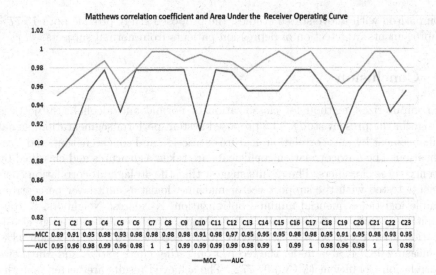

Fig. 5. MCC and AUC results for proposed framework

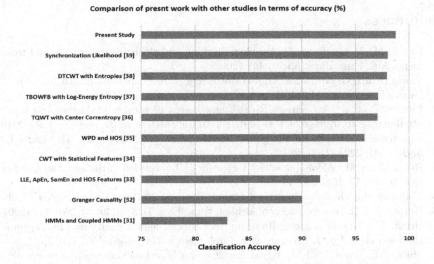

Fig. 6. Comparison of proposed framework with available literature

The proposed study classification accuracy results are compared with other available literature as shown in Fig. 6. It is understood from studies [12,31–38] that all these students require signal decomposition approaches, non-linear features and higher-order statistical features, which suffer mode mixing, complexity and noise artifact issues. On contrary the proposed auto-correlation coefficients based features are relatively simple and help to reduce noise artifacts. In comparison with above-stated studies, the proposed study provide upto 15.77% improvements in detection of depression patients from normal subjects.

5 Conclusion

A computerized method for classification of normal and alcoholic subjects is design in the present study. The proposed system perform segmentation, signal enhancement by autocorrelation, feature extraction and concatenation, and classification. The autocorrelation coefficients are taken as features and classified by twenty-three classifiers. The results suggest that the 40-lag autocorrelation coefficients tested with the support vector machine, logistic, multilayer perceptron, simple logistic, sequential minimal optimization, K-Nearest Neighbors, K star, LogitBoost, rotation forest, and Logistic Model Trees results in average classification accuracy of 98.75%, sensitivity 100%, specificity 97.5%, precision 98%, F-measure 98.9%, area under the receiver operating curve 98.7%, and Matthews Correlation Coefficient (MCC) 97.77%. The achieved results are better than the state-of-the art.

References

1. Enoch, M.-A., Goldman, D.: Problem drinking and alcoholism: diagnosis and treatment. Am. Fam. Phys. **65**(3), 441 (2002)
2. World Health Organization: Global status report on alcohol and health 2018, World Health Organization (2019)
3. Lim, S.S., et al.: A comparative risk assessment of burden of disease and injury attributable to 67 risk factors and risk factor clusters in 21 regions, 1990–2010: a systematic analysis for the global burden of disease study 2010. The LANCET **380**(9859), 2224–2260 (2012)
4. Rehm, J., et al.: Alcohol as a risk factor for global burden of disease. Eur. Addict. Res. **9**(4), 157–164 (2003)
5. Multicultural Organization Development Strategy, National drug strategy (2006)
6. Harper, C.: The neurotoxicity of alcohol. Hum. Exp. Toxicol. **26**(3), 251–257 (2007)
7. Brust, J.: Ethanol and cognition: indirect effects, neurotoxicity and neuroprotection: a review. Int. J. Environ. Res. Publ. Health **7**(4), 1540–1557 (2010)
8. Siuly, Y.L., Wen, P.: EEG signal classification based on simple random sampling technique with least square support vector machine. Int. J. Biomed. Eng. Technol. **7**(4), 390–409 (2011)
9. Acharya, U.R., Bhat, S., Adeli, H., Adeli, A., et al.: Computer-aided diagnosis of alcoholism-related EEG signals. Epilepsy Behav. **41**, 257–263 (2014)
10. Ehlers, C., Havstad, J.: Characterization of drug effects on the EEG by power spectral band time series analysis. Psychopharmacol. Bull. **18**(3), 43–47 (1982)
11. Kannathal, N., Acharya, U.R., Lim, C.M., Sadasivan, P.: Characterization of EEG-a comparative study. Comput. Methods Programs Biomed. **80**(1), 17–23 (2005)
12. Acharya, U.R., Sree, S.V., Chattopadhyay, S., Suri, J.S.: Automated diagnosis of normal and alcoholic EEG signals. Int. J. Neural Syst. **22**(03), 1250011 (2012)
13. Faust, O., Acharya, R., Allen, A.R., Lin, C.: Analysis of EEG signals during epileptic and alcoholic states using AR modeling techniques. IRBM **29**(1), 44–52 (2008)

14. Yazdani, A., Ataee, P., Setarehdan, S.K., Araabi, B.N., Lucas, C.: Neural, fuzzy and neurofuzzy approach to classification of normal and alcoholic electroencephalograms. In: 5th International Symposium on Image and Signal Processing and Analysis, pp. 102–106. IEEE (2007)

15. Sun, Y., Ye, N., Xu, X.: EEG analysis of alcoholics and controls based on feature extraction. In: 2006 8th International Conference on Signal Processing, vol. 1. IEEE (2006)

16. Akbari, H., Ghofrani, S., Zakalvand, P., Sadiq, M.T.: Schizophrenia recognition based on the phase space dynamic of EEG signals and graphical features. Biomed. Sig. Process. Control **69**, 102917 (2021)

17. Snodgrass, J.G., Vanderwart, M.: A standardized set of 260 pictures: norms for name agreement, image agreement, familiarity, and visual complexity. J. Exp. Psychol. Hum. Learn. Memory **6**(2), 174 (1980)

18. Acharya, J.N., Hani, A.J., Cheek, J., Thirumala, P., Tsuchida, T.N.: American clinical neurophysiology society guideline 2: guidelines for standard electrode position nomenclature. Neurodiagnostic J. **56**(4), 245–252 (2016)

19. Semmlow, J.: Signals and Systems for Bioengineers: A MATLAB-Based Introduction. Academic Press, Cambridge (2011)

20. Akbari, H., et al.: Depression recognition based on the reconstruction of phase space of EEG signals and geometrical features. Appl. Acoust. **179**, 108078 (2021)

21. Hussain, W., Sadiq, M.T., Siuly, S., Rehman, A.U.: Epileptic seizure detection using 1 d-convolutional long short-term memory neural networks. Appl. Acoust. **177**, 107941 (2021)

22. Akbari, H., Sadiq, M.T., Rehman, A.U.: Classification of normal and depressed EEG signals based on centered correntropy of rhythms in empirical wavelet transform domain. Health Inf. Sci. Syst. **9**(1), 1–15 (2021)

23. Yu, X., Aziz, M.Z., Sadiq, M.T., Fan, Z., Xiao, G.: A new framework for automatic detection of motor and mental imagery EEG signals for robust BCI systems. IEEE Trans. Instrum. Meas. **70**, 1–12 (2021). https://doi.org/10.1109/TIM.2021.3069026

24. Sadiq, M.T., Yu, X., Yuan, Z., Aziz, M.Z., Siuly, S., Ding, W.: A matrix determinant feature extraction approach for decoding motor and mental imagery EEG in subject specific tasks. IEEE Trans. Cogn. Dev. Syst. 1 (2020). https://doi.org/10.1109/TCDS.2020.3040438

25. Akbari, H., Sadiq, M.T.: Detection of focal and non-focal EEG signals using nonlinear features derived from empirical wavelet transform rhythms. Phys. Eng. Sci. Med. **44**(1), 157–171 (2021)

26. Fan, Z., Jamil, M., Sadiq, M.T., Huang, X., Yu, X.: Exploiting multiple optimizers with transfer learning techniques for the identification of Covid-19 patients. J. Healthc. Eng. **2020** (2020)

27. Akhter, M.P., Jiangbin, Z., Naqvi, I.R., Abdelmajeed, M., Sadiq, M.T.: Automatic detection of offensive language for Urdu and roman Urdu. IEEE Access **8**, 91213–91226 (2020)

28. Akhter, M.P., Jiangbin, Z., Naqvi, I.R., Abdelmajeed, M., Mehmood, A., Sadiq, M.T.: Document-level text classification using single-layer multisize filters convolutional neural network. IEEE Access **8**, 42689–42707 (2020)

29. Sadiq, M.T., et al.: Motor imagery EEG signals decoding by multivariate empirical wavelet transform-based framework for robust brain-computer interfaces. IEEE Access **7**, 171431–171451 (2019)

30. Sadiq, M.T., et al.: Motor imagery EEG signals classification based on mode amplitude and frequency components using empirical wavelet transform. IEEE Access **7**, 127678–127692 (2019)

31. Zhong, S., Ghosh, J.: HMMs and coupled HMMs for multi-channel EEG classification. In: Proceedings of the 2002 International Joint Conference on Neural Networks. IJCNN 2002 (Cat. No. 02CH37290), vol. 2, pp. 1154–1159. IEEE (2002)

32. Bae, Y., Yoo, B.W., Lee, J.C., Kim, H.C.: Automated network analysis to measure brain effective connectivity estimated from EEG data of patients with alcoholism. Physiol. Meas. **38**(5), 759 (2017)

33. Upadhyay, R., Padhy, P., Kankar, P.: Alcoholism diagnosis from EEG signals using continuous wavelet transform. In: Annual IEEE India Conference (INDICON), pp. 1–5. IEEE (2014)

34. Faust, O., Yu, W., Kadri, N.A.: Computer-based identification of normal and alcoholic EEG signals using wavelet packets and energy measures. J. Mech. Med. Biol. **13**(03), 1350033 (2013)

35. Patidar, S., Pachori, R.B., Upadhyay, A., Acharya, U.R.: An integrated alcoholic index using tunable-q wavelet transform based features extracted from EEG signals for diagnosis of alcoholism. Appl. Soft Comput. **50**, 71–78 (2017)

36. Sharma, M., Deb, D., Acharya, U.R.: A novel three-band orthogonal wavelet filter bank method for an automated identification of alcoholic EEG signals. Appl. Intell. **48**(5), 1368–1378 (2018)

37. Sharma, M., Sharma, P., Pachori, R.B., Acharya, U.R.: Dual-tree complex wavelet transform-based features for automated alcoholism identification. Int. J. Fuzzy Syst. **20**(4), 1297–1308 (2018)

38. Mumtaz, W., Kamel, N., Ali, S.S.A., Malik, A.S., et al.: An EEG-based functional connectivity measure for automatic detection of alcohol use disorder. Artif. Intell. Med. **84**, 79–89 (2018)

39. Sadiq, M.T., Yu, X., Yuan, Z., Aziz, Z., Siuly, S., Ding, W.: Towards the development of versatile brain-computer interfaces. IEEE Trans. Artif. Intell. 1 (2021). https://doi.org/10.1109/TAI.2021.3097307

40. Khare, S.K., Bajaj, V.: Constrained based tunable q wavelet transform for efficient decomposition of EEG signals. Appl. Acoust. **163**, 107234 (2020)

41. Sadiq, M.T., et al.: Exploiting feature selection and neural network techniques for identification of focal and nonfocal EEG signals in TQWT domain. J. Healthc. Eng. **2021**, 24 (2021)

42. Supriya, S., Siuly, S., Wang, H.,Zhang, Y.: Eeg sleep stages analysis and classification based on weighed complex network features. IEEE Trans. Emer. Topics Comput. Intell. **5**(2), 236–246, (2018)

43. Sarki, R., Ahmed, K., Wang, H., Zhang, Y.: Automated detection of mild and multi-class diabetic eye diseases using deep learning. Health Inf. Sci. Syst. **8**(1), 1–9 (2020)

An Automatic Scheme with Diagnostic Index for Identification of Normal and Depression EEG Signals

Hesam Akbari[1], Muhammad Tariq Sadiq[2,3]([⊠]) [ID], Siuly Siuly[4], Yan Li[5], and Paul Wen[5]

[1] Islamic Azad University, Tehran, Iran
st_h.akbari@azad.ac.ir
[2] School of Automation, Nothwestern Polytechnical University, Xi'an, China
[3] Department of Electrical Engineering, The University of Lahore, Lahore, Pakistan
muhammad.sadiq1@ee.uol.edu.pk
[4] Victoria University, Melbourne, VIC 3011, Australia
siuly.siuly@vu.edu.au
[5] University of Southern Queensland, Toowoomba, Australia
{Yan.Li,Paul.Wen}@usq.edu.au

Abstract. Detection of depression utilizing electroencephalography (EEG) signals is one of the major challenges in neural engineering applications. This study introduces a novel automated computerized depression detection method using EEG signals. In proposed design, firstly, EEG signals are decomposed into 10 empirically chosen intrinsic mode functions (IMFs) with the aid of variational mode decomposition (VMD). Secondly, the fluctuation index (FI) of IMFs is computed as the discrimination features. Finally, these features are fed into cascade forward neural network and feed-forward neural network classifiers which achieved better classification accuracy, sensitivity, and specificity from the right brain hemisphere in a 10-fold cross-validation strategy in comparison with available literature. In this study, we also propose a new depression diagnostic index (DDI) using the FI of IMFs in the VMD domain. This integrated index would assist in a quicker and more objective identification of normal and depression EEG signals. Both the proposed computerized framework and the DDI can help health workers, large enterprises and product developers to build a real-time system.

Keywords: EEG · Depression · Variational mode decomposition · Fluctuation index · Depression diagnostic index · Classification

1 Introduction

Depression is a mental illness with a prevalence of 264 million people worldwide, and if left untreated, it can lead to self-harm or suicide. Every year, about 800,000 people die due to suicide, which is the second leading cause of death among young

Supported by organization x.

people [1]. The unavailability of psychologists in most developing countries is the main cause of the lack of diagnosis of depression. Thus, an automatic method for the detection of depressed subjects is desirable [2–4]. Magnetic resonance imaging (MRI) and positron emission tomography (PET) scan can be used as a clinical tool for detecting several brain disorders including depression [7], however, the electroencephalogram (EEG) is the most common strategy for such purposes due to its portable, cheap, and non-invasive characteristics [5,6].

Most of the proposed methods for depression detection are based on time frequency analyzing of EEG signals, various nonlinear feature extraction and machine learning techniques and summery of them have been written subsequently. In a time frequency method based on discrete wavelet transform (DWT) [8], the relative wavelet energy (RWE) of sub-bands are extracted as features and fed to an artificial neural network (ANN) classifier, which resulted in 98.11% classification accuracy (ACC). In a fractal based method [9], Katz's and Higuchi's fractal dimensions (KFD and HFD) of DWT coefficients have been extracted as features. These features have been input to a probabilistic neural network (PNN) classifier, which resulted in the classification ACC of 91.30%. The correlation between gender, and depression has been analyzed by wavelet-chaotic based methods [10], which reveal that there is a connection between gender and depression. In another work [11], a combination of linear and nonlinear features extracted from 19 channels has been given to a logistic regression (LR) classifier. They reported the maximum classification ACC of 90%. In an entropy based method [12], sample, approximate, renyi and bispectral phase entropies have been computed in wavelet packet decomposition (WPD) domain as discrimination feature, and fed to a PNN classifier and the maximum classification ACC of 99.5% was reported.

The correlation of rhythms in empirical wavelet transform (EWT) domain has been measured by computing centered correntropy as features for detection of depressed EEG signals, which achieved the classification ACC of 98.76% [13]. Recently, nonlinear behaviors of EEG signals have been quantified as discrimination features by analyzing the 2D shape of EEG signals made by the second order difference plot and phase space reconstruction with several graphical features for the classification of the normal and depressed subjects which resulted in the classification ACC of 98.79% by second order difference plot [14] and 99.30% by phase space reconstruction [15]. In research [16], first depression diagnostic index (DDI) has been developed by combining several nonlinear features, which was the main advantage of their framework. Furthermore, they fed these features into a support vector machine (SVM), which resulted in classification ACC of 98%.

A method based on the synchronization likelihood feature of nineteen channels has been developed in [17], which achieved the classification ACC of 98%. In [18], higher-order spectra based features have been used in bag tree classifier, which achieved 94.30% classification ACC. In another fractal based analyzing method [19], the HFD and the spectral asymmetry index of EEG signals have been extracted as discrimination features, which achieved classification ACC of

94%. In [20], a deep learning method has been developed for the classification of normal and depressed EEG signals based on 13-layer deep convolutional neural network (CNN) which resulted in 95.96% classification ACC. In [21], a new three-channel orthogonal wavelet filter bank has been designed for the detection of normal and depressed EEG signals. They decomposed EEG signals into seven sub-bands, then computed L2 norm entropy as features which resulted in 99.58% classification ACC.

Several time-frequency representations have been proposed to analyze the depressed EEG signals based on Fourier transform and wavelet variants. The traditional methods decompose the EEG signals using fixed filter banks i.e. they do not decompose the EEG signals according to their frequency components or they are non-adaptive decomposition methods [28]. Empirical mode decomposition (EMD) was proposed as an adaptive decomposition method, however, the major defect of EMD were mode mixing, sensitivity to noise, end-effects artifacts, and lack of closed-form mathematical expression [12,29]. Recently, variational mode decomposition (VMD) has been proposed as an adaptive method to analyze the nonlinear and non-stationary signals. The VMD method decomposes the input signals according to frequency components density and provide noise-free spectrum. The VMD eliminates the mode mixing and end-effects problems deliver by the EMD method [24]. Owing to the significance of the VMD, this work provides a new paradigm for the identification of EEG depression signals by the extraction of fluctuation index (FI) in VMD domain and neural network classifiers. The main contributions of this study are listed as below:

- A novel framework is proposed for EEG depression signals detection.
- The proposed framework provides a new depression diagnostic index for the medical team.
- The proposed framework can be installed in hospitals as an inexpensive and available tool for depressed subjects detection.
- The proposed framework achieved perfect classification accuracy, sensitivity, and specificity of 100% in a 10-fold cross-validation (CV) strategy that is higher than previous works.

To the best of the author's knowledge, the VMD and FI have not previously been employed for depression detection. Besides, we presented a new depression diagnostic index (DDI) based on the FI of Intrinsic mode functions (IMFs).

2   Proposed Methodology

The proposed framework comprise of several blocks which are shown in the Fig. 1, and summarized subsequently.

2.1   Data Acquisition

The proposed method is evaluated by self recorded EEG signals of 22 normal subjects and 22 depressed patients. The EEG signals were recorded with a bipolar montage from the left and right halves of the brain. For each subject, the

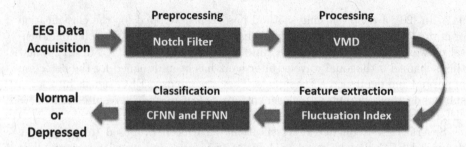

Fig. 1. Block diagram of proposed computerized framework

EEG signals were recorded for 10 min. The power line intrusion and muscle artifacts were discarded by visually and utilizing the notch filter with 0.5 to 150 Hz
band-pass, respectively [12]. The sampling frequency 256 Hz. In this work, the
EEG signals are divided into segments of 500 samples. The data recording experiments were approved by the Research Ethics Committee of AJA University of
Medical Sciences, Iran with approval ID: *IR.AJAUMS.REC.1399.049.*

2.2 Modes Extraction with VMD

The variational mode decomposition (VMD) approach iteratively decomposes
the EEG signal into a N set of modes u_n, compactly supported around their
center frequencies. The VMD constrained problem is mathematically defines as
[24]:

$$
\min_{\{u_n\},\{\Omega_n\}} \left\{ \sum_{n=1}^{N} \left\| \partial_t \left[\left(\delta(t) + \frac{i}{\pi t}\right) * u_n(t) \right] e^{-i\Omega_n t} \right\|_2^2 \right\}
$$
$$
\text{s.t.} \quad \sum_{n=1}^{N} u_n(t) = u(t)
\tag{1}
$$

where $u(t)$ denotes the EEG signal with modes $\{u_n\} := \{u_1, u_2, \ldots, u_N\}$,
$\{\Omega n\} := \{\Omega_1, \Omega_2, \ldots, \Omega_N\}$ reflect the series of each center oscillation referring
to the nth mode., ∂_t represents the differential operator, and $*$. stands for convolution.

The Lagrangian multiplier along with quadratic penalty term help to make
the problem unconstrained and formulation is given as [24]:

$$
\mathcal{L}\left(\{u_n\}, \{\Omega_n\}, \Lambda\right) := \beta \sum_n \left\| \partial_t \left[\left(\delta(t) + \frac{i}{\pi t}\right) * u_n(t) \right] e^{-i\Omega_n t} \right\|_2^2
$$
$$
+ \left\| g(t) - \sum_n u_n(t) \right\|_2^2 + \left\langle \Lambda(t), g(t) - \sum_n u_n(t) \right\rangle
\tag{2}
$$

where $\Lambda(t)$ stands for Lagrangian multiplier, β bandwidth control parameter,
and $\delta(.)$ is the Dirac distribution. An optimization model named as alternate
direction method of multipliers (ADMM) method is used to solve the problem
(2). The frequency domain representation of the obtained modes is formulated
as:

$$\hat{u}_n^{k+1}(\Omega) = \frac{\hat{g}(\Omega) - \sum_{i \neq n} \hat{u}_i(\Omega) + (\hat{\Lambda}(\Omega)/2)}{1 + 2\beta \left(\Omega - \Omega_n\right)^2} \tag{3}$$

Likewise, the frequency representation of the optimization of Ω_n is given as [24]:

$$\Omega_n^{k+1} = \frac{\int_0^\infty \Omega \left|\hat{u}_n(\Omega)\right|^2 \, \mathrm{d}\Omega}{\int_0^\infty \left|\hat{u}_n(\Omega)\right|^2 \, \mathrm{d}\Omega} \tag{4}$$

In this research the 10 modes are empirically utilized for experimentation.

2.3 Fluctuation Index

The fluctuation index (FI) quantifies the oscillations in time series data [25]. The oscillations in EEG signals have a direct relationship with the frequency components obtained by the spectrum of EEG signals. Since the VMD adaptively extracted the 10 modes by obtaining the frequency components density in EEG signals, the FI of modes can assist to obtain good discrimination among normal and depressed groups. Thus in this study FI of modes is used as potential biomarker to classify normal and depressed EEG signals and formulated as follows [25]:

$$FI = \frac{1}{L} \sum_{l=1}^{L-1} |IMF(l+1) - IMF(l)| \tag{5}$$

where L indicates to lengths of IMF.

2.4 Classification

The extracted features are fed to the cascade forward neural network (CFNN) and feed-forward neural network (FFNN) classifiers [30–32]. We use the tan sigmoid transfer function, a single hidden layer with empirically chosen ten neurons, and Levenberg-Marquardt algorithm for fast training as suggested in [26,27]. The normal vs. depression EEG signals classification task is evaluated by the collected EEG signals in ten-fold cross-validation strategy from the left and right hemispheres.

Figure 2 shows a sample of normal and depression EEG signals and their first ten IMFs.

3 Experimental Results

In this section we first explain the results obtained with the proposed framework, subsequently results achieved with depression diagnostic indexes are shown.

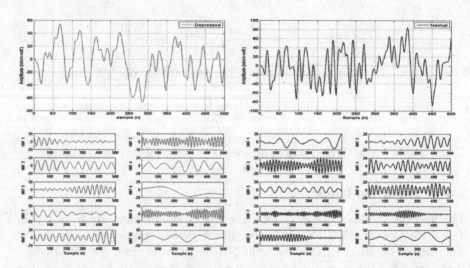

Fig. 2. A sample of depression (red color) and normal (blue color) EEG signals and their 10 IMFs. (Color figure online)

Table 1. Statistical analyzing of features for the left and right hemispheres

IMF no.	Left					Right				
	Normal		Depressed		p-value	Normal		Depressed		p-value
	Mean	Std	Mean	Std		Mean	Std	Mean	Std	
1	0.59	0.28	0.4	0.39	1.78E−08	0.62	0.31	0.47	0.37	1.07E−05
2	2.52	0.71	0.99	0.39	1.15E−31	2.82	0.75	1.27	0.49	1.10E−29
3	2.39	0.55	0.89	0.34	5.09E−33	2.52	0.56	0.96	0.28	9.41E−34
4	2.27	0.57	0.77	0.32	7.46E−33	2.43	0.59	0.82	0.32	2.99E−33
5	1.53	0.46	0.63	0.41	1.33E−26	1.62	0.46	0.55	0.26	2.41E−32
6	0.9	0.48	0.48	0.38	4.48E−11	0.88	0.4	0.58	0.41	3.98E−07
7	0.78	0.7	0.63	0.3	3.00E−10	0.82	0.77	0.88	0.32	1.00E−11
8	1.62	0.67	0.7	0.27	2.20E−22	1.66	0.81	0.75	0.28	5.62E−16
9	1.59	0.86	0.65	0.34	2.93E−14	1.78	0.94	0.63	0.3	2.26E−16
10	1.46	0.75	0.58	0.33	5.75E−18	1.57	0.67	0.53	0.25	3.07E−25

3.1 Results Obtained with the Proposed Framework

The statistical analysis of features for the left and right hemispheres are shown in Table 1. The lesser p-values indicate the better ability of features to discriminate the classes. It is clear from Table 1 that the FI is a pretty good feature for discriminating normal and depression EEG signals. The mean and standard deviation values of FI in the normal group is significantly higher than the depressed group which indicates that depressed EEG signals have lesser non-stationary behaviors than normal. This concept have been reported in previous works by analyzing the nonlinearity of EEG signals with nonlinear features and reporting that normal EEG signals have more complex morphological behavior than depressed EEG signals. This concept has been found out in [14, 15] by reporting that 2D illustration of EEG signals in the depressed group has more regular and simpler shape than the normal.

In Tables 2 and 3, the performance of CFNN and FFNN classifiers in classifying the normal and depression EEG signals is presented respectively. It is noted that the average ACC, SEN, and SPE of 100% is achieved for the right half brain with both classifiers. For the left half hemisphere, the CFNN provides little better results in contrast to the FFNN.

Table 2. Classification results obtained with the CFNN

Evaluation parameters	Hemisphere	
	Left	Right
ACC (%)	99.50	100
SEN (%)	99	100
SPE (%)	100	100

Table 3. Classification results obtained with the FFNN

Evaluation parameters	Hemisphere	
	Left	Right
ACC (%)	99	100
SEN (%)	98.03	100
SPE (%)	100	100

According to Table 4, the proposed framework delivers better results for EEG signals of the right hemisphere and similar results are obtained by other literature [11, 19]. As seen in Table 4, studies [8, 11] achieved good classification outcome but those methods utilized the discrete wavelet transform which results in frequency leakage disadvantages. In addition, several energy or entropy based features are extracted, which make those studies computationally extensive. In study [19], the deep learning based neural network approach is employed but needed a large training time, architecture issues, selecting layers or neuron issues. On the contrary, the proposed framework provides 100% classification ACC with a simple notch filter and a single feature. In comparison with other studies in Table 4, the proposed framework yields up to 6.46% classification ACC improvements. It is also worth mentioning here, the proposed framework are reported in a 10-fold CV strategy for ensuring robust classification performance, while the results in [8, 11] are obtained without any CV technique.

Table 4. The comparison of the proposed method with other studies

Ref	Classification	CV used	ACC	SEN	SPE
[8]	ANN	No	98.11	98.73	97.5
[9]	PNN	No	91.3	Not reported	Not reported
[11]	LR	Leave one out	90.05	Not reported	Not reported
[12]	PNN	No	Left: 98.20	Left: 97.10	Left: 99.40
[12]	PNN	No	Right: 99.50	Right: 99.20	Right: 99.70
[16]	SVM	No	98	97	98.5
[17]	SVM	10-fold	98	96.9	95
[22]	SVM	Leave one out	81.23	Not reported	Not reported
[18]	Bagged tree	Leave one out	94.3	91.46	97.45
[23]	Jackknife replication	No	91.3	Not reported	Not reported
[19]	SVM	No	94%	Not reported	Not reported
[19]	LR	Leave one out	92	Not reported	Not reported
[20]	CNN	10-fold	Left: 93.54	Left: 91.89	Left: 95.18
[20]	CNN	10-fold	Right: 95.96	Right: 94.99	Right: 96.00
[13]	SVM	10-Fold	Left: 98.33	Left: 98.02	Left: 98.65
[13]	SVM	10-Fold	Right: 98.76	Right: 98.47	Right: 99.05
[14]	KNN	10-fold	Left: 97.79	Left: 96.79	Left: 98.79
[14]	KNN	10-fold	Right: 98.58	Right: 97.63	Right: 99.53
[15]	SVM	10-fold	Left: 97.74	Left: 97.81	Left: 97.67
[15]	SVM	10-fold	Right: 99.30	Right: 99.30	Right: 99.30
[21]	SVM	10-fold	Left: 99.02	Left: 98.66	Left: 99.38
[21]	SVM	10-fold	Right: 99.54	Right: 98.66	Right: 99.38
This work	CFNN	10-Fold	Left: 99.50	Left: 99.00	Left: 100
			Right: 100	Right: 100	Right: 100
	FFNN	10-Fold	Left: 99.00	Left: 98.03	Left: 100
			Right: 100	Right: 100	Right: 100

3.2   Results Obtained with Depression Diagnostic Index

Even though the CAD system can be used for diagnosis, it is more convenient for the clinician's use, if we present them with a single integrated index that provides significant differences between the two classes. The excellent performance of the proposed feature motivated us to provide a new DDI based on FI of IMFs in the VMD domain. After hit and trial manner, the developed index is formulated as:

$$DDI = \sqrt{FI_2 + FI_3 + FI_4 + FI_5} \tag{6}$$

where FI_i is computed FI from ith IMF.

To the best of the author's knowledge, there was only one DDI using EEG signals, which is based on laminarity, higher-order spectra parameters, and sample entropy as features that all of them have cumbersome calculations [15]. In contrast, proposed DDI's are based on one feature with very simple and easy

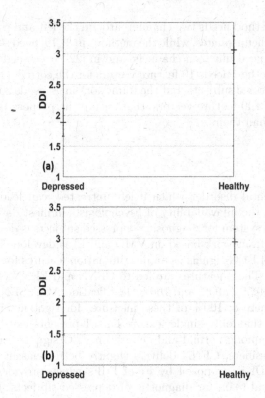

Fig. 3. Depression diagnosis index (a) right hemisphere and (b) left hemisphere.

calculations (i.e. the same FI of IMFs). Besides, the standard deviation of the proposed DDI is around 0.3 and 0.2 in depression and healthy groups while the standard deviation of the proposed DDI in [15] was around 3.5 and 5.5 in depression and healthy groups. In other words, the proposed DDI is more robust and reliable than the DDI proposed in [15]. It should be noted that the p-value of the proposed DDI is 2.6×10^{-34} and 7.8×10^{-34} and for the left and right hemispheres, respectively. The main advantages of the proposed framework are listed as below:

- This is the first time that ability of VMD is evaluated in a depression EEG signals detection.
- The proposed framework provides a new DDI for the medical team.
- The proposed framework can installed on computers of clinics and hospitals as an inexpensive and available tool for depressed subjects identification.
- The proposed framework achieved the perfect classification ACC, SEN, and SPE of 100% in a 10-fold CV strategy that is higher than previous works.
- The effectiveness of the proposed method is evaluated by 44 subjects (22 normal and 22 depressed) while in [12,16,18,20,21] the results reported by 30 subjects (15 normal and 15 depressed), so, the proposed method is more reliable than theirs.

- The proposed method needs two channels around the left and two channels in the right brain's hemispheres, while the methods in [9,19] need seven channels, in [10,11,17,23] need nineteen channels, and in [22], needs eight channels.
- The proposed method needs 10 feature vectors for the correct classification of normal and depressed subjects, but the framework in [8] needs 20, in [11] needs 30, in [17] needs 100 feature vectors, that ensure the proposed framework to be the simpler than theirs.

4   Conclusion

Depression is a mental disorder which if left untreated, can lead to self-harm and suicide. Due to the unavailability of psychologists in most developing countries, an automated system for diagnosing depressed subjects is desirable. In this study, an adaptive framework based on VMD and FI is developed for quantifying the variations of EEG signals as an discrimination features for detecting the depressed subjects. These features are fed to CFNN and FFNN classifiers. The CFNN resulted in 99.50%, 99% and 100% classification ACC, SEN, and SPE for left hemisphere, whereas, 100% of these measures for right hemispheres. This study also suggest that only single feature i.e. FI presents excellent discrimination capabilities among normal and depression EEG signals. Among the two neural network classifiers, CFNN delivers slightly better classification results. At last, a novel DDI is proposed by FI of IMFs which provides a new approach for the medical team for diagnostic of depressed subjects. In the future, the performance of the proposed method can be implemented for other neural diseases.

References

1. World Health Organization Depression Key Facts (2021). https://www.who.int/news-room/fact-sheets/detail/depression
2. Sadiq, M.T., Yu, X., Yuan, Z., Aziz, M.Z.: Identification of motor and mental imagery EEG in two and multiclass subject-dependent tasks using successive decomposition index. Sensors **20**(18), 5283 (2020)
3. Yu, X., et al.: Feasibility evaluation of micro-optical coherence tomography (μoct) for rapid brain tumor type and grade discriminations: μoct images versus pathology. BMC Med. Imaging **19**(1), 1–12 (2019)
4. Jafri, G.A., Rehman, A.U., Sadiq, M.T.: Spectrum sensing and management in cooperative cognitive radio (2011)
5. Sadiq, M.T., et al.: Motor imagery EEG signals decoding by multivariate empirical wavelet transform-based framework for robust brain-computer interfaces. IEEE Access **7**, 171431–171451 (2019)
6. Sadiq, M.T., et al.: Motor imagery EEG signals classification based on mode amplitude and frequency components using empirical wavelet transform. IEEE Access **7**, 127678–127692 (2019)
7. Şengür, D., Siuly, S.: Efficient approach for EEG-based emotion recognition. Electron. Lett. **56**(25), 1361–1364 (2020)

8. Puthankattil, S.D., Joseph, P.K.: Classification of EEG signals in normal and depression conditions by ANN using RWE and signal entropy. J. Mech. Med. Biol. **12**(04), 1240019 (2012)

9. Ahmadlou, M., Adeli, H., Adeli, A.: Fractality analysis of frontal brain in major depressive disorder. Int. J. Psychophysiol. **85**(2), 206–211 (2012)

10. Ahmadlou, M., Adeli, H., Adeli, A.: Spatiotemporal analysis of relative convergence of EEGs reveals differences between brain dynamics of depressive women and men. Clin. EEG Neurosci. **44**(3), 175–181 (2013)

11. Faust, O., Ang, P.C.A., Puthankattil, S.D., Joseph, P.K.: Depression diagnosis support system based on EEG signal entropies. J. Mech. Med. Biol. **14**(03), 1450035 (2014)

12. Akbari, H., Sadiq, M.T., Rehman, A.U.: Classification of normal and depressed EEG signals based on centered correntropy of rhythms in empirical wavelet transform domain. Health Inf. Sci. Syst. **9**(1), 1–15 (2021)

13. Akbari, H., Sadiq, M.T., Payan, M., Esmaili, S.S., Baghri, H., Bagheri, H.: Depression detection based on geometrical features extracted from SODP shape of EEG signals and binary PSO. Traitement du Sig. **38**(1) (2021)

14. Akbari, H., et al.: Depression recognition based on the reconstruction of phase space of EEG signals and geometrical features. Appl. Acoust. **179**, 108078 (2021)

15. Acharya, U.R., et al.: A novel depression diagnosis index using nonlinear features in EEG signals. Eur. Neurol. **74**(1–2), 79–83 (2015)

16. Mumtaz, W., Xia, L., Ali, S.S.A., Yasin, M.A.M., Hussain, M., Malik, A.S.: Electroencephalogram (EEG)-based computer-aided technique to diagnose major depressive disorder (MDD). Biomed. Sig. Process. Control **31**, 108–115 (2017)

17. Bairy, G.M., et al.: Automated diagnosis of depression electroencephalograph signals using linear prediction coding and higher order spectra features. J. Med. Imaging Health Inform. **7**(8), 1857–1862 (2017)

18. Bachmann, M., Lass, J., Suhhova, A., Hinrikus, H.: Spectral asymmetry and Higuchi's fractal dimension measures of depression electroencephalogram. Comput. Math. Methods Med. **2013** (2013)

19. Acharya, U.R., Oh, S.L., Hagiwara, Y., Tan, J.H., Adeli, H., Subha, D.P.: Automated EEG-based screening of depression using deep convolutional neural network. Comput. Methods Programs Biomed. **161**, 103–113 (2018)

20. Sharma, M., Achuth, P., Deb, D., Puthankattil, S.D., Acharya, U.R.: An automated diagnosis of depression using three-channel bandwidth-duration localized wavelet filter bank with EEG signals. Cogn. Syst. Res. **52**, 508–520 (2018)

21. Liao, S.-C., Wu, C.-T., Huang, H.-C., Cheng, W.-T., Liu, Y.-H.: Major depression detection from EEG signals using kernel eigen-filter-bank common spatial patterns. Sensors **17**(6), 1385 (2017)

22. Knott, V., Mahoney, C., Kennedy, S., Evans, K.: EEG power, frequency, asymmetry and coherence in male depression. Psychiatry Res. Neuroimaging **106**(2), 123–140 (2001)

23. Bachmann, M., et al.: Methods for classifying depression in single channel EEG using linear and nonlinear signal analysis. Comput. Methods Programs Biomed. **155**, 11–17 (2018)

24. Dragomiretskiy, K., Zosso, D.: Variational mode decomposition. IEEE Trans. Sig. Process. **62**(3), 531–544 (2013)

25. Hwa, R.C.: Fluctuation index as a measure of heartbeat irregularity. Nonlinear Phenomena Compl. Syst.-MINSK **3**(1), 93–98 (2000)

26. Yu, X., Aziz, M.Z., Sadiq, M.T., Fan, Z., Xiao, G.: A new framework for automatic detection of motor and mental imagery EEG signals for robust BCI systems. IEEE Trans. Instrum. Meas. **70**, 1–12 (2021). https://doi.org/10.1109/TIM.2021.3069026

27. Sadiq, M.T., Yu, X., Yuan, Z., Aziz, M.Z., Siuly, S., Ding, W.: A matrix determinant feature extraction approach for decoding motor and mental imagery EEG in subject specific tasks. IEEE Trans. Cogn. Dev. Syst. 1 (2020). https://doi.org/10.1109/TCDS.2020.3040438

28. Hussain, W., Sadiq, M.T., Siuly, S., Rehman, A.U.: Epileptic seizure detection using 1 d-convolutional long short-term memory neural networks. Appl. Acoust. **177**, 107941 (2021)

29. Akbari, H., Sadiq, M.T.: Detection of focal and non-focal EEG signals using nonlinear features derived from empirical wavelet transform rhythms. Phys. Eng. Sci. Med. **44**(1), 157–171 (2021)

30. Fan, Z., Jamil, M., Sadiq, M.T., Huang, X., Yu, X.: Exploiting multiple optimizers with transfer learning techniques for the identification of Covid-19 patients. J. Healthc. Eng. **2020** (2020)

31. Akhter, M.P., Jiangbin, Z., Naqvi, I.R., Abdelmajeed, M., Sadiq, M.T.: Automatic detection of offensive language for Urdu and roman Urdu. IEEE Access **8**, 91213–91226 (2020)

32. Sadiq, M.T., et al.: Exploiting feature selection and neural network techniques for identification of focal and nonfocal EEG signals in TQWT domain. J. Healthc. Eng. **2021**, 24 (2021)

ADHD Children Identification Based on EEG Using Effective Connectivity Techniques

Mingkan Shen[1]($\boxtimes$), Peng Wen[1], Bo Song[1], and Yan Li[2]

[1] School of Mechanical and Electrical Engineering, University of Southern Queensland, Toowoomba, QLD, Australia
{Mingkan.Shen,Paul.Wen,Bo.Song}@usq.edu.au
[2] School of Science, University of Southern Queensland, Toowoomba, QLD, Australia
Yan.Li@usq.edu.au

Abstract. This paper presents a novel method to identify the Attention deficit hyperactivity disorder (ADHD) children using electroencephalography (EEG) signals and effective connectivity techniques. In this study, the original EEG data is pre-filtered and divided into Delta, Theta, Alpha and Beta bands. And then, the effective connectivity graphs are constructed by applying independent component analysis, multivariate regression model and phase slope index. The measures of clustering coefficient, nodal efficiency and degree centrality in graph theory are used to extract features from these graphs. Statistical analysis based on the standard error of the mean is employed to evaluate the performance in each frequency band. The results show a decreased average clustering coefficient in Delta band for ADHD subjects. Also, in Delta band, the ADHD subjects have increased nodal efficiency and degree centrality in left forehead and decreased in forehead middle.

Keywords: ADHD · EEG · Effective connectivity · Multivariate regression model · Phase slope index · Graph theory

1 Introduction

Attention deficit hyperactivity disorder (ADHD) is a heterogeneous disease with a high prevalence. The prevalence in children worldwide is estimated to be 8%-12%, and about 60% of symptoms and their effect continue into adulthood [1]. In recent years, researchers have used brain Computed Tomography (CT), magnetic resonance imaging (MRI), functional magnetic resonance imaging (fMRI), magnetoencephalography (MEG), electroencephalography (EEG) and other methods to conduct in-depth research on the microstructure of the brain [2–5]. The development of the detection method encouraged researchers to gain further information about ADHD. EEG is a popular and widely used technique for obtaining information from brain. It also is a non-invasive nerve discharge detection technology with millisecond-level high time resolution. Currently, visual inspection of the EEG signal is the most popular method to detect the ADHD, and auto-detect technology is investigated intensively [6].

Majority of the recent papers proposed the complex brain networks analysis method focus on the ADHD research based on the EEG signal. In complex brain network analysis,

S. Siuly et al. (Eds.): HIS 2021, LNCS 13079, pp. 71–81, 2021.
https://doi.org/10.1007/978-3-030-90885-0_7

one of the methods for auto-detecting ADHD is functional connectivity. The functional connectivity represents the statistical correlation of the functional activities of different brain regions in time courses, and the statistical calculation is performed based on EEG signal [7]. Chen et al. highlighted the mutual information (MI) functional connectivity method to classify the ADHD subjects and health control (HC) subjects [8]. Weighted phase lag index (WPLI) connectivity method is reported by Furlong et al. to analysis resting-state EEG data in young children with ADHD [1]. Based on the functional connectivity, the factor the connectivity direction is proposed to analysis ADHD problem, this kind of method also called effective connectivity. Abbas et al. proposed transfer entropy (TE) effective connectivity to detect ADHD [9]. In addition, phase transfer entropy (PTE) connectivity is used to explore the brain activity before and after neurofeedback for ADHD children by Wang et al. [10]. The phase slope index (PSI) as the non-linear measure which can infer dominant unidirectional interactions in brain connectivity analysis is proposed in this paper.

Many methods in time, frequency, time-frequency and phase domain have been developed to address brain connectivity graph construction issue. MI as the time domain measure, Fast Fourier Transform in frequency domain, Wavelet Transform in time-frequency domain, and Phase Locking Value (PLV) in phase domain is used widely in ADHD connectivity analysis [9, 11–13].

Graph theory is the main mathematical tools used in the brain connectivity analysis, the measures of the graph theory describe the local and global features of the brain network [14]. Most of the brain connectivity in ADHD children were focused on the degrees, clustering coefficient, shortest path length, centrality and efficiency [1, 15].

In this study, we used the PSI algorithm based on the multivariate autoregressive (MVAR) model to construct the effective connectivity. We applied the connectivity matrix as the graph to extract the features by three graph theory measures clustering coefficient, nodal efficiency and degree centrality. At last we used the standard error of the mean (SEM) to get the statistical results between ADHD and HC.

2 Method

The framework of the proposed method is shown in Fig. 1, which indicates how to use effectivity connectivity to detect the ADHD and HC progress. The EEG data for ADHD and HC are obtained from IEEE Data port (https://doi.org/10.21227/rzfh-zn36). The 19 channels EEG raw data is collected from ADHD and HC subjects during a visual attention task. Then, the pre-processing is conducted to remove the artifacts and noise from the raw data. The MVAR model and PSI algorithm are applied to construct a connectivity matrix ($19 \times 19 \times 4$) in delta (0.5–4 Hz), theta (4–8 Hz), alpha (8–13 Hz) and beta (13–30 Hz) frequency bands for each subject. Furthermore, graph theoretical analysis is proposed to extract the features from the connectivity matrix (graph) as global efficiency and clustering coefficient. At last, we conducted the statistical analysis by applying the SEM algorithm.

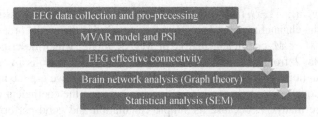

Fig. 1. A framework of effective connectivity analysis in ADHD and HC

2.1 Dataset

According to DSM-IV, there were 60 subjects, children with ADHD (15 boys and 15 girls, ages 7–12) provided by Roozbeh hospital in Tehran, Iran, and 30 HC (15 boys and 15 girls, ages 7–12) collected from a primary school. All children of HC group have not got a history of psychiatric brain disorder such as epilepsy, major medical illness or any report of high-risk behaviours.

The EEG raw data was collected from a 10–20 standard 19 channels electrode cap which correspond to FP1, FP2, F3, F4, C3, C4, P3, P4, O1, O2, F7, F8, T7, T8, P7, P8, Fz, Cz, Pz respectively. The data has a 128 Hz sample rate and with two reference electrodes A1 and A2.

According to the characteristics of ADHD with cognitive impairment, all participants were tested visual attention task which showed the subjects pictures of a set of cartoon characters. Children had been asked to answer the numbers of the characters in the task. All the size of images was large enough to make sure all subjects could see and count clearly, and each image would appear 5 to 16 times randomly. In order to extract features more clearly in the EEG signal, each image will be displayed immediately and will not be interrupted after the subjects responds. Therefore, the duration of EEG recording in the entire visual attention task depends on the subjects' performance.

2.2 EEG Pre-processing

EEG signals were filtered in bandpass frequency between 0.5 Hz to 50 Hz using a zero-phase finite impulse response (FIR) filter. Independent component analysis (ICA) is used to assume statistically independent sources, in addition, removing the blinks, eye-movements and artifacts. Then, we re-referenced the data to the average of all scalp channels.

2.3 Multivariate Autoregressive Model

MVAR model can infer directivity and the causal relationship between brain connections based on effective connectivity methods which is an extension of autoregressive model on multi-dimensional variables [16]. The algorithm of MVAR model is shown as follow:

$$X(n) = \sum_{k=1}^{p} A(k) \times X(n-k) + W(n) \tag{1}$$

$X(n) = [x_1(n), \ldots, x_M(n)]^T$ is the current value of EEG pro-processing signal in time n. M is the channel number, here M equals to 19. p is the model order, $A(k), k = 1, \ldots, p$, are $M \times M$ coefficient matrix of MVAR model which describe the linear interaction at lag k from $x_j(n-k)$ to $x_i(n)$, $(i, j = 1, \ldots, M)$. $W(n)$ is a vector of zero-mean Gaussian noise process with covariance matrix Σ. Here we use the multichannel Yule-Walker equation to describe the relationship between the coefficient matrix $A(k)$ and covariance matrix Σ because its simple calculation and good performance [17]. Thus, the output of the $X(n)$ is the $19 \times 19 \times p$ matrix of each subject.

Another key parameter of the MVAR model is the order of the MVAR model. The choice of order is closely related to the fitting effect of the model. The small order cannot make full use of the information of the observation data for accurate fitting. The large order would cause the phenomenon of overfitting and would increase the expense of calculation.

In this study, Akaike Information Criterion (AIC) equation is provided to assess the order of MVAR model [18].

$$AIC(p) = In|\Sigma(p)| + \frac{2}{N}mp^2 \tag{2}$$

where $\Sigma(p)$ represents the covariance matrix of the fitting error of the p-order model, and N represents the total number of settlements used for model fitting. Thus, p = 5 was selected as the model order according to the AIC equation.

We also need to obtain frequency domain data through coherent spectrum estimation, where the MVAR model is converted to frequency domain form through Fourier transform. The transfer matrix of MVAR model $H(f)$, and cross-spectrum matrix $S(f)$ are estimated as follow:

$$H(f) = (\sum_{k=0}^{p} -A_k e^{-jk2\pi f})^{-1} \tag{3}$$

$$S(f) = H(f)\Sigma\left(H^H(f)\right) \tag{4}$$

where $H^H(f)$ is the conjugate transpose of $H(f)$. Σ is the noise covariance matrix. A_k is the parameter of $M \times M$ coefficient matrix and the p is the model order.

We use the MVAR model to obtain more refined spectral analysis results, which is conducive to more accurate calculation of effective connectivity coefficients. The spectrum power values were calculated in whole frequency band. After the MVAR model fitting, we got a $19 \times 19 \times 128$ matrix for each subject, this is also the input of the PSI algorithm in Eq. 6.

2.4 Effecitve Connectivity Analysis

Phase slope index measure is used in our study. The PSI between two given components signals i and j is defined as:

$$PSI_{ij} = \Im(\sum_{f\in F} C_{ij}^*(f)C_{ij}(f + \delta_f)) \tag{5}$$

where F is the set of frequencies of interest, F equals to half-bandwidth of the integration across frequencies. C is the normalized coherent spectrum and δ_f is an incremental step in the frequency domain. The normalized coherent spectrum C is defined as:

$$C_{ij}(f) = \frac{|S_{ij}(f)|}{\sqrt{S_{ii}(f)S_{jj}(f)}} \qquad (6)$$

The definition of $S_{ij}(f)$ means the cross-spectrum between i and j, and it is the output of the Eq. 4.

According to the definition in Eq. 6, the imaginary part of coherent spectrum is used in this algorithm. Because the imaginary part information of the coherent spectrum would not change due to aliasing between the signals [19]. In other words, PSI can avoid erroneous estimation in effective connectivity caused by signal aliasing.

In this study, we construct the effective connectivity in four frequency bands delta (0.5–4 Hz), theta (4–8 Hz), alpha (8–13 Hz) and beta (13–30 Hz) respectively. An average effective matrix for an ADHD subject and a HC subject of delta band was shown in Fig. 2 and Fig. 3.

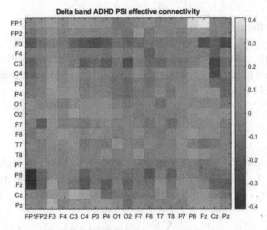

Fig. 2. PSI effective connectivity matrix in delta band (0.5–4Hz) for ADHD subject

2.5 Graph Theoretical Analysis

To detect the ADHD, we use three graph theory measures: clustering coefficient, nodal efficiency and degree centrality.

1) Threshold Method

Regarding to not all connection is necessary to be calculated in the graph theory, threshold method is used in weighted graph analysis. But threshold method has issue with threshold selection. A higher threshold may cause the problem of not being able to

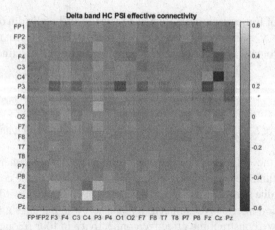

Fig. 3. PSI effective connectivity matrix in delta band (0.5–4Hz) for HC subject

construct a brain network and a lower threshold may cause the problem of no meaningful connectivity measures. Empirically, selecting threshold as 0.2 produced the best results.

2) Clustering Coefficient

Clustering coefficient is proposed to assess the ability of segregation in graph which is the most important measures in researching cognitive problem of brain. The algorithm is shown as follow [14]:

$$c^W = \frac{1}{N} \sum_i \frac{2t_i^w}{k_i(k_i - 1)} \tag{7}$$

The t_i^w is the number of triangles around a node i, a subgraph with three nodes and three edges is called a triangle. k_i is the degree of a node i. N is the numbers of nodes, here N equals to 19. The algorithm of the t_i and k_i is described in Eq. 8 and 9.

$$t_i^w = \frac{1}{2} \sum_{j,h \in N} \left(w_{ij} w_{ih} w_{jh} \right)^{\frac{1}{3}} \tag{8}$$

$$k_i = \sum_{j \in N} w_{ij} \tag{9}$$

where w_{ij} is the connection weights between node i and node j. When the measures of edges from the graph are greater than the threshold value, the connection is defined existed and w_{ij} equals to the value of the edges, otherwise $w_{ij} = 0$.

Object to extract the relatively obvious feature, we also compared the performance of clustering coefficient in different thresholds and the details of delta band and alpha band were shown in the Fig. 4 and Fig. 5.

According Fig. 4 and Fig. 5, we selected the threshold as 0.2 to conduct further analysis. To get more information from the graph to detect the ADHD, the nodal efficiency and degree centrality were also considered in our study.

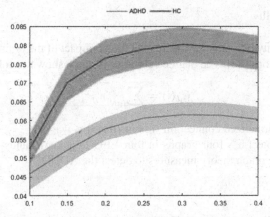

Fig. 4. Threshold comparison of clustering coefficient in delta band (0.5–4Hz)

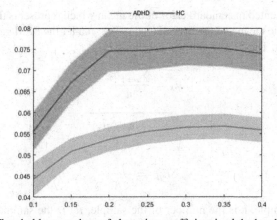

Fig. 5. Threshold comparison of clustering coefficient in alpha band (8–13Hz)

3) Nodal Efficiency

Nodal efficiency of a graph measures the ability of each node to exchange information, and is defined as [14]:

$$E_{nodal}(i) = \frac{1}{N-1} \sum_{i \neq j} \frac{1}{l_{ij}} \tag{10}$$

where N is the number of the nodes in the graph, and l_{ij} is a path between nodes i and j with the minimum number of edges.

4) Degree Centrality

Degree centrality of a graph measures the direct impact of the brain region on other adjacent brain regions [22]. The degree centrality formula shown as follow:

$$C_d(i) = \sum_{j \in N} w_{ij} \tag{11}$$

where w_{ij} is the normalized connection weights that $0 \leq w_{ij} \leq 1$.

Thus, each subject has four graphs in four EEG frequency bands, and each graph has extracted three graph theory measures to detect the ADHD.

3   Results

3.1   Statistical Analysis

All data were presented in standard error of the mean which represents the relative error between the sample mean and the overall mean. The smaller the SEM value, the smaller the sampling error. The SEM is shown as follow:

$$\mu_x = \frac{\sum_{i=1}^n x_i}{n} \tag{12}$$

$$s = \sqrt{\frac{\sum_{i=1}^n (x_i - \mu_x)^2}{n - 1}} \tag{13}$$

$$SE_{\mu_x} = \frac{s}{\sqrt{n}} \tag{14}$$

where x is the sample, n is the number of the sample, μ_x is the sample mean, s is the sample standard deviation and the SE_{μ_x} is the SEM result.

3.2   Clustering Coefficient

Using SEM to do the statistical analysis for the average clustering coefficient, the result is shown as Table 1. Here we found the HC groups is greater than the ADHD groups obviously in each frequency band.

Table 1. The Statistical results of average clustering coefficient between ADHD and HC

	Delta band	Theta band	Alpha band	Beta band
ADHD	0.058 ± 0.003	0.056 ± 0.003	0.054 ± 0.003	0.060 ± 0.003
HC	0.077 ± 0.005	0.074 ± 0.005	0.075 ± 0.005	0.088 ± 0.004

3.3 Nodal Efficiency

Nodal Efficiency is a measure of the network ability to exchange information in each component. Here we found in F3 and P3, the nodal efficiency is increased in ADHD groups, and the difference changeable in F3 and P3 in four frequency bands were shown in Table 2. In addition, the nodal efficiency is decreased in AHDH groups in Fz, Cz and Pz, and at the Fz, the measure changes the most.

Table 2. The Statistical results of nodal efficiency between ADHD and HC

	Delta band	Theta band	Alpha band	Beta band
F3 - ADHD	0.079 ± 0.008	0.086 ± 0.009	0.089 ± 0.008	0.103 ± 0.008
F3 - HC	0.063 ± 0.008	0.066 ± 0.008	0.071 ± 0.008	0.094 ± 0.011
P3 - ADHD	0.072 ± 0.006	0.087 ± 0.008	0.095 ± 0.010	0.120 ± 0.013
P3 - HC	0.062 ± 0.009	0.068 ± 0.009	0.071 ± 0.009	0.108 ± 0.015
Fz - ADHD	0.014 ± 0.004	0.015 ± 0.005	0.014 ± 0.004	0.026 ± 0.006
Fz - HC	0.031 ± 0.009	0.031 ± 0.009	0.034 ± 0.009	0.057 ± 0.011
Cz - ADHD	0.018 ± 0.003	0.016 ± 0.003	0.020 ± 0.003	0.029 ± 0.006
Cz - HC	0.029 ± 0.005	0.029 ± 0.005	0.030 ± 0.005	0.048 ± 0.012
Pz - ADHD	0.014 ± 0.003	0.012 ± 0.002	0.014 ± 0.003	0.029 ± 0.007
Pz - HC	0.026 ± 0.006	0.026 ± 0.006	0.025 ± 0.006	0.039 ± 0.009

According to Table 2, we found in delta band the nodal efficiency provided the most different features and the least error because the mean value between the ADHD and HC, and the smallest value of the SEM. Focus on this frequency band, the F3 and Fz points which represent the left forehead and the forehead midline point have significant differences. Comparing the healthy children, the ADHD children has very high ability of exchange information in left forehead but poor at the forehead middle part.

3.4 Degree Centrality

Similarly, F3, P3, Fz, Cz and Pz were used to assess in the four frequency bands between ADHD groups and HC groups using SEM algorithm. In this part, we found the measures increased in F3 and P3 and decreased in Fz, Cz and Pz for ADHD groups. The details of degree centrality of ADHD and HC were shown in Table 3.

In Table 3, Delta band also proposed a least error. Comparing the HC groups, we found that ADHD groups has most difference in F3 and Fz in measure of degree centrality. That means the left forehead of ADHD children has more correlation with other brain regions, but this ability is poor in the forehead middle part.

Table 3. The Statistical results of degree centrality between ADHD and HC

	Delta band	Theta band	Alpha band	Beta band
F3 - ADHD	1.238 ± 0.153	1.341 ± 0.172	1.359 ± 0.158	1.475 ± 0.145
F3 - HC	0.896 ± 0.129	0.939 ± 0.129	0.997 ± 0.133	1.306 ± 0.198
P3 - ADHD	1.056 ± 0.115	1.300 ± 0.152	1.434 ± 0.170	1.781 ± 0.240
P3 - HC	0.855 ± 0.151	0.955 ± 0.163	0.994 ± 0.165	1.539 ± 0.253
Fz - ADHD	0.134 ± 0.056	0.143 ± 0.065	0.135 ± 0.056	0.263 ± 0.065
Fz - HC	0.378 ± 0.145	0.378 ± 0.144	0.398 ± 0.142	0.764 ± 0.191
Cz - ADHD	0.210 ± 0.049	0.193 ± 0.047	0.205 ± 0.046	0.335 ± 0.072
Cz - HC	0.310 ± 0.068	0.299 ± 0.067	0.295 ± 0.067	0.618 ± 0.200
Pz - ADHD	0.115 ± 0.024	0.117 ± 0.023	0.121 ± 0.022	0.319 ± 0.091
Pz - HC	0.267 ± 0.086	0.264 ± 0.088	0.252 ± 0.087	0.455 ± 0.132

4   Conclusions

In this study, we constructed the brain network using effective connectivity technique to describe the brain activity in whole brain network.

The PSI method (Fig. 2 and 3) is used to combine information about different frequencies. The classic PSI measure is based on the power spectrum in frequency domain, here we used MVAR model to represent the power spectrum. The MVAR model overcomes the limitation of the classic PSI method that has poor resolution in frequency domain for short time dataset. We used the MVAR-PSI method constructed the effective connectivity in each frequency band.

This research proposed a new method to identify the ADHD children using EEG signals and effective connectivity techniques. The original EEG data is pre-filtered and divided into Delta, Theta, Alpha and Beta bands. And then, the effective connectivity graphs are constructed by applying ICA, MVAR model and PSI. The measures of clustering coefficient, nodal efficiency and degree centrality in graph theory are used to extract features from these graphs. Statistical analysis based on the SEM are employed to evaluate the graph theory measures in each frequency band. The results show a decreased average clustering coefficient in whole frequency bands for ADHD subjects. Also, in Delta band, ADHD children has very high ability of exchange information in left forehead but poor at the forehead middle part. Moreover, left forehead of ADHD children has more correlation with other brain region, but this ability is poor in the forehead middle part.

Acknowledgment. We acknowledge the material support by Ali Motie Nasrabadi, Armin Allahverdy, Mehdi Samavati, Mohammad Reza Mohammadi shared on the IEEE Data port (https://doi.org/10.21227/rzfh-zn36).

References

1. Furlong, S., et al.: Resting-state EEG connectivity in young children with ADHD. J. Clin. Child Adolesc. Psychol. 1–17 (2020)
2. Fair, D.A., et al.: Distinct neural signatures detected for ADHD subtypes after controlling for micro-movements in resting state functional connectivity MRI data. Front. Syst. Neurosci. **6**, 80 (2012)
3. Sato, J.R., et al.: Abnormal brain connectivity patterns in adults with ADHD: a coherence study. PloS one **7**(9), e45671 (2012)
4. Heinrichs-Graham, E., et al.: Pharmaco-MEG evidence for attention related hyper-connectivity between auditory and prefrontal cortices in ADHD. Psychiatry Res. Neuroimaging **221**(3), 240–245 (2014)
5. Pereda, E., et al.: The blessing of Dimensionality: feature Selection outperforms functional connectivity-based feature transformation to classify ADHD subjects from EEG patterns of phase synchronization. PloS one **13**(8), e0201660 (2018)
6. Mohammadi, M.R., Khaleghi, A., Nasrabadi, A.M., Rafieivand, S., Begol, M., Zarafshan, H.: EEG classification of ADHD and normal children using non-linear features and neural network. Biomed. Eng. Lett. **6**(2), 66–73 (2016). https://doi.org/10.1007/s13534-016-0218-2
7. Lee, D., et al.: Effects of an online mind-body training program on the default mode network: an EEG functional connectivity study. Sci. Rep. **8**(1), 16935–16938 (2018)
8. Chen, H., Song, Y., Li, X.: A deep learning framework for identifying children with ADHD using an EEG-based brain network. Neurocomputing **356**, 83–96 (2019)
9. Abbas, A.K., et al.: Effective connectivity in brain networks estimated using EEG signals are altered in children with attention deficit hyperactivity disorder. Comput. Biol. Med. 104515 (2021)
10. Wang, S., et al.: A study on resting EEG effective connectivity difference before and after neurofeedback for children with ADHD. Neuroscience **457**, 103–113 (2021)
11. Michelini, G., et al.: Atypical functional connectivity in adolescents and adults with persistent and remitted ADHD during a cognitive control task. Transl. Psychiatry **9**(1), 1–15 (2019)
12. Gabriel, R., et al.: Identification of ADHD cognitive pattern disturbances using EEG and wavelets analysis. In: 2017 IEEE 17th International Conference on Bioinformatics and Bioengineering (BIBE). IEEE (2017)
13. Jang, K.-M., Kim, M.-S., Kim, D.-W.: The dynamic properties of a brain network during spatial working memory tasks in college students with ADHD traits. Front. Hum. Neurosci. **14** (2020)
14. Liu, J., et al.: Complex brain network analysis and its applications to brain disorders: a survey. Complexity (New York, N.Y.) **2017**, 1–27 (2017)
15. Cao, J., et al.: Investigation of brain networks in children with attention deficit/hyperactivity disorder using a graph theoretical approach. Biomed. Signal Process. Control **40**, 351–358 (2018)
16. Pagnotta, M.F., Plomp, G.: Time-varying MVAR algorithms for directed connectivity analysis: critical comparison in simulations and benchmark EEG data. PloS one **13**(6), e0198846 (2018)
17. Seppanen, J.M., et al.: Analysis of electromechanical modes using multichannel Yule-Walker estimation of a multivariate autoregressive model, pp. 1–5. IEEE (2013)
18. Lei, C.L., et al.: Thermal error robust modeling for high-speed motorized spindle, pp. 961–965 (2012)
19. Gomez, C., et al.: Assessment of EEG connectivity patterns in mild cognitive impairment using phase slope index. In: 2018 40th Annual International Conference of the IEEE Engineering in Medicine and Biology Society (EMBC), vol. 2018, pp. 263–266 (2018)

A Novel Alcoholic EEG Signals Classification Approach Based on AdaBoost k-means Coupled with Statistical Model

Mohammed Diykh[2], Shahab Abdulla[1,4(✉)], Atheer Y. Oudah[2,4],
Haydar Abdulameer Marhoon[4,5], and Siuly Siuly[3]

[1] Open Access College, University of Southern Queensland, Toowoomba, Australia
{Shahab.Abdulla,Mohammed.Diykh}@usq.edu.au
[2] College of Education for Pure Science, University of Thi-Qar, Nasiriyah, Iraq
Mohammed.Diykh@utq.edu.iq, Atheer@alayen.edu.iq
[3] Institute for Sustainable Industries and Liveable Cities, Victoria
University, Footscray, Australia
siuly.siuly@vu.edu.au
[4] Information and Communication Technology Research Group, Scientific Research Centre,
Al-Ayen University, Nasiriyah, Iraq
Haydar@alayen.edu.iq
[5] Department of Information Technology, Computer Science and Information Technology,
University of Karbala, Karbala, Iraq

Abstract. Identification of alcoholism is an important task because it affects the operation of the brain. Alcohol consumption, particularly heavier drinking is identified as an essential factor to develop health issues, such as high blood pressure, immune disorders, and heart diseases. To support health professionals in diagnosis disorders related with alcoholism with a high rate of accuracy, there is an urgent demand to develop an automated expert systems for identification of alcoholism. In this study, an expert system is proposed to identify alcoholism from multi-channel EEG signals. EEG signals are partitioned into small epochs, with each epoch is further divided into sub-segments. A covariance matrix method with its eigenvalues is utilised to extract representative features from each sub-segment. To select most relevant features, a statistic approach named Kolmogorov–Smirnov test is adopted to select the final features set. Finally, in the classification part, a robust algorithm called AdaBoost k-means (AB-k-means) is designed to classify EEG features into two categories alcoholic and non-alcoholic EEG segments. The results in this study show that the proposed model is more efficient than the previous models, and it yielded a high classification rate of 99%. In comparison with well-known classification algorithms such as K-nearest k-means and SVM on the same databases, our proposed model showed a promising result compared with the others. Our findings showed that the proposed model has a potential to implement in automated alcoholism detection systems to be used by experts to provide an accurate and reliable decisions related to alcoholism.

Keywords: Alcoholism · EEG · AdaBoost k-means · Covariance matrix · Kolmogorov–Smirnov

© Springer Nature Switzerland AG 2021
S. Siuly et al. (Eds.): HIS 2021, LNCS 13079, pp. 82–92, 2021.
https://doi.org/10.1007/978-3-030-90885-0_8

1 Introduction

The human brain receives signals from the body's organs and sends information to the muscles [1]. The effects of consuming alcohol on the nervous system make human suffering from long- and short-term issues such as impaired vision, impaired hearing [2]. Alcoholism is a type of neurological disorder resulted from excessive and repetitive drinking of alcoholic beverages. The dangerous impacts of drinking alcoholic beverages could be physical and mental [3, 4]. The consuming of alcohol disturbs the entire nervous system, especially the brain. It weakens the brain neurons and leads to cognitive and mobility weakness [5]. According to the latest reports released by the World Health Organization around three million people lost their life because of heavy consumption of alcohol. In addition, more than 200 diseases - and injuries are caused by the excessive use of alcohol. Developing an expert system of Identification of alcoholism may decrease unnecessary economic losses and social problems as well as expedite diagnosis in clinical settings.

Electroencephalogram (EEG) technology has become an important tool in the identification of brain disorders [6]. Developing an expert system based on EEG signals can assist experts in determining alcoholic from non-alcoholic subjects. As a result, a number of methods has been developed based on EEG signals for alcoholism identification using different techniques including Fast Fourier transform (FFT) Tunable-Q Wavelet Transform (TQWT), and Wavelet transforms. For example, Faust et al. [7] classified alcoholic EEG signals using FF, and AR techniques. Their results demonstrated that the power spectral density of EEG signals varied and reflected the abnormalities in alcoholic EEGs. Patidar et al. [8] used TQWT based on PCA to analyse EEG into different bands. The extracted features based on PCA were sent to a least-squares-support-vector machine Shooshtari and Setarehdan [9] developed a reduction technique to select a subset of EEG channels suing spectral analysis and correlation matrices. Their model showed that it had ability to select the optimal channels for Kumar et al. [10] integrated approximate entropy with sample entropy to extract features from EEG. Their findings showed that the value of ApEn and SampEn varied from normal subjects to uncontrol subjects. Cao et al. [11] suggested a synchronization likelihood model to quantify synchronization variations among 28 alcoholics and 28 control participants. Their study revealed that the synchronization for the control group can reflect the levels of the cognitive tasks, while the alcoholics only exhibited erratic changes. Lin et al. [12] studied alcoholic and control EEG signals based on a Hilbert-Huang Transformation technique. Both PCA and WT were integrated and used to analyse EEG data. Kousarrizi et al. [13] showed that power spectrum of the Haar mother wavelet was effective to extract the features. The extracted features were sent to a support vectors machine algorithm and neural network model. Their method achieved a higher rate of classification accuracy than previous developed methods. Sadiq et al., [14] EEG signals were filtered using a multiscale principal component analysis. The denoised EEGs were arranged to form a square matrix of different orders. The determinant matrix was computed for matrix. The extracted features were fed to several machine learning algorithms for classification. Sadiq et al., [15] suggested a technique based on empirical wavelet transform for classification brain signals. The empirical wavelet transform was integrated with four data reduction techniques in that study. For classification, artificial neural networks models were employed to classify brain signals.

According to the review above, it is noticed that the combination of features and machine learning algorithms has become the popular research direction of alcoholism identification using multi-channel EEG signal, however, the effectiveness of reducing the dimensionality of features needs in-depth research. The features selection could have significant effects on alcoholism identification, thus need an effective approach to remove redundant features. A covariance matrix method with its eigenvalues is utilised to extract representative features from EEG and reduce its dimensionality to address this limitation. In addition, to increase the accuracy rate, developing a new classification model has become a vital task to classify non-alcoholic from alcoholic EEG signals with a high rate. In view of these limitation, this paper presents a new classification model called AB-k-means is proposed for alcoholism identification using EEG signals.

2   Methodology

In this paper, a new model is designed to classify alcoholism from EEG signals. To reduce the dimensionality, a covariance matrix method with its eigenvalues is utilised to extract representative is utilised. A set of features to represent EEG data are extracted eigenvalues. A total of ten statistical features are extracted including {mean, *median, maximum, minimum, mode, range, standard deviation, variation, skewness* and *kurtosis}*. The Kolmogorov–Smirnov test (KST) is employed for selecting relevant features. The selected features set is forwarded to AB-k-means to classify alcoholism from EEG signals. Figure 1 describes the proposed model to classify alcoholism from EEG signals.

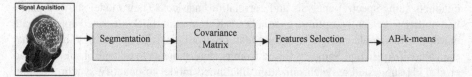

Fig. 1. The proposed methodology for alcoholism classification.

2.1   EEG Dataset

In this paper, a public database known as the UCI Knowledge Discovery in Databases (KDD) Archive from University of California, Department of Information and Computer Science is adopted to evaluate the proposed method [16]. EEG signals were collected from 122 subjects. 120 trials were recorded from each subject using three kinds of stimuli [17]. A total 64 channels were utilised to record EEG signals, two Electrooculography (EOG) channels and one reference electrode. The duration of each trial was one second. The sampling rate of EEG data was 256 Hz. The dataset contains three types of datasets named SMNI CMI TEST, SMNI CMI TRAIN and full dataset. The first two databases were utilised in this paper with a total of 1200 recorded files.

Features Extraction Based on of Covariance Matrix
In this paper, a sliding window technique is used to split the EEG signals into their respective periods. Suppose an EEG signal denoted as: $X = \{x_1, x_2, ..., x_k\}$ with n the data points. The EEG signal X is partitioned into 4 segments [18–20]. Then, each EEG segment is further divided into 32 sub-segments. Then each sub-segment is passed to the determinants of Covariance matrix model to reduce EEGs dimensionality and select the most representative features. The reason behind the use the determinants of Covariance matrix as a data shrinking method is to reduce the dimensionality of the EEG signal and eliminate redundant features. Initially, a time series can be described as a sequential combination of F points or more formally, written as a vector of length $F([x_1, \ldots, x_F])$. The feature candidates, therefore, can be combined in a feature vector set for a point in the EEG time series. Let $\{v_i\}$ be the number of features, defined for a point K. The feature vector for N^{th} point of the subsequence is:

$$a_n = [v_{N1}, \ldots, v_{Nk}] \tag{1}$$

when feature vectors are merged for all points, this ends up with a feature matrix A,

$$A = \begin{bmatrix} v_{11} & \cdots & v_{1k} \\ \vdots & \ddots & \vdots \\ v_{M1} & \cdots & v_{Mk} \end{bmatrix} \tag{2}$$

The covariance of the feature matrix is

$$(H_A) = \frac{1}{F-1} \sum_{i=1}^{F-1} (A_i - m)(A_i - m)^T \tag{3}$$

where μ is the mean vector of feature vectors $\{a_1, \ldots, a_M\}$.

To improve the extraction process, this study aimed to compute the determinant of covariance matrix. Based on essential properties of this covariance matrix, the H_A can be symmetric (*i.e.*, self-adjoint) with the usual inner output its eigenvalues that are all real and positive, and the eigenvectors that belong to distinct eigenvalues orthogonal,

$$H_A = V \wedge V^T \tag{4}$$

Consequently, the determinant of the H_A is:

$$|H_A| = \left| V \wedge V^T \right| = |V||\wedge|\left|V^T\right| = |\wedge||V|\left|V^T\right| = |\wedge|\left|V^T V\right| = |\wedge||I| = \prod_{i=1}^{F} \gamma_i \tag{5}$$

In the proposed technique the matrix elements are chosen to be EEG time series which are one dimensional. Initially, EEG time series were arranged sequentially to form a square matrix based on covariance matrix with the usual inner output its eigenvalues that are all real and positive, and the eigenvectors that belong to distinct eigenvalues orthogonal, and its determinant was estimated. As a result, EEG signals from 61 channels were form as a matrix (15616 × 30). Data set is divided into four segments (n = 4), then, each segment of (3904 × 30) data points is divided into 32 sub-segment to obtain (122 × 30). Each sub-segment is passed to the of Covariance matrix model and its eigen values are investigated. A total of ten statistical features are extracted for each sub-segment to form the final features vector.

Feature Selection

In this section, the extracted features are tested to select the most effective ones. Kolmogorov–Smirnov test (KST) is used in this paper. Below is a summary of the results obtained: In the first experiment, EEG channels were tested and the obtained results showed that the features {*maximum, minimum, mode, range, standard deviation, variation*} are passed the test, and they can be used to discriminate between the alcoholic and non-alcoholic EEG signals with a high rate. Table 1 shows the selected features set based on KST test.

Table 1. Feature set outcome of experiment No. 1

Features	Testing	Training	Compared with the p-values
	Controlled vs Alcohol	Controlled vs Alcohol	
Mean	0.1055	0.1203	Rejected
Max	0.46	0.154	Rejected
Med	0.0017	$2.9480 \times 10{-09}$	Accepted
Min	0.011	0.02	Accepted
Mod	0.011	0.02	Accepted
Range	$1.7552 \times 10{-05}$	0.034	Accepted
Skew	0.1088	0.94	Accepted
Kur	0.1	0.93	Rejected
Std	$2.0212 \times 10{-04}$	0.01088	Accepted
Var	0.1087	0.02003	Accepted

AdaBoost k-Means

AdaBoost classifier is an algorithm utilized to train a set of weak classifiers. According to the AdaBoost classifier mechanism, the alpha (weights) and theta (error rate) values of the training samples are modified after each iteration. The weights of training sets which are misclassified are increased, while the weights of the training sets which are correctly classified are decreased. As a result, the weak classifiers are merged to design a strong classifier as follows:

$$f(x) = max \sum_{i=1}^{n} h_i(v) = max \sum_{i=1}^{n} h(v, f_i, \theta_i, s) \tag{6}$$

The training procedure is carried out according to the following pseudocode [21].

1. Input: a set of training samples consist of by M_1 class_1 sample, and M_2 class_2 samples where, $M = M_1 + M_2$. $(x_1, y_1), (x_2, y_2), \ldots \ldots (x_n, y_n)$.

   where $(x_i)_{i=1}^n$ is the set of input EMG features, and y_i is the number of clusters.
2. Repeat for $s = 0.1$

   2.1. Initialise the weight w_{ij}^s
   2.2. For each cycle $i = 1, 2, \ldots n$

      2.2.1. normalise the weights w_{ij}^s as $w_{ij}^s = \frac{w_{ij}^s}{\sum_{j=1}^n w_{ij}^s}$ for $j = 1, \ldots, n$;
      2.2.2. Define a weak classifier as $h(v, f_i, \theta_i, s) = a\delta(v^f > \theta_i) + b$, where $\delta(x) = 1$ if $\theta > x$ otherwise $\delta(x) = 0$;
      2.2.3. train k-means on the weight training set.
      2.3.4. Assesses the error by $l_i = \sum_{j=1}^n w_{ij}^s (y_j^s - h(v, f_i, \theta_i, s))^2$. where $y_j^s \in [1, -1]$ is the label of each feature;
      2.2.5. Find the best weak classifier $h(v, f_i, \theta_i, s)$ with parameters a, b, f_i, θ_i;
      2.2.6. Update the classifier $H(v, s)$ for class s and weight of the training set $H(v, s) = h(v, f_i, \theta_i, s)$; and
      2.2.7. if $i < n$ increase i by 1 and go to step 2.2.1, otherwise go to step 2.

3. Output the final strong classifier.

Performance Evaluation Methods
To evaluate the performance of the proposed model, a set of metrics was used in this paper, as described below:

a) Accuracy (Acc.): it is utilised to assess the performance of the proposed method depending on the formula as below:

$$\text{Acc.} = (TP + TN)/(TP + TN + FP + FN) \qquad (4.4)$$

b) Sensitivity (Sen.) it is used to measure the rate of the real positive predication. This is defined as follows:

$$\text{Sen.} = TP/(TP + FN) \qquad (4.5)$$

c) Specificity (Spe.) is utilized to measure the proportion of the real negative predication and is defined as follows:

$$\text{Spe.} = TN/(TN + FP) \qquad (4.6)$$

d) Predictive Positive Value (PPV.) is defined as the rate of positives that correspond to the presence of the condition described via the formula as below:

$$PPV. = TP/(TP + FP) \qquad (4.7)$$

e) Predictive Negative Value (PNV.) is the ratio of negatives that correspond to the absence of the condition and is defined as follows:

$$PNV. = TN/(TN + FN) \qquad (4.8)$$

3   Results

The simulation results and findings were presented and discussed in this section. All experiments were run on a computer with 8G Ram, Intel (R) Core (TM) i7-6600U CPU @ 2.60 GHz 2.81 GHz. All experiments were implemented using MATLAB R2019a. To assess the performance of the proposed model in alcoholic EEG signals, a comparison was conducted with SVM, k-means, k-nearest. Table 2 presents the comparison results among the AB-means, k-nearest, k-means and SVM. In this experiment, the extracted features by the covariance matrix were sent AB-means, k-nearest, k-means and SVM. Based on the results, the proposed model AB-k-means obtained higher classification rate than k-nearest, k-means and SVM. However, SVM recorded the second highest classification rate, and it outperformed the k-means, and k-nearest. Our findings showed that integrated AdaBoost with k-means can improve the classification accuracy of EEG signals.

Table 2. Classification accuracy of the comparison among the AB-means, k-nearest, k-means and SVM.

Approach	Accuracy	Sensitivity	Specificity
AB-k-means	99%	99%	98. %
k-means	87%	86%	85%
k-nearest	88%	85%	84%
SVM	94.5%	93%	93%

In this paper, 10-cross validation was also utilised to assess the proposed model, Fig. 2 shows the classification accuracy based on 10-cross validation, in which the proposed model AB-k-means scored an average of 98% while the results of k-means, k-nearest were distributed in the range from 82% to 87%. The SVM gained the second highest rate which ranged from 89% to 93%. As a result, we can notice that the AB-k-means obtained the highest accuracy on each run and the best value is 99%.

3.1 Channel Selection Based on Classification Rate

The accuracy rate of the AB-k-means on 61-channel EEG signals is investigated in this paper. The features were extracted from each channel and forwarded to the AB-k-means. The results demonstrated that not all channels yielded the same classification accuracy. As a result, 13 optimal channels including AF_8, C_1, C_2, C_3, C_4, CP_1, CP_5, CP_6, FC_5, FT_7, P_8, PO_8, P were selected and used to classify EEG signals as shown in Fig. 3. As a result, we invaginated the performance of the proposed method based on the number of channels. Table 3 reports the results based on the number of channels.

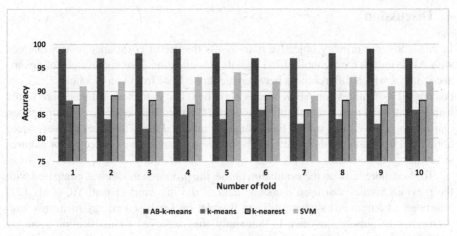

Fig. 2. The classification accuracy of 10 folds.

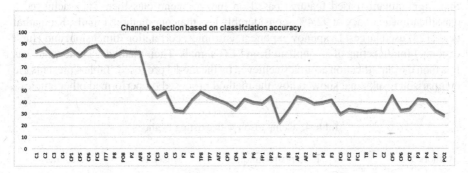

Fig. 3. The classification accuracy based on EEG channels.

Table 3. Presents the classification accuracy based on the number channels.

Channel No	Accuracy	Sensitivity	Specificity
C_1, C_3 and FC_5	85%	83%	82%
AF_8, C_1, C_2, C_3, C_4, CP_1, CP_5, CP_6, FC_5, FT_7, P_8, PO_8, P	99%	98%	99%
All 61 channel	99.5%	98%	99%

4   Discussion

In this study, the primary objective is to assess the use of covariance matrix coupled with AB-k-means for alcoholic EEG signals classification. The eigenvalues of covariance matrix, which differentiates between alcoholic EEG from non-alcoholic EEG, are considered as features for AB-K-means classifier. The extracted features were tested using a statistical metric and the most powerful features were considered in this paper. Our finding showed that not all EEG channels reflected the differences between alcoholic EEG from non-alcoholic EEGs. The optimum channels were selected for features selection.

To shed more light on the evaluation phase, the proposed model was compared with the previous studies that used the same data as did this work. Faust, Yu, et al., [22] improved an automated system utilising wavelet packet based energy measures with a k-nearest neighbour classifier. In that study, they achieved a classification accuracy of 95.8% which is less than the rate obtained by the proposed model. Patidar et al., [8] suggested an automated system for the diagnosis of alcoholism using Tunable Q-wavelet transform. Their results were lower than the results obtained by the proposed method. Patidar et al., 2017 obtained a classification accuracy of 97.02%, which is, again, less than our classification accuracy of 99%. Faust, Yanti, et al., [23] proposed a higher Order Spectra cumulants-based features based on fuzzy sugeno classifier. They achieved a classification accuracy of 92.4%--considerably less than our method. Finally, Kannathal et al., [24] used largest Lyapunov exponent, entropies, correlation dimension, and Hurst exponent for detecting of alcoholism from EEG signals. Their method accuracy rate was less than the classification accuracy achieved by the model proposed. Table 4 presents the comparison results that showed how the method proposed outperformed other studies.

Table 4. Comparison with existing methods

Authors	Features/techniques	Analysis	Accuracy
Faust, Yu, et al. [22]	WPT, energy measures	KNN	95.8%
Patidar et al. [8]	TQWT, CE	LS-SVM	97.02%
Faust, Yanti, et al. [23]	HOS cumulants	FSC	92.4%
Kannathal et al. [24]	CD, LLE, entropy, H	Unique ranges	90%
The proposed model	**Cov-Eig**	**AB-K-means**	**99%**

5   Conclusion

The methodology of using covariance matrix with AB-K-means model for alcoholism identification is proposed in this study. It achieves results competitive to similar studies in the recent past. The current study achieved optimal results in high classification rate based on various metrics including accuracy (ACC), sensitivity (Sen), specificity (Spec).

The proposed model can be used to assist neurologists and other medical specialists in the precise diagnosis of alcoholism EEG signals. Future studies may investigate the improvement of the performance of the proposed model by decreasing the number of features used in this initial study. Furthermore, the AB-k-means model will be evaluated with different EEG datasets such as sleep EEG signals, epileptic EEG signals, aesthetic EEG signals.

References

1. Pelvig, D.P., Pakkenberg, H., Stark, A.K., Pakkenberg, B.: Neocortical glial cell numbers in human brains. Neurobiol. Aging **29**(11), 1754–1762 (2008)
2. Deiner, S., Silverstein, J.: Postoperative delirium and cognitive dysfunction. Br. J. Anaesth. **103**(suppl_1), i41–i46 (2009)
3. Volkow, N.D., Wiers, C.E., Shokri-Kojori, E., Tomasi, D., Wang, G.-J., Baler, R.: Neurochemical and metabolic effects of acute and chronic alcohol in the human brain: studies with positron emission tomography. Neuropharmacology **122**, 175–188 (2017)
4. Lieber, C.S.: Medical disorders of alcoholism. N. Engl. J. Med. **333**(16), 1058–1065 (1995)
5. Oscar-Berman, M., Shagrin, B., Evert, D.L., Epstein, C.: Impairments of brain and behavior: the neurological effects of alcohol. Alcohol Health Res. World **21**(1), 65 (1997)
6. Acharya, U.R., Bhat, S., Adeli, H., Adeli, A.: Computer-aided diagnosis of alcoholism-related EEG signals. Epilepsy Behav. **41**, 257–263 (2014)
7. Faust, O., Acharya, R., Allen, A.R., Lin, C.: Analysis of EEG signals during epileptic and alcoholic states using AR modeling techniques. IRBM **29**(1), 44–52 (2008)
8. Patidar, S., Pachori, R.B., Upadhyay, A., Acharya, U.R.: An integrated alcoholic index using tunable-Q wavelet transform based features extracted from EEG signals for diagnosis of alcoholism. Appl. Soft Comput. **50**, 71–78 (2017)
9. Shooshtari, M.A., Setarehdan, S.K.: Selection of optimal EEG channels for classification of signals correlated with alcohol abusers. In: IEEE 10th International Conference on Signals Processing, pp. 1–4. IEEE, Beijing (2010)
10. Kumar, Y., Dewal, M., Anand, R.: Features extraction of EEG signals using approximate and sample entropy. In: The 2012 IEEE Students Conference on Electrical, Electronics and Computer Science, pp. 1–5, IEEE, Bhopal (2012)
11. Cao, R., Deng, H., Wu, Z., Liu, G., Guo, H., Xiang, J.: Decreased synchronization in alcoholics using EEG. IRBM **38**(2), 63–70 (2017)
12. Lin, C.-F., Yeh, S.-W., Chien, Y.-Y., Peng, T.-I., Wang, J.-H., Chang, S.-H.: A HHT-based time frequency analysis scheme for clinical alcoholic EEG signals. In: The WSEAS International Conference. Proceedings of the Mathematics and Computers in Science and Engineering, no. 9. World Scientific and Engineering Academy and Society (2009)
13. Kousarrizi, M.R.N., Ghanbari, A.A., Gharaviri, A., Teshnehlab, M., Aliyari, M.: Classification of alcoholics and non-alcoholics via EEG using SVM and neural networks. In: 3rd International Conference on Bioinformatics and Biomedical Engineering, pp. 1–4, Beijing. IEEE (2009)
14. Sadiq, M.T., Yu, X., Yuan, Z., Aziz, M.Z., Siuly, S., Ding, W.: A matrix determinant feature extraction approach for decoding motor and mental imagery EEG in subject specific tasks. IEEE Trans. Cogn. Dev. Syst. (2020). https://doi.org/10.1109/TCDS.2020.3040438
15. Sadiq, M.T., Yu, X., Yuan, Z.: Exploiting dimensionality reduction and neural network techniques for the development of expert brain–computer interfaces. Expert Syst. Appl. **164**, 114031 (2020)

16. Hettich, S., Bay, S.: The UCI KDD Archive. University of California, Irvine, CA. Department of Information and Computer Science 152 (1999). http://kdd.ics.uci.edu
17. Zhang, X.L., Begleiter, H., Porjesz, B., Litke, A.: Electrophysiological evidence of memory impairment in alcoholic patients. Biol. Psychiat. **42**(12), 1157–1171 (1997)
18. Diykh, M., Li, Y., Wen, P.: Classify epileptic EEG signals using weighted complex networks-based community structure detection. Expert Syst. Appl. **90**, 87–100 (2017)
19. Diykh, M., Li, Y., Wen, P., Li, T.: Complex networks approach for depth of anesthesia assessment. Measurement **119**, 178–189 (2018)
20. Diykh, M., Miften, F.S., Abdulla, S., Saleh, K., Green, J.H.: Robust approach to depth of anaesthesia assessment based on hybrid transform and statistical features. IET Sci. Meas. Technol. **14**(1), 128–136 (2019)
21. Miften, F.S., Diykh, M., Abdulla, S., Siuly, S., Green, J.H., Deo, R.C.: A new framework for classification of multi-category hand grasps using EMG signals. Artif. Intell. Med. **112**, 102005 (2021)
22. Faust, O., Yu, W., Kadri, N.A.: Computer-based identification of normal and alcoholic EEG signals using wavelet packets and energy measures. J. Mech. Med. Biol. **13**(03), 1350033 (2013)
23. Faust, O., Yanti, R., Yu, W.: Automated detection of alcohol related changes in electroencephalograph signals. J. Med. Imaging Health Inform. **3**(2), 333–339 (2013)
24. Kannathal, N., Acharya, U.R., Lim, C.M., Sadasivan, P.: Characterization of EEG—a comparative study. Comput. Methods Programs Biomed. **80**(1), 17–23 (2005)

Medical Data Analysis

Multi-BERT-wwm Model Based on Probabilistic Graph Strategy for Relation Extraction

Yingxiang Zhang[1,2], Xiangyun Liao[2(✉)], Li Chen[3], Hongjun Kang[4], Yunpeng Cai[2], and Qiong Wang[2]

[1] College of Electronics and Information Engineering, Shenzhen University, Shenzhen, China
[2] Shenzhen Institutes of Advanced Technology Chinese Academy of Sciences, Shenzhen, China
[3] General Medicine Department, Medical School of Chinese PLA, Chinese PLA General Hospital, Beijing, China
[4] Department of Critical Care Medicine, Medical School of Chinese PLA, Chinese PLA General Hospital, Beijing, China

Abstract. As the core work of information extraction, relation extraction aims to find medical entity pairs with relations from the medical records. The current methods of relation extraction either ignore the relevance of entity extraction and relation classification, or fail to solve the problem of multiple relations or entities in one sentence. To handle those problems, this paper proposes a cascading pointer Multi-BERT-wwm model based on the probabilistic graph strategy. The model selects an entity randomly from all the predicted entities each time, then predicts other entities and their relations according to that entity. Meanwhile, the pointer labeling network helps to solve the problem of overlapping entities. The Multi-BERT-wwm model is improved based on BERT, which connects a layer of self-attention to the multi-head attention layer in the first six Encoder modules to strengthen the feature extraction ability. In addition, we add the adversarial training to improve the robustness and generalization ability of the model. The experimental results tested on the CMeIE dataset show that compared with the traditional CNN+Attention and BERT methods, our method improves the F1-score by 4.42% and 1.91% respectively in relation extraction task.

Keywords: Relation extraction · Probabilistic graph · Multi-BERT-wwm · Pointer labeling · Adversarial training

1 Introduction

In recent years, major hospitals have begun to popularize electronic medical records (EMR) with the advancement of medical informationization. There are many entities such as diseases, examinations and treatments in EMR. The relations among these entities reflect the changes of patients' health status and the

© Springer Nature Switzerland AG 2021
S. Siuly et al. (Eds.): HIS 2021, LNCS 13079, pp. 95–103, 2021.
https://doi.org/10.1007/978-3-030-90885-0_9

effects achieved by treatment. So extracting those relational entity pairs is the primary task of structuring EMR, and a large number of relation extraction methods based on neural network structures have been proposed [4,15].

The pipeline method divides relation extraction into entity extraction and relation prediction. The results of relation extraction in this way rely heavily on the results of entity extraction, suffering from the error accumulation problem and neglecting the relevance between the two steps. Therefore, an end-to-end joint extraction method is proposed, which extracts entities and relations from the same model, realizing parameter sharing and reducing the possibility of error accumulation in the pipeline method. However, it cannot solve the problems of overlapping entities and multiple entities or relations in the same sentence. Considering the shortcomings of those methods, this paper adopts the probabilistic graph method and proposes a novel model named Multi-BERT-wwm with cascading pointer labeling. The main contributions of our work are summarized as follows:

1. We adopt the probabilistic graph strategy to extract entities and relations, that is, select an entity randomly from the predicted entities first, and then use this entity to predict its corresponding other entity and their relations.
2. In the proposed Multi-BERT-wwm language model, we design a new Encoder structure, which changes the multi-head attention layer in the first 6 Encoder structures of the BERT model.
3. Adversarial training is added to the training process to regularize the parameters, improving the robustness and generalization ability of the model.

2   Related Work

The purpose of relation extraction is to extract the relational triples (subject, relation, object). With the advance of deep learning and word representation learning, supervised relation extraction method has become a research hotspot, which can be divided into pipeline and joint learning method.

Pipeline approaches recognize entities at first, then choose a relation for every possible pair of extracted entities. Nguyen et al. [8] use character-based word embedding and position embedding to train a CNN model for biomedical relation extraction. Zhang et al. [13] use CNN and RNN for biomedical relation extraction. Since RNN is difficult to deal with long-term dependence, Yan et al. [11] adopt LSTM and merge multiple features for relation extraction.

The joint learning model performs entity recognition and relation extraction simultaneously, which make use of the interaction information between entities and relations. Yu and Lam [12] propose the approach to connect the two models through global probabilistic graphical models. And then Miwa et al. [6] first apply neural network methods to jointly represent entities and relations in 2016. Zheng et al. [14] use a novel labeling strategy which converts the joint extraction to a sequence labeling task and directly obtain relational triples through an end-to-end model. Bekoulis et al. [1] propose a joint neural model, which using the BiLSTM to extract contextual features and conditional random field (CRF) to extract entity boundaries and labels.

3 Proposed Method

3.1 Probabilistic Graph Strategy

For relational triples (s, r, o) in current methods of relation extraction, the pipeline method can't handle the case that the same group (s, o) corresponds to multiple r. And the joint model based on sequence labeling also fails to solve the problem of multiple s or o in the sentence simultaneously. To overcome these problems, we can learn from the idea of probabilistic graph in the seq2seq task. In Seq2Seq, the decoder is actually modeling:

$$P(y_1, y_2, \ldots, y_n \mid x) = P(y_1 \mid x)P(y_2 \mid x, y_1) \cdots P(y_n \mid x, y_1, y_2, \ldots, y_{n-1}) \quad (1)$$

That is, when predicting, the first word is predicted by x, and then the second word is predicted by the first word, and so on until the end word. Therefore, for the extraction of triples, we can also consider adopting this method: predict s first, then predict the o according to the s, finally predict the r according to s and o. In addition, we can further combine the predictions of o and r, that is:

$$P(s, r, o) = P(s)P(o, r \mid s) \quad (2)$$

Therefore, only two steps are required. This method is also known as relation extraction based on subject perception [10], which extracts subject first and then extracts the predicate and object.

3.2 Multi-BERT-wwm Language Model

BERT [2] is a language representation model, which uses a bidirectional attention mechanism [5,9] and a large-scale unsupervised corpus to obtain an effective contextual representation of each word. The structure of the Encoder in the BERT model is shown in Fig. 1. Multi-head attention divides the model into multiple heads and forms multiple subspaces, which allows the model to learn relevant information in different presentation subspaces. Each attention focuses on a different part of the input and then splices it together:

$$MultiHead(Q, K, V) = Concat(head_1, \ldots, head_h)W^O \quad (3)$$

As a large number of papers show that specific layers of Transformer or Bert have unique functions. The bottom layer is more focused on syntax while the top is more focused on semantics. Therefore, in order to further improve the performance, we propose a new Multi-BERT model to extract the context features of characters. The Encoder structure of Multi-BERT model (Multi-Encoder) is shown in Fig. 2. We connect self-attention on the multi-head attention layer in parallel for the first 6 layers of Encoder, and the next 6 layers keep the previous single multi-head attention unchanged. The superposition of Attention at the bottom layer can obtain more grammatical and position features, while the upper layer remains unchanged and uses multiple heads to

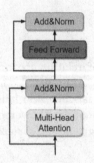

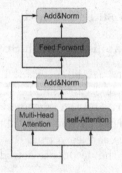

Fig. 1. The Encoder structure of BERT.

Fig. 2. The Encoder structure of Multi-BERT.

obtain semantic information. The experimental results show that the Encoder structure in Multi-BERT can achieve better results than that in BERT. Figure 3 shows the overall structure of the 12-layer Encoder in Multi-BERT.

3.3 Pointer Labeling and Adversarial Training

Cascading Pointer Labeling. For the selection of tag framework in relation extraction, the commonly used framework of sequence labeling is to mark each sequence position as a label one by one, such as labeling according to BIO. However, there are many nested and overlapping entities in medical cases.

As shown in Fig. 4, the cascading pointer labeling we used is to mark the start and end of each span, and the labeling of multiple entity do not interfere with each other. If multiple categories are involved, it can be converted into cascading pointer labeling (C pointer networks, C is the total number of categories). In this way, the problem of overlapping entities is well solved.

Adversarial Training. Adversarial training in NLP is more regarded as a regularization method to reduce overfitting, improve the generalization ability and robustness of the model. Goodfellow et al. [3] put forward the concept of

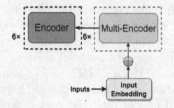

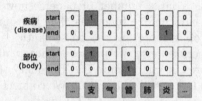

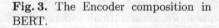

Fig. 3. The Encoder composition in BERT.

Fig. 4. The framework of cascading pointer labeling.

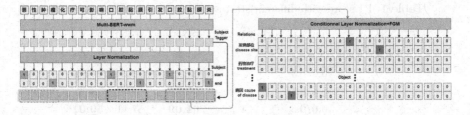

Fig. 5. An overview of the proposed cascading pointer relation extraction framework based on probability graph strategy.

adversarial training in 2014. It is to add a perturbation r_{adv} to the original input sample x, and use it for training after obtaining the adversarial sample.

According to Goodfellow, neural networks are vulnerable to linear perturbation due to their linear characteristics. Fast Gradient Method (FGM) [7] proposed by Goodfellow later scales according to specific gradients to get better countermeasure samples:

$$r_{adv} = \epsilon \cdot \nabla_x L\left(\theta, x, y\right) / \left\| \nabla_x L\left(\theta, x, y\right) \right\|_2 \tag{4}$$

Therefore, we add FGM to the model training. In order to further improve the Chinese natural language processing tasks, BERT-wwm is subsequently opensourced. BERT-wwm uses the whole word mask and more data for training to bring further performance improvements. In summary, the architecture of our proposed model is shown in Fig. 5.

4 Experiments

Dataset and Evaluation Metrics. The dataset used in this paper is the schema-based Chinese Medical Information Extraction (CMeIE) dataset. The dataset includes pediatric and common diseases training corpus, nearly 75,000 triple data, 28,000 disease sentences, and 53 defined schemas.

The task requires to output all the SRO triples [(s1, r1, o1), (s2, r2, o2)...] that meet the schema constraints, and then accurately match the real label results on the test set. If the relation type of a triple and two related entities are correct (in terms of scope and type), the relation extraction result is considered correct. Precision, Recall and F1 score are used as evaluation indexes.

Results. For the decoding process of the model, we choose the pointer network combined with the sigmoid activation function to mark the head and tail of the entity. An appropriate threshold should be set for optimal decoding. That is, the entity is considered appeared when the scores of head or tail beyond the threshold. We try different threshold combinations of head and tail based on 0.5. Table 1 shows that the recall is higher when the threshold is set lower, and a higher threshold will bring higher accuracy. To obtain the best F1 score of

Table 1. F1 score with different start and end thresholds in the model

Model	Threshold (Start/End)	Precision	Recall	F1
BERT-wwm	0.5/0.4	59.09	57.75	58.41
	0.5/0.5	59.29	**57.79**	58.53
	0.6/0.4	61.01	57.07	58.92
	0.6/0.5	**61.09**	57.11	**59.01**

Table 2. The F1 score of different benchmark models on the dataset. DGCNN(E1) represents 6-layer DGCNN with expansion rate of $[1, 2, 4, 1, 2, 4]$, DGCNN(E2) represents 9-layer DGCNN with expansion rate of $[1, 2, 4, 1, 2, 4, 1, 1, 1]$

Model	Precision	Recall	F1
BERT-wwm	**61.09**	57.11	**59.01**
BERT-wwm+BiLSTM	60.34	56.85	58.54
BERT-wwm+CNN	60.47	57.21	58.79
BERT-wwm+DGCNN(E1)	59.53	57.34	58.42
BERT-wwm+DGCNN(E2)	59.54	**57.92**	58.72

decoding result, we set the threshold of head as 0.6 and the tail as 0.5 according to the experiment.

In order to further explore the influence of different neural network layers on the results of relation extraction, we add CNN, DGCNN and LSTM layers before predicting the subject respectively. It can be seen from Table 2 that the addition of these networks fail to increase the F1 score of the model on the basis of BERT-wwm, and it also take more time during training. Therefor, we use BERT-wwm as our experimental benchmark model.

In the improvement of the multi-head attention layer in Encoder, we try two approaches: connecting a self-attention layer on the multi-head attention in parallel (Multi-BERT-wwm) or connecting another multi-head attention (Mix-BERT-wwm). In addition, for the 12-layer Encoder in BERT-wwm, we choose to change all Encoder (all) and only the first 6 layers of Encoder (half) 2 options. With other parameters remaining the same, the results of relation extraction for each combination are provided in Table 3. The effect of Mix-BERT-wwm stacking more multi-head attention seems not better, as some papers point out that multi-head is not necessary. That is to say, multiple heads of multi-head attention do not always pay attention to different aspects of information as we expect, the effect can still be good if some heads are removed. These heads already have the ability to pay attention to position information, grammatical information and rare words when heads are enough, more heads are nothing more than an enhancement or noise. It can be seen from the results that Multi-BERT-wwm(half) works best.

Table 3. Comparison of various improvement effects of multi-head attention layer

Model	Precision	Recall	F1
BERT-wwm	61.09	**57.11**	59.01
Mix-BERT-wwm (all)	61.28	56.37	58.72
Mix-BERT-wwm (half)	62.01	55.77	58.86
Multi-BERT-wwm (all)	61.32	56.86	58.99
Ours (Multi-BERT-wwm (half))	**63.42**	56.23	**59.30**

Table 4. Comparison results of our model with different relation extraction methods

	Model	Precision	Recall	F1
Pipeline	BERT	57.49	50.79	53.13
	BERT-wwm	57.85	51.02	53.51
Joint	CNN+Attention	62.04	50.82	55.77
	Roformer	59.07	56.61	57.81
	BERT	60.07	56.60	58.28
	BERT+CNN	60.47	57.21	58.79
	BERT-wwm	61.09	57.11	59.01
	BERT-wwm+BiLSTM	60.34	56.85	58.54
	BERT-wwm+DGCNN	59.54	**57.92**	58.72
Ours	Multi-BERT-wwm	63.42	56.23	59.30
	Multi-BERT-wwm+FGM	**64.67**	56.30	**60.19**

To evaluate the performance of our relation extraction model, we compare it with other reference models on the CMeIE dataset. These models include the pipeline and joint learning method based on CNN+Attention, BERT, CNN, BiL-STM and their various improved models. As shown in Table 4, the F1 score of the BERT joint learning model using our probabilistic graph strategy is much higher than the BERT model of the pipeline method, with an increase from 53.13% to 58.28%. The model we proposed achieves the best F1 score of 60.19% compared with the existing method, which is 1.18% higher than that of the BERT-wwm model. Compare with the Multi-BERT-wwm model which not adding adversarial training (FGM), the F1 score increased from 59.30% to 60.19%, an increase of 0.89%. It can be seen that adversarial training can not only improve the robustness and generalization ability of the model, but also has a certain effect on improving the accuracy of relation extraction.

5   Conclusion

In this paper, we propose a Multi-BERT-wwm model with cascading pointer network and probabilistic graph strategy for relation extraction. The model effectively solves the situation where there are multiple entities or relations in a sentence and the problem of overlapping entities. At the same time, the improved Multi-BERT-wwm model based on BERT obtains more grammatical and position features. We also use the adversarial training in the training process and achieve higher F1 score. Compared with the current BERT and CNN+Attention methods, this model can more accurately extract entities and relations from medical records. The effectiveness of our method is verified by experimental results on the CMEIE dataset. In the future, we will continue to explore the tag framework of multi-head selection in relation extraction and add lexicon information to improve the existing performance.

Acknowledgment. This work is supported by multiple grants, including: The National Key Research and Development Program of China (2020YFB1313900), National Natural Science Foundation of China (61902386, 62072452), Shenzhen Science and Technology Program (JCYJ20180507182415428), and Research on digital battlefield rescue integrated command Platform and auxiliary Equipment (CX19024).

References

1. Bekoulis, G., Deleu, J., Demeester, T., Develder, C.: Joint entity recognition and relation extraction as a multi-head selection problem. Expert Syst. Appl. **114**, 34–45 (2018)
2. Devlin, J., Chang, M.W., Lee, K., Toutanova, K.: Bert: pre-training of deep bidirectional transformers for language understanding. arXiv preprint arXiv:1810.04805 (2018)
3. Goodfellow, I.J., Shlens, J., Szegedy, C.: Explaining and harnessing adversarial examples. STAT **1050**, 20 (2015)
4. Kumar, S.: A survey of deep learning methods for relation extraction. arXiv preprint arXiv:1705.03645 (2017)
5. Lin, Y., Shen, S., Liu, Z., Luan, H., Sun, M.: Neural relation extraction with selective attention over instances. In: Proceedings of the 54th Annual Meeting of the Association for Computational Linguistics: Long Papers, , vol. 1, pp. 2124–2133 (2016)
6. Miwa, M., Bansal, M.: End-to-end relation extraction using LSTMs on sequences and tree structures. arXiv preprint arXiv:1601.00770 (2016)
7. Miyato, T., Dai, A.M., Goodfellow, I.: Adversarial training methods for semi-supervised text classification. arXiv preprint arXiv:1605.07725 (2016)
8. Nguyen, D.Q., Verspoor, K.: Convolutional neural networks for chemical-disease relation extraction are improved with character-based word embeddings. arXiv preprint arXiv:1805.10586 (2018)
9. Vaswani, A., et al.: Attention is all you need. In: Advances in Neural Information Processing Systems, pp. 5998–6008 (2017)
10. Wei, Z., Su, J., Wang, Y., Tian, Y., Chang, Y.: A novel cascade binary tagging framework for relational triple extraction. arXiv preprint arXiv:1909.03227 (2019)
11. Xu, Y., Mou, L., Li, G., Chen, Y., Peng, H., Jin, Z.: Classifying relations via long short term memory networks along shortest dependency paths. In: Proceedings of the 2015 Conference on Empirical Methods in Natural Language Processing, pp. 1785–1794 (2015)

12. Yu, X., Lam, W.: Jointly identifying entities and extracting relations in encyclopedia text via a graphical model approach. In: Coling 2010: Posters, pp. 1399–1407 (2010)
13. Zhang, Y., et al.: A hybrid model based on neural networks for biomedical relation extraction. J. Biomed. Inform. **81**, 83–92 (2018)
14. Zheng, S., Wang, F., Bao, H., Hao, Y., Zhou, P., Xu, B.: Joint extraction of entities and relations based on a novel tagging scheme. In: ACL, no. 1 (2017)
15. Zhou, Z.H.: A brief introduction to weakly supervised learning. Natl. Sci. Rev. **5**(1), 44–53 (2018)

Personalized Skin Care Service Based on Genomics

Jitao Yang[✉]

School of Information Science, Beijing Language and Culture University,
Beijing 100083, China
yangjitao@blcu.edu.cn

Abstract. The condition of people's skin is not only affected by environmental and psychological factors such as diet, sports, sleep and mood, genetic factors also play a very important role. Numerous genes have been identified to have associations with people's skin color, skin inflammation, skin type, sensitivity, and so on; and many genes are connected to the regulation of the synthesis of functional proteins which are related to the skin condition such as inflammation sensitivity, anti-oxidation, anti-glycosylation, aging, collagen regeneration, moisturizing and etc. In addition, loci polymorphisms are important contributors to the occurrence, development and prognosis of various skin diseases. In terms of skin nutrition, vitamins play an important role in maintaining skin balance, and the deficiency of vitamins may cause dull complexion, lack of luster and the other skin problems. In this paper, we first describe the genes (such as *MC1R*, *ASIP* and *BNC2*) that are related to skin conditions including sun sensitivity, skin moisturizing function, oxidative stress, stretch marks, and skin inflammation. Then we describe the relationships between nutrients (such as vitamin A and vitamin C) and healthy skin. Finally, we design and implement a personalized skin care service consists of genetic testing, personalized nutrition for healthy skin, and personalized skin care cosmetics recommendation.

Keywords: DNA testing · Skin care · Personalized nutrition · Personalized recommendation

1 Introduction

A person's skin health is affected by environmental, psychological, and genetic factors, therefore, apart from paying attention to our diet, sports, sleeping, mood, and cosmetics to improve our skin's health, we also need to know our skin's genetic factors, so that to maintain and promote our skin's health more precisely and personalized. Many genes related to people's skin color [1], skin inflammation [2], skin aging [3], and the other skin conditions have been identified, and those genes are connected to the regulation of the synthesis of functional proteins which have associations with skin's inflammation sensitivity, anti-oxidation, anti-glycosylation, aging, collagen regeneration, and moisturizing conditions. Studies

© Springer Nature Switzerland AG 2021
S. Siuly et al. (Eds.): HIS 2021, LNCS 13079, pp. 104–111, 2021.
https://doi.org/10.1007/978-3-030-90885-0_10

have also found that gene loci's polymorphisms play an important role in the occurrence, development and prognosis of different kinds of skin diseases.

Sufficient nutrition is necessary for skin to keep in good condition, vitamins are vital contributors to maintain skin balance, and the lack of vitamins may cause dull complexion, lack of luster and the other skin problems. For example, vitamin C synthesizes healthy collagen by combining with certain enzymes responsible for the effectiveness of collagen molecules, therefore, it provides support for connective tissue and promotes the healing of wounds and blemishes on the skin.

2   Skin and Genes

Numerous genes have been identified to have connections with people's skin conditions, such as sun sensitivity, moisturizing capability, oxidative stress, skin inflammation, and etc.

2.1   Sun Sensitivity

Sunshine can have either beneficial or harmful effects on people's skin health. In front of ultraviolet radiation (UVR), people with pale skin are more at risk of suffering from one of the photodermatoses [4], people with dark skin are more at risk of suffering from vitamin D deficiency [5]. For example, the *MC1R* gene's mutations can impair melanin synthesis and reduce melanin synthesis, resulting in lighter skin and hair color [6]. The genes *IRF4*, *MC1R*, *ASIP* and *BNC2* have genome wide associations with visible skin characteristics, including facial pigmented spots [7], pigmentation (eye, hair and/or skin color) [8], freckling [9], tanning response [10], and skin cancer (such as basal cell carcinoma, squamous cell carcinoma, and melanoma) [11–13].

2.2   Skin Moisturizing

Skin's moisturizing factor has the capacity of maintaining normal skin's elasticity and permeability, stratum corneum can reduce skin moisture loss, and prevent the invasion of harmful substances [14]. The *FLG* gene is related to skin's natural moisturizing ability, and mutations in the *FLG* gene and the loss of gene function will decrease the expression of filaggrin and skin moisturizing ability, resulting in more risk of dry skin [14].

2.3   Oxidative Stress

The proliferation of oxidative free radicals in the body is the root cause of dryness, dullness, ageing, and spots on skin, and damages the structure and function of skin [15]. The antioxidant capacity of skin is related to genetic factors, such as the peroxidase gene *CAT* participates in maintaining the balance of oxidation in the body [16]. The locus rs1050450 $(C > T)$ is located in the gene *GPX1*, compared with CC genotype carriers, CT and TT genotype carriers have more weaker antioxidant capacity [17].

2.4 Stretch Marks

Stretch marks are a pathological skin change that occurs during pregnancy [18]. In recent years, studies have pointed out that gene mutations can cause a decrease in the expression of fibrin and elastin, which affects skin elasticity, leading to an increased risk of stretch marks.

The rs7787362 in *ELN* gene has been identified to be associated with stretch marks, individuals with CC and CT genotypes have a lower and average risk of stretch marks, while individuals with TT genotypes have a higher risk of stretch marks [19].

2.5 Skin Inflammation

Skin inflammation mainly refers to reactions to the substances causing abnormal phenomena such as redness, swelling, itching or peeling when the skin's external environment has been changed.

The loci mg874146 and mg222425177 are located between the *HLA-DRA* and *BTNL2* genes. Individuals carrying mg874146 AG or AA genotype will have a risk of 1.18 times to have rosacea, individuals carrying mg222425177 AT or TT genotype will have a risk of 1.15 times to have rosacea [20]. Individuals carrying *IL12B* (rs2082412) locus of AG or GG genotype can induce the production of a large amount of inflammatory molecules which will result in a higher risk of psoriasis [21].

3 Nutrients for Healthy Skin

At present, a new concept has emerged in the cosmetics market, namely "nutritional cosmetics". Nutrition has a good positive effect on improving skin condition. Vitamins play a pivotal role in maintaining normal body operation. In terms of skin nutrition, vitamins play a positive role in anti-oxidation, scavenging free radicals, and maintaining skin balance. The micro-nutrients currently known to improve skin conditions include but not limited to vitamin A, vitamin B2, vitamin B_6, vitamin B_{12}, vitamin C, vitamin D, vitamin E, folic acid, omega-3, and omega-6.

For instance, vitamin A plays an important role in the growth and differentiation of tissue cells. The deficiency of vitamin A can cause dry skin, wrinkles, rough skin, scaling, or atrophy of sweat glands. The *BCMO1* gene encodes beta-carotene oxygenase 1, which is closely related to the synthesis of vitamin A. The mutations of the rs7501331 and rs12934922 on the *BCMO1* gene will reduce the enzyme activity of beta-carotene to synthesize vitamin A, and the absorption capacity of vitamin A will be weak [22].

Vitamin C is an effective antioxidant, therefore, it is an good choice for treating and preventing the effects of photoaging. Vitamin C is also helpful to refine skin, reduce skin damage, prevent ultraviolet rays from harming skin, and reduce pigmentation. The genetic polymorphism of the rs33972313 in the

SLC23A1 gene is related to the level of vitamin C in blood, individuals carrying TT or CT genotype will affect the transportation of vitamin C in the body, resulting in the un-effective absorption and utilization of vitamin C [23].

4   Personalized Skin Care Service

To help people improve skin conditions, we designed and implemented a personalized skin care service including genetic testing, personalized nutrition for healthy skin, and personalized cosmetics recommendation.

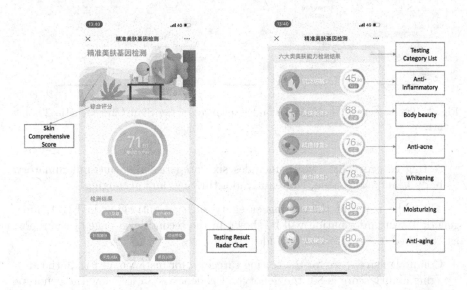

Fig. 1. The screen shots of the home page of the Skin Care Genetic Testing report.

4.1   Genetic Testing

As shown in Fig. 1, the home page of the Skin Care Genetic Testing Report is composed by three modules:

- skin comprehensive score, which calculates the comprehensive score of each person based on all the genetic testing items (such as anti-oxidant capacity, anti-aging ability and etc.): 1) if the comprehensive score is less than 60, then the customer's skin condition is poor, 2) the score between 60 and 80 means the customer's skin condition is normal, 3) if the score is higher than 90, then the customer's skin condition is excellent.
- genetic testing result radar chart, which displays the strong and weak parts of the customer's skin condition.

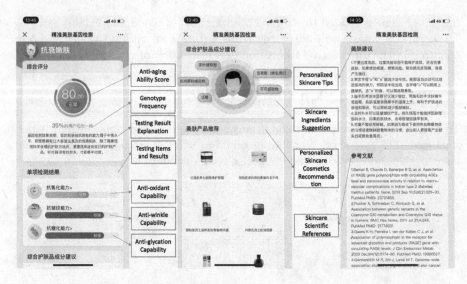

Fig. 2. The screen shots of the second level page of the Skin Care Genetic Testing report.

- testing category list, which includes six categories, *i.e.* anti-inflammatory, body beauty, anti-acne, whitening, moisturizing, and anti-aging.

Click the name of the testing category such as anti-aging in Fig. 1, more genetic testing information will be shown in the second level page of the report as described in Fig. 2, which includes six modules:

- Comprehensive score for the testing category: for instance, in Fig. 2, the anti-aging ability score is 80, the genotype frequency is 35%, below the genotype frequency is the comprehensive explanation for the testing result.
- Testing items and results: each testing category includes multiple testing items, such as the anti-aging category includes the items of anti-oxidant capability, anti-winkle capability, and anti-glycation capability.
- Skin care ingredients suggestion: based on the genetic testing results, the report will give suggestions on the ingredients that can help the customer to improve skin condition.
- Personalized skin care cosmetics recommendation: based on the ingredients the customer's skin required, the report recommends the suitable skin care cosmetics for the customer.
- Personalized skin care tips: based on the genetic testing result, the report will provide personalized skin care tips for the customer to improve the customer's skin condition.
- Skin care scientific references: this module lists some of the scientific evidences that support the genetic interpretation and personalized skin care solutions.

The skin care genetic testing report includes the testing items of: anti-tanning ability, anti-sunburn ability, anti-sunspots ability, anti-photoaging ability, antiox-

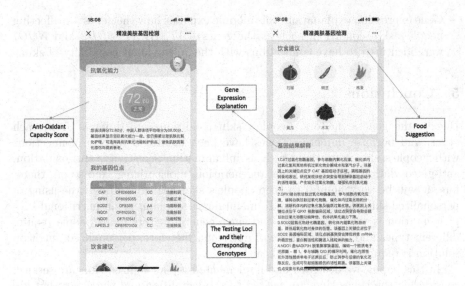

Fig. 3. The screen shots of the third level page of the Skin Care Genetic Testing report.

idant capacity, anti-glycation ability, anti-wrinkle ability, anti-inflammatory ability, skin protection ability, skin moisturizing ability, skin nutrition absorption, anti-stretch marks ability, anti varicose veins ability, anti-cellulite ability, skin repair ability, and anti-acne ability.

4.2   Personalized Nutritional Supplements

Skin nutrition plays an important role in keeping skin in good condition, however, because different people have different nutrition absorption, transformation and metabolism capabilities due to genetic factors, therefore, it's necessary to customize nutrition supplement solutions for different people.

Click the testing item name (*e.g.*, anti-oxidant capability) in Fig. 2, a third level page as described in Fig. 3 will be opened to give more detail information for the genetic testing item, the single genetic testing item (*e.g.*, anti-oxidant capability) report is composed by four modules:

- Testing item score and testing result explanation: for instance, in Fig. 3, the anti-oxidant capability score is 72, below the score is the summary and explanation about the testing result.
- Testing loci and their corresponding genotypes: this module lists the testing loci that related to the genetic testing item (*e.g.*, anti-oxidant capability), and gives the corresponding detected genotypes.
- Food suggestion: as described in Sect. 3, sufficient nutrient supplementation is very important for healthy skin, therefore, this module gives food suggestions based on the genetic testing result.

– Gene expression explanation: this module explains how the genes are affecting people's skin condition, such as the genes *CAT, GPX1, SOD2* and *NQO1* were identified to have connections with the anti-oxidant capability of skin.

5 Conclusions

Due to the genetic factors, people's skin conditions are different from each other, and because numerous genes have been identified to have connections with people's skin conditions such as inflammation sensitivity, anti-oxidation, anti-glycosylation, aging, collagen regeneration, moisturizing, and so on, therefore, it will be very helpful to keep people's skin healthy through the using of personalized skin care solutions. To maintain skin balance, skin nutritional supplementation is very important, and since genetic factors make people require different types and different doses of nutrients, therefore, personalized nutrition solution is required to keep skin healthy.

In this paper, we designed and implemented a personalized skincare service, considering the genes that are related to skin condition and the genes that are associated with skin nutrition to our data model, so that to compute different skin care solutions for different people. Our personalized skin care service has been delivered online and used by tens of thousands of persons, and played a very effective role in skin care industry.

Concerning further studies, more data will be integrated into our data model, such as we may use multi-spectral imaging analysis equipment and technology to test and analyze people's visible spots, ultraviolet spots, brown spots, wrinkles, textures, and pores conditions, so that to further support our personalized skin care nutrition and cosmetic solutions.

Acknowledgment. This research project is supported by Science Foundation of Beijing Language and Culture University (supported by "the Fundamental Research Funds for the Central Universities") (Approval number: 21YJ040002).

References

1. Pavan, W.J., Sturm, R.A.: The genetics of human skin and hair pigmentation. Annu. Rev. Genom. Hum. Genet. **20**, 41–72 (2019)
2. Marzano, A.V., Ortega-Loayza, A.G., et al.: Mechanisms of inflammation in neutrophil-mediated skin diseases. Front. Immunol. **10**, 1059 (2019)
3. Rinnerthaler, M., Streubel, M.K., et al.: Skin aging, gene expression and calcium. Exp. Gerontol. **68**, 59–65 (2015)
4. Rees, J.L.: The genetics of sun sensitivity in humans. Am. J. Hum. Genet. **75**(5), 739–751 (2004)
5. Holick, M.F.: Sunlight "D"ilemma: risk of skin cancer or bone disease and muscle weakness. Lancet **357**(9249), 4–6 (2001)
6. Bastiaens, M., Huurne, J.T., et al.: The melanocortin-1-receptor gene is the major freckle gene. Hum. Mol. Genet. **10**(16), 1701–1708 (2001)

7. Jacobs, L.C., Hamer, M.A., et al.: A genome-wide association study identifies the skin color genes IRF4, MC1R, ASIP, and BNC2 influencing facial pigmented spots. J. Investig. Dermatol. **135**(7), 1735–1742 (2015)

8. Han, J., Kraft, P., et al.: A genome-wide association study identifies novel alleles associated with hair color and skin pigmentation. PLoS Genet. **4**(5), e1000074 (2008)

9. Eriksson, N., Macpherson, J.M., et al.: Web-based, participant-driven studies yield novel genetic associations for common traits. PLoS Genet. **6**(6), e1000993 (2010)

10. Nan, H., Kraft, P., et al.: Genome-wide association study of tanning phenotype in a population of European ancestry. J. Investig. Dermatol. **129**(9), 2250–2257 (2009)

11. Demenais, F., Bishop, D.T., et al.: Genome-wide association study identifies three loci associated with melanoma risk. Nat. Genet. **41**(8), 920–925 (2009)

12. Nan, H., Xu, M., et al.: Genome-wide association study identifies novel alleles associated with risk of cutaneous basal cell carcinoma and squamous cell carcinoma. Hum. Mol. Genet. **20**(18), 3718–3724 (2011)

13. Stacey, S.N., Sulem, P., et al.: New common variants affecting susceptibility to basal cell carcinoma. Nat. Genet. **41**(8), 909–914 (2009)

14. Flohr, C., England, K., et al.: Filaggrin loss-of-function mutations are associated with, early-onset eczema, eczema severity and transepidermal, water loss at 3 months of age. Br. J. Dermatol. **163**(6), 1333–1336 (2010)

15. Shekar, S.N., Luciano, M., et al.: Genetic and environmental influences on skin pattern deterioration. J Invest Dermatol. **125**(6), 1119–1129 (2005)

16. Gromadzka, G., Kruszynska, M., et al.: Gene variants encoding proteins involved in antioxidant defense system and the clinical expression of Wilson disease. Liver Int. **35**(1), 215–222 (2015)

17. Tang, T.S., Prior, S.L., et al.: Association between the rs1050450 glutathione peroxidase-1 (C>T) gene variant and peripheral neuropathy in two independent samples of subjects with diabetes mellitus. Nutr. Metab. Cardiovasc. Dis. **22**(5), 417–425 (2012)

18. Garcia Hernandez, J.A., Madera Gonzalez, D., et al.: Use of a specific anti-stretch mark cream for preventing or reducing the severity of Striae gravidarum. Randomized, double-blind, controlled trial. Int. J. Cosmet. Sci. **35**(3), 233–237 (2013)

19. Tung, J.Y., Kiefer, A.K., et al.: Genome-wide association analysis implicates elastic microfibrils in the development of Nonsyndromic Striae Distensae. J. Investig. Dermatol. **133**(11), 2628–2631 (2013)

20. Chang, A.L.S., Raber, I., et al.: Assessment of the genetic basis of rosacea by genome-wide association study. J. Investig. Dermatol. **135**(6), 1548–1555 (2015)

21. Lee, Y.H., Choi, S.J., et al.: Genome-wide pathway analysis of a genomewide association study on psoriasis and Behcet's disease. Mol. Biol. Rep. **39**(5), 5953–5959 (2012)

22. Leung, W.C., Hessel, S., et al.: Two common single nucleotide polymorphisms in the gene encoding beta-carotene15,15'-monoxygenase alter beta-carotene metabolism in female volunteers. FASEB J. **23**(4), 1041–1053 (2009)

23. Timpson, N.J., Forouhi, N.G., et al.: Genetic variation at the SLC23A1 locus is associated with circulating concentrations of L-ascorbic acid (vitamin C): evidence from 5 independent studies with >15,000 participants. Am. J. Clin. Nutr. **92**(2), 375–382 (2010)

Empowering Patients with HIPAA Aware Personal Health Libraries

Hasan M. Jamil[1](✉) ⓘ, Evanthia Bernitsas[2] ⓘ, Alexandar Gow[2] ⓘ,
and Berhane Seyoum[2] ⓘ

[1] Department of Computer Science, University of Idaho, Moscow, ID, USA
jamil@uidaho.edu
[2] School of Medicine, Wayne State University, Detroit, MI, USA
{ebernits,agow,bseyoum}@med.wayne.edu

Abstract. One of the most difficult issues that confronts clinicians and patients alike is sharing EHRs across service providers. While HIPAA grants ownership of EHR data to patients, the information is not easily shareable. At times, doctors cannot access their own patients' EHR in two different medical systems even when the record keeping systems are the same and patients grant consent. The onus of sharing falls on the patient who must physically acquire the necessary record. Such a policy hinders quality of service, causes delays and higher costs for all involved. In this paper, we introduce a new data sharing protocol aimed at reducing this hurdle, using a personal health library architecture being encouraged by National Institutes of Health in the USA.

Keywords: EHR · Data integration · Privacy and sharing · Access rights · Personal health library · HIPAA · Distributed database · Middleware

1 Introduction

In an increasingly mobile society, patients move from place to place for various reasons. Even within a single location, they seek medical services from multiple providers often for overlapping medical conditions. In such cases, they need to share their electronic health records (EHR) with multiple providers which will avoid unnecessary repetition of that incurs avoidable costs and time for both patients and physicians. Even when they are visiting clinicians for completely different medical conditions, having a global knowledge of the patient's medical history may aid clinicians to arrive at a more accurate and appropriate diagnosis and treatment.

Currently, all patient medical records are kept in individual provider data silos to which patients presumably have unfettered access since the Affordable Cares Act was passed in March 2010. While most providers have instituted remote access to individual EHRs and now allow patients to access them at varying levels of granularity, compiling a unified view of all accessible records is difficult if not impossible. For example, Moscow Medical, Idaho, uses the HealOW

S. Siuly et al. (Eds.): HIS 2021, LNCS 13079, pp. 112–123, 2021.
https://doi.org/10.1007/978-3-030-90885-0_11

system from eClinicalWorks as their EHR patient portal. They routinely refer patients to the Gritman Medical Center and Hospital for various tests and procedures. Gritman uses FollowMyHealth system from AllScripts Healthcare as their EHR solution and patient portal. Unfortunately, even though Gritman serves Moscow Medical patients and treats them, FollowMyHealth does not recognize the referring practice as a partner in their portal because they can only communicate with other FollowMyHealth clients or users. Finally, Moscow Medical has an in-house pathology lab run by LabCorp and they perform almost all tests recommended by the clinicians at Moscow Medical. Yet, the LabCorp reports are not integrated with the HealOW EHR system at the clinic.

The EHR debacle above points to a larger problem patients and physicians face all the time. Given the fact that these three establishments in a small American town work so closely together, yet are unable to share patient EHRs, it is not unfathomable to realize that a patient referred to the University of Michigan Health Systems (UMHS) was unable to share her EHRs from these three establishments with UMHS. In particular, patient request for information release works promptly and electronically within the same establishment, not across establishments. Thus, a request for EHRs must go out from UMHS to all these medical service providers for a physical record that would arrive by mail. Alternately, the patient could potentially print the records from the individual patient portal and hand them over to the UMHS clinicians for manual integration – largely defeating the purpose of the very idea of EHRs.

Perhaps the more critical failure of these EHRs is that low level data from which a clinician draws medical conclusions remain with the system, sequestered deep in the lab results – DNA information generated from ordered test panels, ultrasound and MRI imaging data, device data, etc. Without access to such detailed data, clinicians routinely order new tests, even within the same service providers because physicians prefer to get an accurate picture of the state of the medical condition of their patients quickly and cannot afford to wait. In the case of the patient referred to UMHS, a highly costly new ultrasound of the wrist was ordered again since the test results with the image was not made available with the referrals, and the patient initiated record transfer will need more than a few weeks, if not months.

We believe that the core of the problem is not related to the technology using which the EHR systems are designed, but the HIPAA data sharing policies themselves. In our view, while HIPAA addressed the digitization of the medical records and empowered patients to access their own records, it failed to address EHR integration and information sharing dimensions of health record management. Privacy regulations under HIPAA prevents EHR systems from sharing data easily by assigning patients as the main vehicle for transferring records rather than the systems. For example, a doctor at UMHS cannot access the EHR at Cleveland Clinic for the patient she treats at both systems even with the consent of the patient, and when both establishments use Epic EHR system as their medical record keeping databases.

In this paper, we recognize this limitation of contemporary EHR systems and introduce a new access rights protocol for improved data sharing based on the recently proposed Personal Health Library (PHL) architecture being encouraged by the National Institutes of Health in the USA. The preliminary idea of our PHL, called *PerHL* (Personal Health Library, and pronounced "pearl") was introduced in [9] where we have discussed the features of PerHL query capabilities. In this paper, we present the contours of the data sharing capabilities of PerHL to complement its novel conversational querying capabilities in natural language.

2   An Illustrative Example

Consider a patient Fiia, 37 year old woman, college graduate, who has hypertension and progressive-relapsing multiple sclerosis (PRMS) diagnosed about 15 years ago. Fiia has two younger sisters – Enni, 26 and Elli, 23. Her father has Insulin dependent diabetes mellitus (IDDM), or type 1 diabetes and maternal aunt has multiple sclerosis (MS). She recently moved to Idaho from Michigan where she lives with her husband. She prefers to follow up with her neurologist in Michigan when she routinely visits family in Michigan. This means that she must share all her medical records with the establishment in Idaho and her previous primary care physicians (PCPs) at UMHS in Michigan.

Recently, she has been experiencing some pain in a lump on her wrist and consulted her new PCP in Moscow Medical in Idaho who ordered an ultrasonographic diagnostic test at the Gritman Medical Center and Hospital. It was found to be a dupuytren's contracture and was recommended that it be removed. She was referred to an orthopedic surgeon in Michigan at her request so that she can be close to her family during the surgery and also because there was no qualified surgeon in Moscow who can perform the surgery.

Fiia had previously manually shared all her medical records with all her physicians in Michigan because she could not share her EHRs electronically (meaning in a machine readable way), and the shared EHRs do not update when new entries are made in any of her EHRs at any of the provider's network. However, most of her EHR data are nearly universally shared across all Michigan clinics and hospitals she goes to, because of her personal effort to make them available to all her doctors.

After her recent move to Moscow, Idaho, she faced serious complications with her PRMS and new symptoms of weakness and numbness on the right arm and leg. Since her Michigan system EHRs are not available in Idaho yet, miscommunication among the physicians at both states, and conflicting diagnostic tests followed by emergency department visits made it a nightmarish experience for Fiia which could have been avoided if the EHRs were electronically shared instantly. However, eventually her treatment was successful.

The strong family history of autoimmune diseases raises critical questions for her sisters which could be addressed if the EHR is shared properly. For example, although not a standard of care, genetic analysis could be helpful as it can predict risk, alert patient and clinicians for early treatment, encourage healthy life style and administration of a high dose of Vitamin D3 that can decrease the risk of developing MS and/or slow down disability. At this point, genetic analysis is done only in research studies aimed at assessing the risk in families with high frequency of autoimmune diseases.

As a routine procedure, Enni and Elli participated in clinical genetic studies for relatives of MS patients. Elli was found to have the HLA-DRB1*15:01 allele, and the test results were reported to her primary care doctor. Even if Elli did not share her EHRs with Fiia's doctors, because of the family connections, Fiia or Elli could initiate an exploratory collaboration between their respective physicians, and Fiia's neurologist could recommend Elli to start a high dose vitamin D3 treatment and ways to modify other risk factors for MS, such as weight management and physical activity. However, this is not possible under the current HIPAA practices, at least not automatically.

3   An Architecture for EHR Data Sharing in PHLs

As noted earlier, the recently proposed idea of personal health libraries [1] can potentially address most of these data sharing concerns only if there is a HIPAA compliant privacy protocol that would allow patient controlled EHR data sharing fully electronically. Theoretically, PHLs consolidate patients' EHR data in a single library and provide a global view of their health information. However, such consolidated EHR data may not be shareable in its entirety with legitimate entities – physicians, hospitals, labs, insurance companies, clinic or hospital staff, nurses or lab technicians. A patient may wish to provide access to someone to a certain part of her medical history and another part to someone else. She might also want to share a portion with someone temporarily and revoke the access privilege after certain period or action. Such a nuanced and advanced data sharing model quickly becomes complicated and demands a privacy model based data sharing approach. In this section, we present a minimally invasive privacy aware and HIPAA compliant data sharing model and declarative access control language for PHLs.

3.1   Privacy Model

The PerHL PHL data model $\mathcal{M} = \langle E, R, H, L, P \rangle$ consists of i) a set of active entities E such as patients Fiia, Enni and Elli; doctors Alan and Rama, lab technicians Sayed and so on; ii) a set of defined relationships R that associates entities with other entities such as Fiia who is a patient at UMHS and Gritman; iii) a set of EHRs H that described patients' health history and diagnoses, iv) L is a set of access rights organized in a lattice with defined LUB and GLB, and finally, v) a set of permissions P granted by entities to arbitrary entities – related or not.

Entities. Entities can be simple or complex. Individual actors such as Fiia, Alan and Sayed are simple entities, while institutions such as diagnostic labs (e.g., Lab-Corp, Syneos, Parexel, Quest, etc.), hospital systems (e.g., Henry Ford Health Systems, UMHS, Gritman Medical Center and Hospital, Pullman Regional Hospital, etc.), and medical practices (e.g., Moscow Medical, Detroit Health Professionals, Spokane Cancer Center, etc.) are complex entities as they cluster simple and other complex entities into one. Entities are identified with a globally unique ID similar to ORCID IDs [5]. It is possible that each of these entities will have other unique IDs but for our model, we will identify them using our unique ID called *PerHLID*, represented by the set $I = I_s \cup I_c \cup I_o$, where I_s, I_c and I_o respectively represent simple and complex entities, and ordinary identifiers.

Relationships. Relationships among entities are of two types – lateral and hierarchical and are a subset of $I \times I \times I \times \rho$ such that $\rho = \rho_l \cup \rho_h$ where ρ_l is a set of lateral relationship roles and similarly ρ_h is a set of hierarchical roles. A triple $<i_1, i_2, i_3, r_1>$ implies $<i_2, i_1, i_3, r_1>$ only when $r_1 \in \rho_l$, and $i_1, i_2, i_3 \in I$. In other words, lateral relationships are symmetric but hierarchical relationships are not. In a hierarchical relationship, i.e., $<i_1, i_2, i_3, r_1>$ where $r_1 \in \rho_h$, the entity i_1 is called a parent, and i_2 is a child, and the relationship is a DAG (directed acyclic graph). A further distinction is that in a hierarchical relationship, a child entity's properties become part of the parent (also ancestors) entities, but in a lateral relationship it does not. For example <Fiia, Moscow Medical, 22961, Patient>[1] is a lateral relationship, while <Fiia, Elli, $\perp$, Sibling> is a hierarchical relationship assuming "Patient" $\in \rho_l$ and "Sibling" $\in \rho_h$.

In all these relationships, i_3 is an identifier in I that is unique for the relationship $<i_1, i_2>$ and $<i_2, i_1>$. In practice, i_3 is intended to be a patient ID assigned to a patient which could potentially be the patients PerHLID itself, i.e., i_1, including the distinguished ID $\perp \in I_o$ which signifies no assigned ID or *nil*, and $i_3 \notin I_h$. The roles in the relationships are also interpretive, meaning that these are not merely labels and that the relationships are defined by these labels semantically. For example, the label "Patient" associates a person with a clinic in a certain way, and this label may be interpreted differently by different pairs of associations. Similarly, the label "Insured" may have multiple different connotations for each combination of a person and an insurance company. In other words, there is an interpretive function associated with each label that assigns the meaning of these labels in the context of the entities involved. For example, for the pairs (Fiia, Aetna) and (Joe, Aetna), the label "insured" may mean health coverage, and third part assurance of coverage, respectively.

Universal Patient IDs and Health Information of Patients. Each patient has a health history at each of the health services provider and insurance agencies where they maintain their insurances. We call them respectively EHRs and EIRs

---

[1] Note that in these examples, we are abusing our notations and using entity names directly as their unique PerHLID, which is not exactly unnatural.

(electronic insurance record). In each of these agencies with whom the patients have a lateral relationship, a unique patient or subscriber ID is assigned which may be, but not necessarily, distinct from the PerHLID. In case a local ID is used, PerHLID is included in the EHR/EIR. Additionally, in the event the PerHLID is not included in the EHR/EIR, a separate relationship is created to associate the patient's PerHLID with the EHR/EIR ID. This separate association is required to be minimally invasive to the current practice of EHR/EIR system and yet remain compliant with the HIPAA provisions.

Permission Lattice and Access Rights. The HIPAA Privacy Rule[2] delineates standards to protect individuals' medical records and other personal health information. These standards apply to health plans, health care clearinghouses, and health care providers serving patients. The rule mandates appropriate safeguards to protect the privacy of personal health information, and establishes limits and conditions on the uses and disclosure of such information to someone who needs to know without patient consent. The rule also grants patients rights over their health information, including rights to examine and obtain a copy of their health records, and to request corrections.

Most of the HIPAA compliant EHR systems assign the patient as the owner of her EHR data and the controller of disclosures – legally mandated access rights as the lowest level of electronic user service. Unfortunately, the current setup for most EHR systems do not allow patients electronic control of the disclosures they would like to make as outlined in the examples earlier. Since interoperability among the EHR systems and consented disclosures are not currently easily supported and these systems are slow to change, we approach these two issues by designing a PHL as an umbrella system under patient control as follows.

Under the current system, most HIPAA compliant health service portals allow patients to access their EHRs electronically with wide ranging sophistication and ease. For example, Fiia has access to her EHR at LabCorp diagnostic lab, Moscow Medical, Gritman and UMHS systems via a secure login. Most of them allow her to download the EHRs in PDF. In Fiia's particular case, though LabCorp uses Moscow Medical's patient ID for her EHR, the recent blood test results in LabCorp EHR showing high fasting glucose levels was not included in her Moscow Medical EHR. Nor did the diagnostic results of her wrist contracture from Gritman make it to the EHR which was also ordered by her PCP at Moscow Medical. Furthermore, the detailed and raw lab test data that Lab-Corp carried out and the imagery from which Gritman summarised the findings which Fiia has access to, were not included in respective EHRs at LabCorp and Gritman.

Our goal is to allow Fiia to integrate, not just manually send the PDF of a EHR, any subset of her EHRs including the raw data and imagery with any of the EHRs she owns or shares. Figure 1 captures the data integration and sharing model for Fiia's EHRs we capture in PerHL. In this figure, Elli made a portion of her EHR accessible to Fiia, which is part of Fiia's EHR via the

---

[2] https://www.hhs.gov/hipaa/for-professionals/privacy/laws-regulations/index.html.

part of relationship. The way Fiia can use the part shared by Elli, called "Elli's White EHR" depends on what rights Elli grants Fiia. In a similar way, Gritman, Moscow Medical and LabCorp all shared Fiia's EHR they respectively maintain with Fiia who virtually and computationally consolidated all the records into one giant EHR – called "Fiia's Consolidated EHR".

Note that Fiia's Consolidated EHR is not really materialized. Actually it does not exist as stored data. Rather it is a process or query that generates the EHR when referred to. This approach of generating the EHR on the fly has several advantages. First, it allows updates at the lower level and thus always presents the most recent view of the EHR. Second, it does not duplicate information in multiple repositories and invite inconsistency. Finally, since most patients will most likely install their PHLs on their smartphones, a virtual EHR will require much less device memory which many phones may not have. Instead, the precious storage can be used to save a needed PHL toolbox that contains patient selected analytic tools for various services she wishes to use.

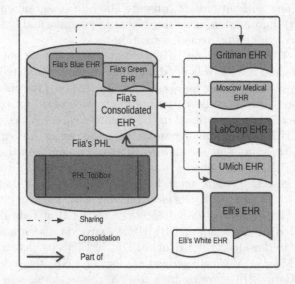

Fig. 1. Fiia's PHL and EHR relationships. (Color figure online)

For example, a file conversion tool set and a query engine are standard entries in this toolbox. Since PerHL adopts a minimally disruptive architecture, it does not insist the individual EHRs in a specific format. Instead, it just requires that access be allowed to "all" data, not just the summarized notes. It will, however, accept all it is granted access to, for example, image data and low level DNA analyses data, and that the data be made available in some form of machine readable format instead of PDF. PerHL then converts the EHRs into a canonical format for sharing and integration purposes. Individual patients, however, may have a large number of other analytic tools for specific heath issues such as heart rate monitoring or diabetes related apps.

Researchers have proposed methods to standardize clinical data for sharing purposes [3] already, and to convert data descriptions [4] to facilitate their use. The easiest and most common form of standardization is file format conversion [11] which we also adopt. For our purpose, we use a two step process, a first step is to convert all EHR data into an intermediate step [2,12], and then make a final representation in HTML for client visualization or into a target format for onward sharing. For example, all EHR data is first converted in JSON, and then to HTML for visualization by Fiia, or conversion of the Blue EHR to CSV format for Gritman, and the Green EHR to line format for UMHS.

Figure 2 depicts the outlines the other essential component of PerHL, the query engine. This engine serves as a smart conversational and contextual natural language question answering platform of PerHL based on a declarative query language called HQL. We do not discuss this component of PerHL in this paper for the sake of brevity, and refer interested readers to [9] for a more detailed introduction. However, we just note that this engine is capable of responding to two common types of queries – *what* and *why* queries, while additional query types are being actively contemplated.

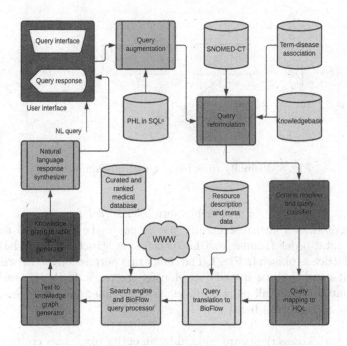

Fig. 2. Query processing in PerHL.

Permission Lattice. Not all data owned by an entity are shareable with another entity, and it is necessary to spell out what the recipient may be able to do with the shared data – terms of use. This type of relationship is usually based on the intended roles of the association, e.g., patient, sibling, insured, etc. For example, patient Fiia cannot update the EHR at Gritman, except perhaps the personal information part of it. Similarly, the internal electronic discussions among the physicians about Fiia's ER visit may not be shared with Fiia or the insurance provider.

The global and corporate nature of the health care system adds new wrinkles to the already complicated privacy enforcement rules of HIPAA. For example, both Moscow Medical and Pullman Regional Hospital use LabCorp as their diagnostic partner. Fiia was assigned two different patient IDs by the referring practices (Moscow Medical and Pullman Regional Hospital). The question is, if Fiia is to share some medical information using permission level *edit* with Moscow Medical and *view* with Pullman Regional Hospital, which permission should be assigned to LabCorp? Because the patient IDs assigned are immaterial to Fiia and should be allowed to be abstract. This becomes complicated in particular when Fiia had already assigned a *copy* permission to LabCorp sometime ago.

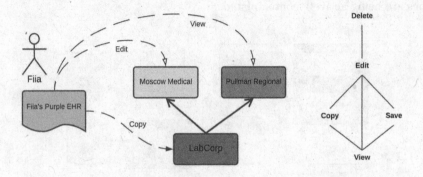

Fig. 3. Visibility rules based on permission lattice.

In Fig. 3, we show a set of possible permissions (*delete, edit, view, copy* and *save*) organized as a lattice structure. We do not make a choice of the lattice type, i.e., total order (similar to Unix permission structure), semi-lattice or a complete lattice as shown in Fig. 3. The choice of a permission lattice will depend on the PHLs and the anticipated data sharing protocols. In PerHL, we choose a complete lattice where all pairs of nodes have a defined join and meet, making it definitive as explained below.

Access Rights. Access rights are granted by an entity to another entity for a part of the EHR. The subset is computed as a qualitative specification, or a query, that extracts it from the EHR and assigns a single permission level from the lattice to another entity. If the receiver is a simple entity, it is all set. However, if the receiver is a complex entity, the assigned permission flows down (or is inherited) to the sub-ordinate or child entities, all of them. Such a large scale permission assignment may be counter productive or even unwanted. Therefore, some form of revision, or overriding is essential if the parent-child relation of the complex entities cannot be altered. From this viewpoint, overriding and non-monotonic inheritance in object-oriented systems appear pertinent.

In Fig. 3, the permission copy should override the other two permissions inherited down the parent child association. In this event, where the copy permission was not assigned, we face the much-researched issue of multiple-inheritance in object-oriented (OO) systems. The absence of a suitable resolution method makes it necessary for imperative languages such as C++ to disallow multiple inheritance by allowing only tree-like subclass relationships. In some logic-based languages though, multiple-inheritance conflict is resolved based on model selection [10]. Such an approach would make PHL permission structure uncertain because in model selection the allowed permission is randomly chosen.

In PHLs, a more definitive determination of access rights is necessary so that we are able to predict what permission will hold in advance, at least to know what the model will choose. A more definitive resolution model was proposed in [6] which rejects all conflicting permissions in multiple inheritance hierarchies in case a single source of inheritance cannot be computed. An extension of this conflicting overriding has been addressed using parameterization of inheritance mode [8] and further leveraged to support security permission in multi-level secure databases [7]. For the purpose of PHL, we introduce a new idea of *permission preference*, and use a much simpler method for conflict resolution based on permission lattice's meet and join operation.

In our model, we inherit all permission as a set. We let entities choose a preference – *permissive* or *restrictive*. If a permissive mode is chosen, we take the meet of all permission to assign an access right. For example, in the case of Fiia, the access right LabCorp will be assigned is edit since it is the meet of copy, view, edit. If a restrictive preference is chosen, the permission assigned will be view, the join of the three permissions.

3.2   A Declarative Privacy-Aware EHR Sharing Language

PerHL's existing query language HQL (which stands for Health Query Language) is geared toward conversational querying. In this language, a contextual exploration of structured and unstructured health information can be set up and the responses can be iteratively filtered assuming all necessary health data are in the patient's EHR or are online. The existing design does not consider the privacy consideration of HIPAA. In this section, we introduce an extension of HQL to account for its missing privacy features with the aim of making it HIPAA compliant.

We develop a privacy language along the lines of SQL's grant revoke statement structure. Since we plan to regard all access as stored procedure which will execute when referred, we choose the style of SQL view definition as follows.

```
set permission mode restrictive;
create view blueEHR as diagnosis, recommendation, comment
where date = 6/20/ 2021 and pcp = "Moscow Medical";
```

create permission *labcorp* allow copy on *blueEHR* revoke never;
create permission *moscowmedical* allow edit on *blueEHR* revoke after *8/30/2021*;
create permission *pullmanregional* allow view on *blueEHR* revoke never;

The simple definition above supports several features that make EHR data sharing possible as outlined in Sect. 3.1. First, the set permission statement establishes a global privacy mode for a PHL, for example, Fiaa's. The two choices as discussed before are *permissive* and *restrictive*, Fiia chose to be conservative in her permissions.

Second, the create permission statement separates the permission assignment from the content, but associates the content using a named reference. The reference can be any named view or procedure that is not a query which cannot be named and returns a table. Finally, the permission statement includes a permission level and an active period of the permission using the revoke option. The statements above captures the scenario presented in Fig. 3 with a restrictive view. While Fiia is allowed to change her permission mode, changing it could have unwanted consequences on the permission eventualities as discussed. An extended and parameterized mode assignment is required to support access right assignment in multiple permission modes and left as future research.

4   Conclusion

The proposed EHR data sharing approach in PerHL relies on a distributed database model integrated using a middleware with no disruption of existing systems. Actually, it leverages the delegation of access rights to the patients as the owner of the EHRs granted in HIPPA, and delegates the visibility to the target entities with whom the EHRs or the part thereof need to be shared. PerHL also ensures that all updates in the parent EHRs are delegated to the providers of healthcare with whom the EHRs are shared on a dynamic basis. This currency of EHR is achieved by accessing the EHR data at the source using a computational code similar to a database query or methods in OO systems. Appropriate apps or analytics are included in the PHLs to support intelligent health information queries, and to provide an illusion of the PHL as a giant personalized virtual health database.

While the model and the theoretical underpinning of the privacy query language are available, the implementation of PerHL is currently ongoing. We must note that the proper implementation of the proposed language will require a model for EHR document engineering that we did not consider in this paper. For example, an EHR has numerous components – diagnoses, test results, raw diagnostic data, summaries and findings, medication, medical advises, personal information, and so on. A query language to extract appropriate portions of an EHR needs to be developed based on the document engineering model, e.g., how to create the Blue EHR of Fiia from the EHRs in Moscow Medical and UMHS that only includes all relevant information on the dupuytren's contracture, and nothing else? We plan to investigate this issue and a more refined and practical permission lattice in our future research.

References

1. Ammar, N., Bailey, J.E., Davis, R.L., Shaban-Nejad, A.: The personal health library: a single point of secure access to patient digital health information. In: Pape-Haugaard, L.B., Lovis, C., Madsen, I.C., Weber, P., Nielsen, P.H., Scott, P. (eds.) Digital Personalized Health and Medicine - Proceedings of Medical Informatics Europe, Geneva, Switzerland, 28 April–1 May 2020. Studies in Health Technology and Informatics, vol. 270, pp. 448–452. IOS Press (2020)

2. Dang, T.K., Ta, M.H., Hoang, N.L.: Intermediate data format for the elastic data conversion framework. In: Lee, S., Choo, H., Ismail, R. (eds.) 15th International Conference on Ubiquitous Information Management and Communication, Seoul, South Korea, 4–6 January 2021, pp. 1–5 (2021)

3. Freedman, H.G., Williams, H., Miller, M.A., Birtwell, D., Mowery, D.L., Stoeckert, C.J.: A novel tool for standardizing clinical data in a semantically rich model. J. Biomed. Inform. X **8**, 100086 (2020)

4. Gancheva, V., Shishedjiev, B., Kalcheva-Yovkova, E.: An approach to convert scientific data description. In: IEEE 6th International Conference on Intelligent Data Acquisition and Advanced Computing Systems: Technology and Applications, Prague, Czech Republic, 15–17 September 2011, vol. 2, pp. 564–568 (2011)

5. Haak, L.L., Fenner, M., Paglione, L., Pentz, E., Ratner, H.: ORCID: a system to uniquely identify researchers. Learn. Publ. **25**(4), 259–264 (2012)

6. Jamil, H.M.: Implementing abstract objects with inheritance in Datalog^{neg}. In: International Conference on Very Large Databases, Athens, Greece, pp. 56–65, August 1997

7. Jamil, H.M.: Belief reasoning in MLS deductive databases. In: SIGMOD Conference, Philadelphia, PA, pp. 109–120, June 1999

8. Jamil, H.M.: A logic based language for parametric inheritance. In: Proceedings of the Seventh International Conference on Principles of Knowledge Representation and Reasoning, Breckenridge, CO, pp. 611–622, April 2000

9. Jamil, H.M.: Architecture of an intelligent personal health library for improved health outcomes. In: Proceedings of the IEEE International Conference on Digital Health, 5–10 September 2021, Held Online, USA (2021)

10. Kifer, M., Lausen, G., Wu, J.: Logical foundations of object-oriented and frame-based languages. J. ACM **42**(4), 741–843 (1995)

11. Neudert, G., Klebe, G.: fconv: Format conversion, manipulation and feature computation of molecular data. Bioinformatics **27**(7), 1021–1022 (2011)

12. van Horik, R., Roorda, D.: Migration to intermediate XML for electronic data (MIXED): repository of durable file format conversions. Int. J. Digit. Curation **6**(2), 245–252 (2011)

Automatic Breast Lesion Segmentation Using Continuous Max-Flow Algorithm in Phase Preserved DCE-MRIs

Dinesh Pandey[1], Hua Wang[1](✉), Xiaoxia Yin[2], Kate Wang[3], Yanchun Zhang[1], and Jing Shen[4]

[1] Victoria University, Melbourne, Australia
hua.wang@vu.edu.au
[2] Guangzhou University, Guangzhou, China
[3] RMIT University, Melbourne, Australia
[4] Radiology Department, Affiliated Zhongshan Hospital of Dalian university, Dalian, China

Abstract. In this work, we propose a framework for the automatic and accurate segmentation of breast lesions from the Dynamic Contrast Enhanced (DCE) MRI. The framework is built using max flow and min cut problems in the continuous domain over phase preserved denoised images. The proposed method is achieved via three steps. First, post-contrast and pre-contrast images are subtracted, followed by image registrations that benefit to enhancing lesion areas. Second, a phase preserved denoising and pixel-wise adaptive Wiener filtering technique is used, followed by max flow and min cut problems in a continuous domain. A denoising mechanism clears the noise in the images by preserving useful and detailed features such as edges. Then, lesion detection is performed using continuous max flow. Finally, a morphological operation is used as a post-processing step to further delineate the obtained results. The efficiency of the proposed method is verified with a series of qualitative and quantitative experiments carried out on 21 cases with two different MR image resolutions. Performance results demonstrate the quality of segmentation obtained from the proposed method.

Keywords: Automatic lesion segmentation · DCE MRI · Phase preservation denoising

1 Introduction

Breast cancer is due to the abnormal growth of cells around breast lobules or ducts [1]. The growth of cells is uncontrollable and can spread to other parts of body. After lung cancer, it is the cancer most commonly diagnosed in women resulting in death. Early diagnosis and treatment is essential to improving the survival rate. Several medical imaging modalities are used to diagnose breast cancer, including mammography [2], ultrasound [3], biopsy CT scan [4] and

MRI scan [5]. Among the imaging techniques, dynamic contrast-enhanced magnetic resonance imaging (DCE-MRI) provides three-dimensional high resolutions images with accurate anatomical information that is not available with the other two widely used techniques: mammography and ultrasound. Therefore, it is the most common and important tool for breast cancer diagnosis which provides relatively accurate results. However, manual segmentation of these imaging techniques for suspicious breast lesions is a tedious and time-consuming task due to the large amount of data required [6,7].

Many segmentation techniques discussed in the existing literature fall under supervised and unsupervised learning approaches [8–10]. The goal of supervised learning is to develop a trained model to classify different object labels [11–13]. Some popular supervised approaches in the literature are K-Nearest Neighbors (KNN) [14], random forests (RF) [15], SVM [16], Bayesian, and deep learning which is one of the advance supervised technique [17–19].

Since large labelled datasets are required in supervised methods, they are a complex and computationally expensive means of achieving an efficient result [20,21]. Furthermore, supervised learning approaches are limited to the size and quality of datasets, and possess the limitation of overfitting. Furthermore, in real clinical applications, it is challenging to obtain sufficient labelled data due to limited patient numbers and time constraints [22,23]. It is also likely that neighboring pixels take the same label or have a low number of connected components.

In contrast, an unsupervised method requires prior knowledge of required segmentation labels which relies on different features such as region, boundary texture and image edges [24,25]. Unsupervised techniques rely on patterns (feature vectors) belonging to the same object. These features can be studied and defined as per requirements. Moreover, unsupervised machine learning models learn from unlabelled data without human interaction. Once results are achieved, they can be used as labelled data to train supervised learning models that produce more resilient results. Unsupervised segmentation techniques are considered useful for handling more complicated cases [26,27]. Among several unsupervised segmentation techniques, continuous max flow min cut algorithm has been successfully applied in a wide class of application such as image segmentation [28,29]. However, simply using a continuous max flow min cut algorithm on MRI images will produce a less efficient result due to existing noise, and slow down the convergence without a multigrid and parallel implementation [30]. To solve the aforementioned challenges, we propose a fully automatic and unsupervised framework that is able to produce accurate lesion segmentation. The framework incorporates a graph method (solved by formulating max flow and min cut problems in the continuous domain) with denoising methods and morphological operations. It is observed that, although the continuous max flow (CMF) algorithm is able to reduce the iterations avoiding the computational load, the segmentation quality heavily depends upon the denoising process prior to the execution. Hence, prior to the segmentation process, a good denoising algorithm is needed to eliminate noise while preserving useful information and structure.

Lesion segmentation begins with a pre-processing step to eliminate common background signals and improve the contrast of breast lesions. This step is carried out using image registration followed by subtraction between pre- and post-contrast images. Next, we use the phase preserved denoising and adaptive Weiner filtering, which significantly reduces noise and unwanted artifacts while preserving important features such as edge and boundary required for segmentation. This process is followed by a CMF algorithm to obtain the segmentation. Finally, we use a morphological operation on the resulting image to remove the unwanted region and obtain the final result.

The remainder of the paper is organized as follows. A detailed review of methods used for breast lesion segmentation is discussed in Sect. 2. In Sect. 3, the proposed lesion segmentation method is explained. Section 4 analyses the experimental results and provides a detailed discussion, and a concluding remark is given in the final section.

2   Materials and Methods

2.1   Image Subtraction After Registration

The important and primary step in our algorithm is the subtraction between pre- and post-contrast images [31]. This process makes it easier to characterize lesions by eliminating common background signals [32,33]. The resultant image is obtained with the improved contrast in breast lesion. However, the performance of subtraction depends upon the image pre and post images acquisition. A patient should not move between the whole imaging session, which is not always feasible. These unintended movements create a misalignment of images sequence [34]. Hence, it requires image registration prior to the image subtraction. Image registration is the geometrical transformation of one image to another. The normalized image is obtained from the subtraction of pre-contrast image from the post-contrast image after the registration.

2.2   Local Phase-Preserved Denoising of DCE-MRI

Denoising of DCE-MR images is an important process during lesion segmentation [35]. Denoising is a process in which the image is transformed into some domain such that the noise component is easily identified. The noise is then removed and transformed back into a noise-free image. Among several denoising algorithms, wavelet transformation is considered very efficient to distinguish between the signal and noise in the image. Also, the image is consist of two important information, magnitude and phase. It is seen that the previous denoising mechanism on breast DCE-MR images has not considered this important information, phase i.e. phase information is not preserved [36]. Phase information is important not only for perception but also for image enhancement.

The phase preserved denoising methodology utilizes a log Gabor wavelet filter. The image is initially decomposed into amplitude and phase information at each point of slices in of DCE-MRI. The observation shows that most of the amplitude information is concentrated on the center and the phase information is distributed throughout the image. It is seen that amplitude or phase information alone is not sufficient in reconstructing a noise-free image while preserving important image features. Hence, we design a phase preserved technique for breast DCE-MRI image that shrinks the amplitude information in different scaling factors and orientations.

2.3 CMF Based Lesion Segmentation

Continuous max flow (CMF) [37] method is a graph-based approach and found to be very effective to label important regions in an image.

Let us consider a problem of partitioning continuous image domain Ω to partition for $i = 1..........n$ region or label. There are three concerning flows : $F_s(x), F_i(x)$ and $r_i(x)$ are the source, sink and spatial flow as shown in the Fig. 1. Let x be the image position and each image position $x \in \Omega$. In n label max flow model of Ω_i where $i = 1...n$ are given in parallel.

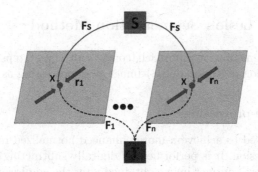

Fig. 1. Continuous max flow with n labels.

At each position $x \in \Omega$, $F_s(x)$ stream from s to x for each label $i = 1.......n$ Hence, the source field is same and there is no constraint for the source flow $F_s(x)$ for n label partition.

$F_i(x)$ and $r_i(x)$ are constrained by the capacities $\rho(L_i, x)$ and $C_i(x)$, $i = 1.....n$.

The flow are conserved as

$$(divr_i - F_s + F_i)(x) = 0, i = 1......n \tag{1}$$

Hence, the max flow problem for the total flow from source to sink for n labels is given by

$$\max_{F_s, F, r} \{P(F_s, F, r) \int_\Omega F_s dx\} \tag{2}$$

Potts model is considered as a powerful tool for image segmentation. The multi region segmentation through potts model can be mathematically expressed as shown in equation

$$\min_{\Omega_{i}{}_{i=1}^{n}} \sum_{i=1}^{n} \int_{\Omega_i} C_i(x)dx + \alpha \sum_{i=1}^{n} |\partial\Omega_i| \tag{3}$$

where $|\partial\Omega_i|$ is the perimeter of each disjoint sub domain Ω_i, $i = 1...n$. $C_i(x)$, $i = 1...n$ is the cost of assigning the specified position $x \in \Omega$ to the region Ω_i. The segmentation problem can be solved using convex relaxation potts model derived from Eq. 3 as shown in Eq. 4

$$\min_{u \in S} \sum_{i=1}^{n} \int_{\Omega} u_i(x)C_i(x)dx + \sum_{i=1}^{n} \int_{\Omega} \omega(x)|\nabla u_i|dx \tag{4}$$

where $u_i(x), i = 1....n$ defines the function of the segmented region Ω_i. S is the convex constrained set of $u(x) = (u_1(x), ...u_n(x))$.

3   Proposed Lesion Segmentation Method

The proposed segmentation approach consists of three steps: 1) Image pre-processing 2) Lesion detection and 3) Image post-processing as shown in Fig. 2.

3.1   Image Pre-processing

This process is used to achieve a more enhanced normalized image to ease the detection of the lesion. It is performed by digitally subtracting the pre-contrast image from the post-contrast image obtained after the admission of the contrast agent. Prior to the image subtraction, image registration should be carried out. Image registration resolves the misalignment of the pre and post contrast image originated due to the unintentional movement during imaging. Furthermore, the image subtraction operation removes native T1 signal and hence the remaining enhancement is effective to accurately detect the lesion. This process is seen competent to the image where enhancement is critical to detect the complicated cysts. The figure illustrates the effectiveness of image subtraction. Figure 3 (a) (d) are the pre-contrast, (b), (e) are the post-contrast and (c), (f) are the resultant image after the image subtraction respectively.

3.2   Lesion Segmentation

DCE-MRI contains noise due to the fluctuations in the receiver coil and from the electrically conducting tissue. The presence of noise in the DCE-MRI image increases the complexity and leads towards the misinterpretation. It is necessary to remove this noise, minimize the new artifacts and preserve kinetic

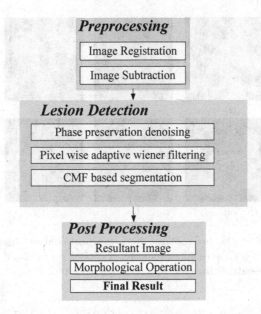

Fig. 2. The proposed functional diagram of retinal vessel segmentation.

enhancement information and fine structural details. Therefore following the pre-processing step, the phase preserved denoising method is applied. Also, it is essential to smoothen the image while sharpening the edges during the lesion segmentation. Hence, after phase preserved denoising, we apply an adaptive Wiener filtering technique.

The process of denoising begins with the construction of Gabor features using wavelet filters. The slices of DCE-MRI is then involved with the constructed Gabor features. AS a result feature vector response will be generated. Hence, the final denoised image is obtained by summing responses over all scales and orientations. Figure 4 show the image with or without using phase preserved denoising and bilateral filtering. The image is denoised to some extent however, smoothing is required before the application of CMF to achieve the accurate segmentation. At this point, smoothing is required while preserving edges as well as the boundary. Edges and boundaries are the high-frequency areas and bilateral filtering is efficient to remove noise in these areas. Hence, we applied bilateral filtering to preserve edges and boundaries while smoothing the images.

The continuous max-flow algorithm is performed on the denoised MRI image obtained from the phase preserved denoising. Initially, each pixel of each slice in the DCE-MRI is connected to the source S and sink T in the continuous plane. Also, we consider that each pixel is associated with three flows: source, sink and spatial flow. The source flow is directed from source S towards sink T. The spatial flow is determined by the strength of interaction with its neighborhood pixels. For a noisy image with low SNR, the capacity values of all the pixels would confine solutions within local minimal thus failing to determine the global

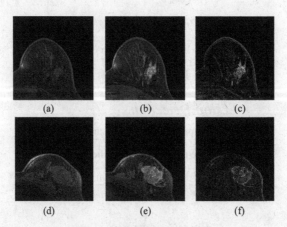

Fig. 3. Subtraction of the pre-contrast from the post-contrast image. (a), (d) Pre-contrast image. (b), (e) Post-contrast image. (c), (f) The resultant image after subtraction of the pre-contrast image from post-contrast image

optimum. Hence, prior to the application of CMF method, the phase preserved denoise is used that clears the noise of the image and preserve the important features of image. Additionally, the use of bilateral filtering on the phase preserved image will smoothen the image while preserving edges.

3.3   Image Post-processing

Based on the observed result from the earlier section, post-processing of the image are required. Morphological erosion and dilation operation are used to remove the boundary of edges. Secondly, the nearby components are connected together and the biggest area among the connected component are searched and preserved. Rest of the areas are considered as noise and removed. The obtained segmented image are compared with manually drawn available ground truth image from the expert. Figure 5, show resultant images obtained after the post-processing. It is observed that post-processing plays a vital role to further precisely segment lesions.

4   Performance Evaluation and Results

4.1   Data Acquisition and Evaluation Criteria

The experiment is conducted on Windows 10 (x64), with Intel Core i5 CPU, 2.9 GHZ and 8 GB RAM. We validate the proposed algorithm on the image generated from 1.5T scanner. The imaging parameters for DCE-MRI were: TR/TE = 4.5/1.8 ms, a matrix size = 512×512, with the number of signal averages set to 1, a field of view of 30 cm, and a slice thickness of 1.5 mm. The gray-level range of MRIs is 0–255. There are total 23 cases in which 19 cases with the size

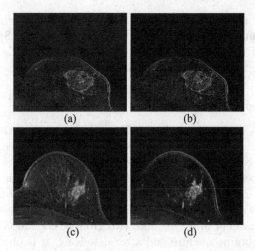

Fig. 4. Illustration of resultant images obtained with and without phase-preserved denoising and bilateral filtering. (a) and (c) are the resultant image after the subtraction of the pre-contrast from the post-contrast image without using phase-preserved denoising and bilateral filtering. (b) and (d) are the resultant image after the subtraction of the pre-contrast from the post-contrast image using phase-preserved denoising and bilateral filtering

of $512 \times 512 \times 96$ and 4 cases with the size of $480 \times 480 \times 160$. All cases have one pre-contrast and 4 post-contrast imaging frames were acquired. Ground truth images are available for all the cases which is manually labeled by qualified doctors. The result for the lesion segmentation is acquired from 2464 scans of 23 cases. For the experiment, we have divided the images into two groups: G1 and G2. G1 includes images with resolution of $512 \times 512 \times 96$ and G2 with resolution of $480 \times 480 \times 160$.

Initially, the performance of a denoised image before and after phase preserved denoising is demonstrated by calculating the peak signal-to-noise ratios (PSNR). Furthermore, the quantitative assessment of the proposed algorithm is tested with nine metrices: accuracy (Acc), sensitivity (Se) or Recall and Specificity (Sp). These parameters are based on pixel-based classification technique where each pixel on the slice of DCE-MRI is classified as lesion or background. In the pixel-based classification technique, there are four combinations: two classifications and two mis-classifications. Under classification, true positive (TP) and true negative (TN) refers to the pixels which are correctly identified. Misclassification refers to the false positive (FP) and false negative (FN) which are incorrectly identified as a lesion. SG signify the segmentation's obtained from the proposed methods and "GT" signify the ground truth which is manually segmented. These metrics are defined as the following equations.

$$\text{Acc} = \frac{\text{TP+TN}}{\text{TP+FP+TN+FN}}, \text{Se} = \frac{\text{TP}}{\text{TP+FN}}, \text{Sp} = \frac{\text{TN}}{\text{TN+FP}}$$

Acc is defined as the total number of classified pixels which are correctly identified to the number of total pixels in an image. Se and Sp are the metrics which are derived from the proportion of positive and negative pixels in the ground truth image that is truly identified.

4.2 Results and Discussion

The original DCE-MRI image is noisy. The segmentation of the lesion from the noisy image degrades the performance of the algorithm. Hence, phase preserved denoising is used to remove the unwanted noise and artifacts from the image. The image enhancement can be observed visually as shown in Fig. 4 and is also tested by calculating the PSNR value before and after denoising as shown in Table 1. Since the data set consist of an image with two resolution, we have divided the total number of images into two groups (G1 and G2) and calculated the PSNR value obtained before and after denoising. It is observed that PSNR value in both the group has a significant improvement as shown in Table 1.

The obtained segmentation results can be observed visually. Figure 5 show that the post-processing step is able to remove most of the unwanted areas from the obtained resultant images. The method while compared with the ground-truth image, show that the proposed method is able to efficiently segment the lesion as depicted in Fig. 6. Figure 6 (a, d and g) are the manually segmented ground truth image by an expert radiologist. Figure 6 (b, e, and h) are the final result obtained from the proposed method. Figure 6 (c, f and i) shows that the overlap between the lesion area in the original image and the result obtained from the proposed method. The result shows that the proposed method is able to segment the lesion area accurately, which is further validated by the quantitative analysis as shown in Table 2. In this paper, we have used nine parameters to analyze the effectiveness of the proposed work.

The experiments show that the results obtained from the proposed methods when compared with the results obtained from the recent methods outperform or highly comparable as shown in Table 3. It is observed that Acc, Se and Sp obtained from the proposed method are above 90%, proving the effectiveness of the proposed algorithm. When comparing with the result obtained from the recently proposed method, Accuracy was observed to be better than all of the other methods except Marrone et al. 2013. However, the result is highly comparable.

Segmentation of lesion from breast DCE-MR image is a significant and challenging job. To achieve the level of accuracy as mentioned before we went through several experiments and finally came across the presented solution. The lesion can be found in various shapes and intensity in different slices of DCE-MRI. Moreover, DCE-MRI images are populated with noises during image acquisition because of untended movement of the object. To overcome this problem, we concluded that image registration is required as the initial step. Furthermore, it is observed that the segmentation process is further complicated by geometric distortion and non-uniform illumination in the tissues. Hence, to preserve most of the useful information of the image while removing the noise, we utilized the

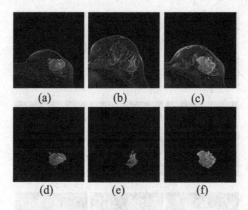

Fig. 5. Illustration of resultant lesion segmentation obtained by using the proposed method after post-processing. First row (a, b, c) represents the original image and second row (d, e, f) represents the final result i.e. segmented lesions.

Table 1. Comparison of PSNR values before and after the phase preserved denoising.

Dataset	Average PSNR	
	Subtracted image	After denoising
G1	21.36 ± 0.7	32.54 ± 0.42
G2	20.82 ± 0.21	34.19 ± 0.53

Table 2. Quantitative comparison of performance of lesion segmentation using the proposed method with the ground-truth image.

	Acc	Se	Sp
Cases(G1)			
1	0.9933	0.9081	0.9968
2	0.9921	0.9152	0.9841
3	0.9789	0.9231	0.9799
-	-	-	-
-	-	-	-
-	-	-	-
15	0.9898	0.909	0.9798
16	0.9632	0.8821	0.9712
17	0.9787	0.8928	0.9912
18	0.9963	0.9181	0.9963
19	0.9879	0.9099	0.9874
Avg	**0.9845**	**0.9076**	**0.9877**

	Acc	Se	Sp
Cases(G2)			
1	0.9674	0.9191	0.9926
2	0.9874	0.9221	0.9874
3	0.9742	0.8989	0.9858
4	0.9931	0.9182	0.9745
Avg	**0.9805**	**0.9145**	**0.9850**

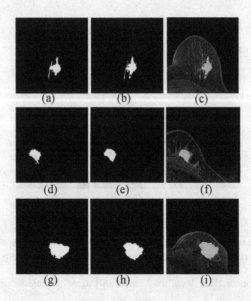

Fig. 6. Results of lesion segmentation on the MRI images with different levels of BD and different breast shapes. The images in the first column are the manually segmented ground truth images. Similarly, second and third columns are the automatically segmented results with the proposed method and its mask on the original image to visually inspect the accuracy.

Table 3. Quantitative comparison of performance of lesion segmentation using the proposed method with the recently developed other approaches.

	Acc	Sp	Se
Conte et al. 2020	x	x	0.75
Vogl et al. 2019	x	0.93	0.94
Li et al. 2018	x	x	0.88
Rasti et al. 2017	0.9639	0.9487	0.9773
Jayender et al. 2014	0.9	x	x
Marrone et al. 2013	0.98	0.989	0.71
Proposed method (G1)	**0.9845**	**0.9873**	**0.9076**
Proposed method (G2)	**0.9805**	**0.985**	**0.9145**

phase preserved denoising algorithm in the registered image followed by pixelwise adaptive Wiener filtering to preserve the sharp edges. Thereafter, we use the graph-based approach i.e. CMF to label the important region of the image. This method is found to be effective to solve the segmentation problem while allocating the minimum parameter. Hence, reducing the iteration time to obtain a faster segmentation.

5   Conclusions

In this paper, we proposed an automatic and fast lesion segmentation method from breast DCE-MRI images. The produced accurate lesion segmentation uses image registration before image subtraction as a pre-processing step. Furthermore, a phase preserved denoising and adaptive Wiener filtering followed by CMF technique (which is a graph-based approach) is applied in the pre-processed image. Finally, post-processing is carried out to remove the unwanted remaining noises except for the lesion. This framework has been tested with 23 different DCE-MRI cases with resolutions. The quantitative analysis, in terms of three metrics, shows significant improvement in segmentation quality compared to recent segmentation techniques. Furthermore, the proposed unsupervised method does not require any prior knowledge and can work with most medical images with a slight modification of the parameters.

References

1. Akram, M., Iqbal, M., Daniyal, M., Khan, A.U.: Awareness and current knowledge of breast cancer. Biol. Res. **50**(1), 33 (2017)
2. Welch, H.G., Prorok, P.C., O'Malley, A.J., Kramer, B.S.: Breast-cancer tumor size, overdiagnosis, and mammography screening effectiveness. N. Engl. J. Med. **375**(15), 1438–1447 (2016)
3. Abdel-Nasser, M., Melendez, J., Moreno, A., Omer, O.A., Puig, D.: Breast tumor classification in ultrasound images using texture analysis and super-resolution methods. Eng. Appl. Artif. Intell. **59**, 84–92 (2017)
4. Cheng, J.Z., et al.: Computer-aided diagnosis with deep learning architecture: applications to breast lesions in US images and pulmonary nodules in CT scans. Sci. Rep. **6**, 24454 (2016)
5. Zhang, J., Saha, A., Zhu, Z., Mazurowski, M.A.: Hierarchical convolutional neural networks for segmentation of breast tumors in MRI with application to radiogenomics. IEEE Trans. Med. Imaging **38**(2), 435–447 (2019)
6. Wan, T., Cao, J., Chen, J., Qin, Z.: Automated grading of breast cancer histopathology using cascaded ensemble with combination of multi-level image features. Neurocomputing **229**, 34–44 (2017)
7. Pandey, D., Yin, X., Wang, H., Su, M.Y., Chen, J.H., Wu, J., et al.: Automatic and fast segmentation of breast region-of-interest (ROI) and density in MRIs. Heliyon. **4**(12), e01042 (2018)
8. Bhattacharjee, R., et al.: Comparison of 2D and 3D U-net breast lesion segmentations on DCE-MRI, p. 10 (2021)
9. Khalil, F., Wang, H., Li, J.: Integrating Markov model with clustering for predicting web page accesses, pp. 63–74 (2007)
10. Hu, H., Li, J., Wang, H., Daggard, G.: Combined gene selection methods for microarray data analysis. In: Gabrys, B., Howlett, R.J., Jain, L.C. (eds.) KES 2006. LNCS (LNAI), vol. 4251, pp. 976–983. Springer, Heidelberg (2006). https://doi.org/10.1007/11892960_117
11. Li, H., Wang, Y., Wang, H., Zhou, B.: Multi-window based ensemble learning for classification of imbalanced streaming data. World Wide Web **20**(6), 1507–1525 (2017). https://doi.org/10.1007/s11280-017-0449-x

12. Khalil, F., Li, J., Wang, H.: An integrated model for next page access prediction. Int. J. Knowl. Web Intell. **1**, 48–80 (2009). https://doi.org/10.1504/IJKWI.2009.027925

13. Sarki, R., Ahmed, K., Wang, H., Zhang, Y., Ma, J., Wang, K.: Image preprocessing in classification and identification of diabetic eye diseases. Data Sci. Eng. (6), 1–17 (2021). https://doi.org/10.1007/s41019-021-00167-z

14. Bzdok, D., Krzywinski, M., Altman, N.: Points of significance: machine learning: supervised methods (2018)

15. Du, S., Zhang, F., Zhang, X.: Semantic classification of urban buildings combining VHR image and GIS data: an improved random forest approach. ISPRS J. Photogramm. Remote Sens. **105**, 107–119 (2015)

16. Fabelo, H., et al.: SVM optimization for brain tumor identification using infrared spectroscopic samples. Sensors **18**(12), 4487 (2018)

17. Kendall, A., Gal, Y.: What uncertainties do we need in Bayesian deep learning for computer vision? In: Advances in Neural Information Processing Systems, pp. 5574–5584 (2017)

18. Conte, L., Tafuri, B., Portaluri, M., Galiano, A., Maggiulli, E., De Nunzio, G.: Breast cancer mass detection in DCE-MRI using deep-learning features followed by discrimination of infiltrative vs. in situ carcinoma through a machine-learning approach. Appl. Sci. **10**(17), 6109 (2020)

19. Sarki, R., Ahmed, K., Wang, H., Zhang, Y.: Automated detection of mild and multi-class diabetic eye diseases using deep learning. Health Inf. Sci. Syst. **8**(1), 1–9 (2020). https://doi.org/10.1007/s13755-020-00125-5

20. Du, J., Michalska, S., Subramani, S., Wang, H., Zhang, Y.: Neural attention with character embeddings for hay fever detection from twitter. Health Inf. Sci. Syst. **7**(1), 1–7 (2019). https://doi.org/10.1007/s13755-019-0084-2

21. He, J., Rong, J., Sun, L., Wang, H., Zhang, Y., Ma, J.: A framework for cardiac arrhythmia detection from IoT-based ECGs. World Wide Web **23**(5), 2835–2850 (2020). https://doi.org/10.1007/s11280-019-00776-9

22. Wang, K., et al.: Use of falls risk increasing drugs in residents at high and low falls risk in aged care services. J. Appl. Gerontol. **40**, 073346481988884 (2019). https://doi.org/10.1177/0733464819888848

23. Wang, K., Bell, J., Tan, E., Gilmartin-Thomas, J., Dooley, M., Ilomaki, J.: Statin use and fall-related hospitalizations among residents of long-term care facilities: a case-control study. J. Clin. Lipidol. **14**. (2020). https://doi.org/10.1016/j.jacl.2020.05.008

24. Aganj, I., Harisinghani, M.G., Weissleder, R., Fischl, B.: Unsupervised medical image segmentation based on the local center of mass. Sci. Rep. **8**(1), 13012 (2018)

25. Ayaz, M., Shaukat, F., Raja, G.: Ensemble learning based automatic detection of tuberculosis in chest x-ray images using hybrid feature descriptors. Phys. Eng. Sci. Med. **44**(1), 183–194 (2021). https://doi.org/10.1007/s13246-020-00966-0

26. Wadhwa, A., Bhardwaj, A., Verma, V.S.: A review on brain tumor segmentation of MRI images. Magn. Reson. Imaging **61**, 247–259 (2019)

27. Siuly, S., Khare, S., Bajaj, V., Wang, H., Zhang, Y.: A computerized method for automatic detection of schizophrenia using EEG signals. IEEE Trans. Neural Syst. Rehabil. Eng. **1**, 1 (2020)

28. Yuan, J., Bae, E., Tai, X.C.A.: Study on continuous max-flow and min-cut approaches. In: IEEE Computer Society Conference on Computer Vision and Pattern Recognition, pp. 2217–2224. IEEE (2010)

29. Jiang, H., Zhou, R., Zhang, L., Wang, H., Zhang, Y.: Sentence level topic models for associated topics extraction. World Wide Web **22**(6), 2545–2560 (2018). https://doi.org/10.1007/s11280-018-0639-1

30. Supriya, S., Siuly, S., Wang, H., Zhang, Y.: Automated epilepsy detection techniques from electroencephalogram signals: a review study. Health Inf. Sci. Syst. **8**(1), 1–15 (2020). https://doi.org/10.1007/s13755-020-00129-1

31. Villringer, K., et al.: Subtracted dynamic MR perfusion source images (sMRP-SI) provide collateral blood flow assessment in MCA occlusions and predict tissue fate. Eur. Radiol. **26**(5), 1396–1403 (2016)

32. Hu, H., Li, J., Wang, H., Daggard, G.E., Shi, M.: A maximally diversified multiple decision tree algorithm for microarray data classification. Intell. Syst. Bioinform. **73**, 35–38 (2006)

33. Khalil, F., Li, J., Wang, H.: Integrating Markov model with clustering for predicting web page accesses. In: AusWeb 2007: 13th Australasian World Wide Web Conference (2007)

34. Brock, K.K., Mutic, S., McNutt, T.R., Li, H., Kessler, M.L.: Use of image registration and fusion algorithms and techniques in radiotherapy: report of the AAPM radiation therapy committee task group no. 132. Med. Phys. **44**(7), e43–e76 (2017)

35. Vaishali, S., Rao, K.K., Rao, G.S.: A review on noise reduction methods for brain MRI images. In: 2015 International Conference on Signal Processing and Communication Engineering Systems, pp. 363–365. IEEE (2015)

36. Pandey, D., Yin, X., Wang, H., Zhang, Y.: Accurate vessel segmentation using maximum entropy incorporating line detection and phase-preserving denoising. Comput. Vis. Image Underst. **155**, 162–172 (2017)

37. Hou, G., Pan, H., Zhao, R., Hao, Z., Liu, W., et al.: Image segmentation via the continuous max-flow method based on Chan-Vese model. In: Wang, Y. (ed.) IGTA 2017. CCIS, vol. 757, pp. 232–242. Springer, Singapore (2018). https://doi.org/10.1007/978-981-10-7389-2_23

Medical Record Mining (I)

Research on Suicide Identification Method Based on Microblog "Tree Hole" Crowd

Xiaomin Jing[1], Shaofu Lin[1(✉)], and Zhisheng Huang[2,3]

[1] Faculty of Information Technology, Beijing University of Technology, Beijing 100124, China
linshaofu@bjut.edu.cn
[2] Department of Computer Science, Vrije University Amsterdam, Amsterdam, The Netherlands
[3] Advanced Innovation Center for Human Brain Protection, Capital Medical University, Beijing, China

Abstract. Suicide has always been a key issue of social and health organizations and research of scholars. In recent years, with the increasing popularity of Internet and social media, more and more people record their lives and feelings in social media, even more, they publish suicide speeches, especially in the youth. The microblog "tree hole" is generated because a depressed patient has left, a large number of potential depression patients or suicide prone people to leave messages under her account until today, including venting negative emotions, suicide messages and even committing suicide together. In view of this situation, the paper analyzes the actual needs and business scenarios of monitoring and identifying online depression suicide messages. Based on the data of "tree hole" message on microblog, this paper designs and implements a multi-channel convolutional neural network social suicide warning model. By mining the time of message of "tree hole" people in microblog, the feature matrix is obtained after quantifying some knowledge elements; After word orientation quantization, word vector matrix and word vector matrix are obtained. Feature matrix and text vector matrix are used as three inputs of convolutional neural network respectively to identify and warn social suicide. The model is proved to be better by experiments and improve the accuracy of early warning.

Keywords: Suicide · Microblog tree hole · Temporal characteristics · Suicide identification · Monitoring and rescue

1 Introduction

Around the world, nearly one million people commit suicide every year [1]. Studies have shown that most suicides have mental diseases, in which depression occupies the main position [2]. In the study of suicidal tendency, most scholars focus on the reasons behind the suicidal tendency and suicide intervention. Ding Ling et al. Studied and analyzed the causes of suicide in patients with depression and related intervention measures and effects [3]; In literature [4], EAP-BiLSTM-CRF method combining conditional random field with bi-directional long-short term memory network was used to identify the suicide causes of suicide prone people in social media.

Although the research on depression and suicidal tendency has been relatively mature, most of them are based on the research and analysis of offline specific groups, and there are few researches on specific users in social media. In order to make up for the lack of this research direction, this paper studies the user message data of online microblog "tree hole", Using artificial intelligence and deep learning method to build algorithm model to mine potential suicidal tendency.

2 Related Work

With the more and more serious phenomenon of suicide, scholars pay more and more attention to the research of suicide warning and intervention. Through literature analysis, the research of suicide intervention can be summarized as the research and analysis of suicide for different groups, and then the specific intervention program and the construction of intervention system can be studied. For example, Pickering Trevor A and others investigated and analyzed the spread of suicidal behavior in 20 schools, and came to the conclusion that network volunteers of the same age as students in school can be cultivated for benign guidance and intervention, which can effectively reduce the spread of suicidal behavior in schools [5]; Literature [6] introduces the suicide intervention of cancer inpatients in a cancer hospital by setting up psychological nurses and establishing suicide prevention workflow.

Suicide early warning is also mostly focused on different warning mechanisms for different groups and different ways to identify and early warn suicide tendency. For example, Lv Juncheng used multiple logistic regression model to screen the suicide factors and then established BP neural network to predict the suicide of rural residents in Shandong Province [7]; Zhang Xuan et al. Discussed and studied the risk factors of suicide, and used the support vector machine algorithm to build a suicide early warning model, which was used for the suicide early warning of people with depression [8].

In this paper, artificial intelligence is used for suicide early warning. The commonly used algorithm models include CNN, LSTM, naive Bayes, random forest and so on. For example, in reference [9], we use the above algorithms to build suicide recognition models for microblog data and compare the results. The results show that the recognition accuracy of multilayer neural network is higher; For another example, Zhang Xuan et al. [10] used a hybrid neural network (NC BiLSTM) combining multi-channel CNN and bidirectional long-term and short-term memory network to identify and early warn the suicide of microblog text, which can better extract the feature words in the text and effectively improve the accuracy of judgment.

At present, there are few researches on suicide warning for online depressed people. Most of the researches on suicide warning focus on offline research data or online social media data, and less on specific online people. At present, the accuracy of suicide warning has not achieved good results. Therefore, a suicide warning model based on knowledge mapping and deep learning is proposed to meet the practical needs of online suicidal tendency mining.

3 Research Contents

In this paper, we study the message time of "tree hole" crowd on microblog and mine the behavior pattern of "tree hole" crowd around time, and use the results of its time feature distribution to support the feature selection of suicide warning model; Combining the characteristics of message time distribution with emotion and suicide tendency, this paper selects the relevant learning and training characteristics of suicide early warning model, and uses multi-channel convolution neural network to identify and early warn suicide tendency.

3.1 Text Vectorization

After studying the characteristics of depression suicide related information and microblog "tree hole" message, this paper will select features from two aspects: the first aspect is the semantic information of microblog "tree hole" message itself, that is, the semantic information of complete message sentence; The second aspect is based on the relevant characteristics of the message information, including the time and length of the message, whether the message contains emotional words and suicidal words.

The first one is vectorization of extended features, that is, vectorization of extended features including message time, message text length, whether there are emotional words and suicide tendency words (emotional words and suicide tendency words are selected by dictionary matching). The rule is: the message time is 1 from 8:00 p.m. to 8:00 a.m. (The study found that suicides were more active during this period), otherwise it is 0; The length of the message is the number of words; The value of negative emotion words is 1, otherwise it is 0; The value of suicide intention words or suicide behavior words is 1, otherwise it is 0.

In this paper, the extended feature is adopted one_ hot. The relevant formula is as follows:

$$u_{time} = \begin{cases} (1, 0), t = [20 : 00, 8 : 00) \\ (0, 1), t = [8 : 00, 20 : 00) \end{cases} \tag{1}$$

$$u_{sui} = \begin{cases} (1, 0), \text{Words with suicide intention} \\ (0, 1), \text{Words without suicide intention} \end{cases} \tag{2}$$

$$u_{sb} = \begin{cases} (1, 0), \text{Words with suicidal behavior} \\ (0, 1), \text{Words without suicidal behavior} \end{cases} \tag{3}$$

$$u_{ew} = \begin{cases} (1, 0), \text{Words with negative emotion} \\ (0, 1), \text{Words with positive emotion} \end{cases} \tag{4}$$

Finally, all the above extended features are spliced to get the microblog "tree hole" extended feature set.

The second is to use word2vec tool to quantify the word orientation of "tree hole" text. In this experiment, the skip gram models of word2vec are selected for training. The parameter settings are shown in Table 1.

Table 1. Parameter setting

Parameter	Value
Sentence	Microblog "tree hole" message text corpus
Size	300
sg	1
Window	4

3.2 Model Building

In this paper, we build a multi-channel fine-grained convolutional neural network (N-CNN) to build a suicide warning model based on the "tree hole" message text of microblog. The fine-grained word vector, word vector and the extended features selected according to the "tree hole" text analysis are used as the input of the model. The model can capture the semantic information between sentences based on the word vector, based on the word vector to extract deeper and more fine-grained information of the text statement, at the same time, the extended features can supplement the features of suicide recognition outside the text statement information, which is more accurate and effective for suicide recognition and early warning. Its structure is shown in Fig. 1.

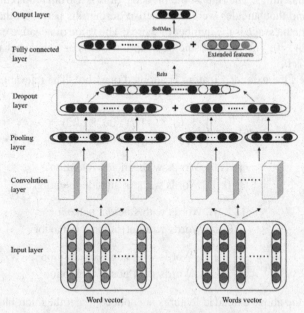

Fig. 1. The model structure diagram

The input layer is to train the word vector and word vector of the microblog "tree hole" message text, and vectorize the extended features in the knowledge map to obtain the vector matrix respectively, which is used as the input of three channels of the suicide warning model.

The convolution layer mainly uses the feature extractor (convolution kernel) to extract local features, and uses the window sliding (convolution operation) convolution operation to enhance the original text features and reduce the noise. The calculation formula is as follows:

$$C_{hi} = f(W_h X_{i:i+h-1} + b) \tag{5}$$

Among them, C_{hi} is the output of convolution layer, h is the size of convolution kernel, W_h is the weight matrix, b is its bias term, and f is its nonlinear activation function. Here, the relu function is used. The convolution calculation process is shown in Fig. 2.

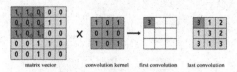

Fig. 2. Convolution process

The pooling layer compresses and reduces the dimension of the message text feature matrix after convolution operation and makes secondary screening to reduce over fitting. In this model, the maximum pooling function is used, that is, the maximum number of the region is taken as the value of the output matrix. The pooling process is shown in Fig. 3, in which 2 × 2 windows is used.

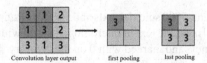

Fig. 3. Pooling process

In the full join layer, the feature matrix extracted from the word vector matrix after convolution pooling, the feature matrix extracted from the word vector after convolution pooling and the extended feature matrix are spliced, and then the classification is performed by softmax function.

4 Experimental Design and Research Results

4.1 Experimental Design

The main structure of suicide early warning model in this paper is shown in Fig. 4, and the experimental process is mainly as follows: text vectorization, model building and parameter setting, model experimental testing. The specific experimental steps are as follows.

Firstly, the text is annotated. With the help of jieba word segmentation tool, the "tree hole" message data is segmented and stop words such as modal particles and connectives are removed. Word2vec is used to train the word vector and generate the word vector matrix, which is used as an input of the multi-channel convolution network model; Secondly, the text is processed into a single word, and the word vector is trained by word2vec to generate the word vector matrix, which is used as another input of the multi-channel convolution network; Thirdly, the extended features beyond the text semantics are vectorized to generate the extended eigenvector matrix as the third input of the multi-channel convolution network. The difference from the first two inputs is that this eigenvector matrix is directly input to the full connection layer of the model to splice with the other two eigenmatrices without convolution and pooling operations; Finally, the model is used for training and the results are analyzed.

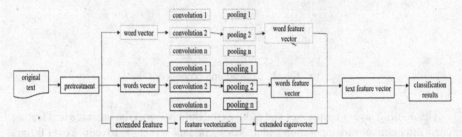

Fig.4. Model architecture

(1) Text Vectorization

In this experiment, 5000 suicidal texts and 5000 non-suicidal texts were selected from the "tree hole" message text of microblog, marked with 0 and 1, marked with 1 with suicidal tendency, and marked with 0 on the contrary. The training set and test set were divided according to the ratio of 8:2, and word2vec was used to quantify word orientation and word orientation, and the extended features were analyzed, Extended feature vectorization is performed.

(2) Model parameter setting

In this paper, the multi-channel convolutional neural network suicide warning model N-CNN is built by tensorflow framework, and the core of the algorithm is CNN. The adaptive momentum estimation method Adam is used to optimize the model, and the learning rate is set to 0.001. The specific parameter settings are shown in Table 2.

4.2   Results Comparison and Analysis

In this chapter, in order to make the effectiveness of the model more convincing, in the case of the same data set, the experimental effect of different models is compared. The model evaluation index still adopts the accuracy P, recall R, F1 value F. The comparison

Table 2. Parameter setting

Parameter	Value
Number of convolution kernels	150
Convolution kernel size	(3, 4, 5)
Number of windows	128
Words vector dimension	256
Word vector dimension	256
Pooling	Max
Dropout	0.7

results are shown in Table 3. At the same time, in order to make the comparison more intuitive, it is designed as a histogram, as shown in Fig. 5.

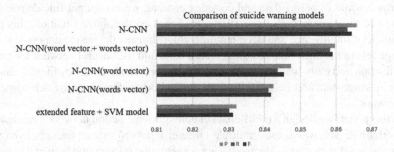

Fig. 5. Model effect comparison chart

Table 3. Model experiment results

Model	P	R	F
Extended feature + SVM model	0.8321	0.8301	0.8311
CNN (words vector)	0.8425	0.8411	0.8418
CNN (word vector)	0.8473	0.8436	0.8454
CNN (word vector + words vector)	0.8597	0.8583	0.8590
N-CNN	0.8657	0.8631	0.8643

It can be seen from Table 3 and Fig. 5 that the multi-channel neural network model used in this paper has good effect on suicide recognition and early warning and can improve the accuracy of recognition and early warning. The accuracy of the N-CNN model used in this paper is higher than that of CNN (word vector + words vector) model, CNN (word vector) model, CNN (words vector) model and extended feature + SVM model. The differences are 0.006, 0.0184, 0.0232 and 0.0336. The experimental results show that the proposed suicide early warning model is better than other commonly used models and can effectively improve the accuracy of suicide recognition.

Through the analysis, it can be concluded that: the fine-grained word vectorization processing of microblog "tree hole" message data is more suitable for mining deep semantic information of message data than word vectorization processing, and the combination of the two can extract more comprehensive and detailed text semantic features. At the same time, the extended features extracted based on knowledge map query analysis are better for suicide recognition and early warning. It can make up for the lack of semantic mining information.

5   Conclusion

At present, the problem of depressive suicide is more and more serious, especially the number of teenagers who die of depressive suicide is increasing year by year; There are more and more suicide messages and suicide users in online social platforms. But at present, there is no mature and perfect rescue intervention mechanism, and because of the large amount of online data and complex content, we cannot get suicide messages in time and take rescue measures. Therefore, based on the above situation, this paper uses artificial intelligence and deep learning algorithms as the basic support, takes the message text in the "tree hole" as the research data, and uses neural network for suicide identification and early warning, so as to promote the suicide tendency identification of online message data and enhance the online monitoring, Speed up the deployment of rescue work.

In this paper, we design a multi-channel convolutional neural network suicide warning model N-CNN, which uses multiple channel inputs to extract features from word vector and word vector, and effectively capture semantic information between sentences and deeper and more fine-grained information of text sentences. Based on the message text time feature distribution extraction and microblog "tree hole" crowd analysis, get the feature relationship of the message text association. At the same time, the semantic features extracted by convolutional neural network CNN and the extended features are combined to form a whole feature to participate in the model training and experiment, and the suicide warning calculation is carried out together. Experiments show that this model has better performance in suicide warning task.

References

1. Palay, J., Taillieu, T.L., Afifi, T.O., et al.: Prevalence of mental disorders and suicidality in Canadian Provinces. Can. J. Psychiatry **64**(11), 761–769 (2019)
2. Dong, X.Q., Chang, E.S., Zeng, P., et al.: Suicide in the global Chinese aging population: a review of risk and protective factors, consequences, and interventions. Aging Dis. **6**(2), 121–130 (2015)
3. Ding, L., Zhang, H., Ye, N., et al.: Analysis of suicide causes of depression patients with suicidal tendency and preventive effect of standardized nursing. China Pract. Med. **14**(10), 138–140 (2019). (in Chinese)
4. Liu, R.: Research on identifying the cause of suicidal tendency for microblog texts. Jiangxi University of Finance and Economics (2020). (in Chinese)

5. Pickering, T.A., Wyman, P.A., Schmeelk-Cone, K., et al.: Diffusion of a peer-led suicide preventive intervention through school-based student peer and adult networks. Front. Psychiatry **9**, 598 (2018)
6. Zhou, Z., Qin, H., Huang, W., et al.: Suicide prevention intervention of cancer inpatients led by full-time psychological nurses in cancer hospital. J. Nurs. **20**(17), 69–71 (2013). (In Chinese)
7. Lv, J.: Construction of BP neural network and index system for suicide attempt early warning of rural residents in Shandong Province. Shandong University (2015). (in Chinese)
8. Zhang, X., Sun, J., et al.: Prediction of suicide risk in depressive disorder population based on support vector machine. J. Hangzhou Normal Univ. (Nat. Sci. Ed.) **18**(02), 219–224 (2019). (In Chinese)
9. Tian, W., Zhu, T.: Suicide risk prediction of microblog users based on deep learning. J. Univ. Chin. Acad. Sci. **35**(1), 131–136 (2018)
10. Zhang, X., Zhao, B., et al.: Suicide risk identification model for microblog texts. Comput. Syst. Appl. **29**(11), 121–127 (2020). (in Chinese)

Strengthen Immune System Based on Genetic Testing and Physical Examination Data

Jitao Yang[✉]

School of Information Science, Beijing Language and Culture University,
Beijing 100083, China
yangjitao@blcu.edu.cn

Abstract. Immune system is the human body's most important defense against pathogenic bacteria attacks so as to avoid diseases. Immunity has the functions of physiological defense, self stability and immune monitoring, if these functions were changed, it will lead to various diseases. Many gene variants have been found to be associated with human immune system, for instance, the polymorphism of the loci in the *AGFG1* gene can affect a person's susceptibility to influenza A viruses, therefore, to strengthen immune system, genetic factors should be considered to evaluate immune capacity. Some physical examination indicators are also connected with immune capacity, for example, if serum 25 (OH)D level is low, this means vitamin D is insufficient, which will lead to the development of respiratory infections and multiple autoimmune diseases, therefore the physical examination data should also be involved in the evaluation model of immune capacity. Nutrition is the material basis to support the normal function of the immune system, for instance vitamin A and zinc can enhance anti-infection ability, therefore, the diet data need to be integrated into the immunity evaluation model. In this paper, we combine the genetic testing data, physical examination data, diet assessment data together to establish an immune capacity evaluation model as well as a personalized nutrition data model to provide personalized nutrition service for strengthening immune system.

Keywords: Immune system · Genetic testing · Physical examination · Personalized nutrition.

1 Introduction

The body has an immune system, which is the human body's most important defense against pathogenic bacteria attacks, and is the body's ability to be free from disease. Immunity is the human body's physiological function to identify self and non-self components, thereby destroying and rejecting the antigens, the damaged cells, the tumor cells, and etc. [1].

© Springer Nature Switzerland AG 2021
S. Siuly et al. (Eds.): HIS 2021, LNCS 13079, pp. 150–159, 2021.
https://doi.org/10.1007/978-3-030-90885-0_14

Immune system includes immune organs (bone marrow, thymus, spleen, lymph node, tonsil, small intestine collecting lymph node, appendix, thymus, and etc.), immune cells (lymphocytes, phagocytes, neutrophils, basophils, eosinophils, mast cells, and etc.), and immune molecules (immunoglobulin, interferon, interleukin, tumor necrosis factor, and etc.).

The immune system [2,3] is divided into:

- Non-specific (innate) immunity. Human skin and mucous membrane constitute the first line of defense, preventing and killing pathogens and cleaning up foreign bodies; bactericides and phagocytes in body fluids form the second line of defense dissolving, swallowing and eliminating bacteria.
- Specific (adaptive) immunity, which is further divided into humoral immunity and cellular immunity. The humoral immunity is targeting extracellular pathogens and toxins; the cellular immunity is targeting intracellular antigens and toxins, as well as cancerous cells.

Immunity has the functions of physiological defense, self stability, and immune monitoring, if these functions were changed, it will lead to various diseases:

- the physiological defense function, protects the body from damage, helps the body eliminate foreign bacteria and viruses, so as to avoid diseases;
- the self stability function, eliminates the aging and dead cells constantly to keep the purification and renewal of the body; and
- the immune monitoring function, identifies and eliminates the chromosomal aberration or gene mutation cells timely to prevent the occurrence of cancer.

Efficient immune response can defense against infections and diseases, too little or wrong immune response will cause diseases, overactive immune response can lead to the happening of autoimmune diseases [4,5].

2 Nutrition and Immunity

Nutrition is the material basis to support the normal function of the immune system [6]. Different nutrients will affect the immune function at different stages:

- Vitamin A and vitamin C can maintain the integrity of skin and mucous membrane. Vitamin C is a water-soluble antioxidant vitamin, its concentration in phagocytes and lymphocytes is much higher than that in plasma. It is widely involved in the functions of the immune system, including enhancing epithelial barrier function, enhancing phagocyte function, promoting antibody production, immune regulation and so on [7]. Vitamin C deficiency often leads to colds or infections, vitamin C supplementation can prevent respiratory tract infection, reduce the severity of cold symptoms and shorten the duration of cold [8].

- Vitamin D supports the production of antimicrobial peptides in macrophages. Vitamin D has a wide range of receptors in human cells, its active form participates in immune regulation in vivo in the form of hormones and can inhibit the generation of interleukin II in activated T lymphocytes, vitamin D supports the production of macrophage antimicrobial peptides stimulated and induced by virus and bacterium [9]. Vitamin D deficiency is prone to have respiratory tract infection and a variety of autoimmune diseases, vitamin D supplementation can promote the control of asthma and the improvement of lung function [10].
- Vitamin A and zinc can enhance anti-infection ability. The balance of zinc in the body is very important to maintain normal immune function. Zinc is involved in regulating innate and adaptive immune responses, resisting pathogen infection, regulating inflammatory response and controlling oxidative stress [11]. Zinc deficiency can lead to diarrhea, poor wound healing, recurrent oral ulcer, decreased immunity and repeated infection [12]. Zinc supplementation can significantly reduce the incidence rate and prevalence of acute respiratory infections and pneumonia in children, and shorten the duration of colds [13].
- Vitamin A, vitamin B_6, and folic acid can promote immune cells to produce antibodies. Folic acid is involved in DNA and protein synthesis, which is closely related to every mechanism of cell proliferation, especially cell-mediated immunity; folic acid deficiency can significantly change the immune response by inhibiting the activity of immune cells and interfering with metabolic processes, including the circulation of methylation, serine, glycine and purine [14].
- DHA, vitamin E, and selenium can regulate inflammatory response. Vitamin E is an effective antioxidant with the ability to regulate host immune function; vitamin E induces the high differentiation of immature T cells by increasing the positive selection of thymic epithelial cells, and participates in cellular immune function; vitamin E has a selective effect on humoral immunity mediated by different antigens in a dose-dependent manner; vitamin E deficiency can lead to downward trend of most of the immune indexes, which is related to the increase of infectious diseases and the occurrence of tumors [15].

Therefore, sufficient nutritional supplementation is necessary for strengthening the immune system.

3   Personalized Nutrition for Strengthening Immunity

3.1   Immunity Genetic Testing

Many gene variants have been identified to be connected with human immune system. For instance, the coding product of the *AGFG1* gene is related to the nucleoporine protein, which is a class of proteins that mediate the transport of nuclei, studies found that the polymorphism of the loci in the *AGFG1* gene can affect a person's susceptibility to influenza A viruses [16]. The coding product of the *AGBL1* gene is glutamate decarboxylase, which catalyzes the deglutylation of polyglutaminated protein, some studies found that the polymorphism of the key locus of the *AGBL1* gene is closely related to the cytomegalovirus (CMV) antibody response [17].

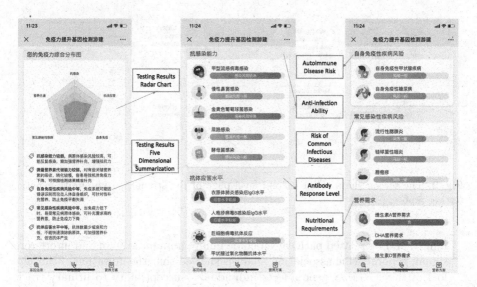

Fig. 1. The screen shots of the home page of the strengthen immunity genetic testing report.

Therefore, we developed a genetic testing service to evaluate a person's immune capacity from the genetic dimension. As described in Fig. 1, in the home page of the strengthen immunity genetic testing report, the first module (in Fig. 1 left) uses a radar chart to express the immune capacity of the customer from five dimensions, and meanwhile summarizes the testing results from the five dimensions, which correspond to the followed five genetic testing categories (in Fig. 1 middle and right):

– Anti-infection Ability, which includes the genetic testing items of: Influenza A Virus Infection, Chronic Sinus Infection, Staphylococcus Aureus Infection, Urinary Tract Infection, and Yeast Infection. Infection generally refers to the local tissue and systemic inflammatory reaction caused by the invasion of pathogens such as bacteria, viruses, fungi and parasites into the human body. Our innate immune protection usually prevents the infection of most of these pathogens into the human body. Our immunity determines the infection risk of these pathogens. For example, urinary tract infection is caused by the direct invasion of bacteria (a few can be caused by fungi, protozoa, and viruses), the protein encoded by the *TRIM38* gene belongs to three domain protein

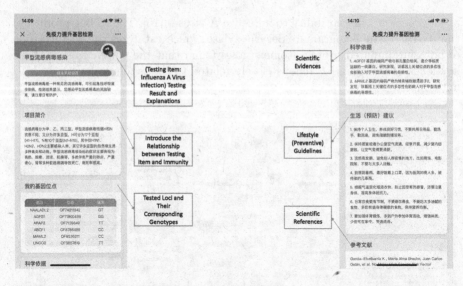

Fig. 2. The screen shots of the second level page of the strengthen immunity genetic testing report.

family, and its related pathways include innate immune system and interferon signal; genome wide association analysis showed that the mutation of the key loci of the *TRIM38* gene affects individual's susceptibility to urinary tract infection [18].

- Antibody Response Level, which includes the genetic testing items of: IgG Level after Chlamydia Pneumonia Infection, The Level of IgG after Human Herpesvirus 8 Infection, Cytomegalovirus Antibody Response, and Thyroid Peroxidase Antibody Level. The antibody level of some common pathogens after infection could be evaluated from the genetic level, and according to some genes' detection results, the immunity level under the infection of the above mentioned pathogens can be reflected. For example, the *BACH2* gene is a protein-coding gene, the *BACH2* gene related diseases include immunodeficiency and chronic granulocytic leukemia, studies have shown that the polymorphism of the loci in the *BACH2* gene is closely related to the level of thyroid peroxidase antibodies [19].
- Autoimmune Disease Risk, which includes the genetic testing items of: Autoimmune Thyroid Disease, and Autoimmune Diabetes Mellitus. Autoimmune disease refers to the disease caused by the body's immune response to its own antigen, which leads to the damage of its own tissue. For instance, autoimmune type 1 diabetes (also known clinically as congenital diabetes) is caused by autoimmune problems, autoimmune type 1 diabetes is incurable, and must be regulated over a long period of time, the *PTPN22* gene encodes a member of non receptor 4 subfamily of protein tyrosine phosphatase family, the encoded protein is a lymphoid intracellular phosphatase associated with molecular adaptor protein *CBL*, which may be involved in regulating

the *CBL* function in T cell receptor signaling pathway, studies have shown that the polymorphism of the key loci of this gene is closely related to the susceptibility of autoimmune type 1 diabetes [20].

– Risk of Common Infectious Diseases, which includes the genetic testing items of: Epidemic Parotitis, Streptococcal Pharyngitis, and Herpes Labialis. When bacteria, viruses and other pathogens infect the human body and break through the three lines of defense of human immunity, they will lead to the corresponding diseases and symptoms. For instance, streptococcal pharyngitis mainly refers to acute pharyngitis, among the streptococcus is a type A B hemolytic streptococcus, which can enter the bloodstream, causing bacteremia, causing purulent infection in other parts of tissues and organs, the polymorphism of the key loci in the *HLA-DQB1* gene are associated with the susceptibility to streptococcal pharyngitis [18].

– Nutritional Requirements, which includes the genetic testing items of: Vitamin A, Vitamin D, Vitamin E, Vitamin C, Vitamin B$_6$, Folic Acid, Magnesium, Iron, Zinc, Selenium, DHA. Nutritional deficiencies are the main cause of low immunity, reasonable and balanced nutritional supplementation is the necessary basis for strengthening immunity [21, 22].

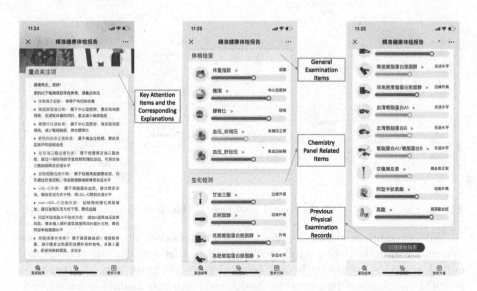

Fig. 3. The screen shots of the home page of the physical examination report.

Click the name of each testing item, the second level page will be opened as demonstrated in Fig. 2. In Fig. 2 left, the first module includes the testing result and its corresponding explanation, such as the testing result of Influenza A Virus Infection is high; the second module explains how the testing item is related to the immune system; the third module lists the tested gene loci and their corresponding genotypes. In Fig. 2 right, the fourth module gives the scientific evidences explaining how the related genes affect immune system; the fifth module provides lifestyle and disease preventive guidelines based on the testing results; the sixth module lists the scientific reference papers and clinical evidences.

3.2 Physical Examination

Most of the people have a physical examination each year, generally, the annual physical examination checks the: Blood Pressure, Heart Rate, Respiration Rate, Temperature, Heart, Throat, Ears, Nose, Sinuses, Eyes, Lymph Nodes, Thyroid, Carotid Arteries, and etc.; and takes the tests of: Complete Blood Count, Chemistry Panel, and Urinalysis (UA).

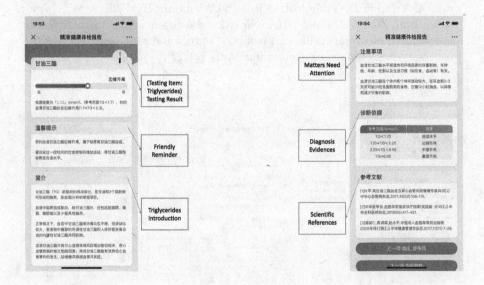

Fig. 4. The screen shots of the second level page of the physical examination report.

Unless symptoms already suggest a problem, however, the physical examination data are unlikely to be fully utilized. To further support our personalized nutrition service for strengthening immunity, we integrate part of customer's physical examination data into our model, the customers can upload or fill their personal physical examination data to our system. Figure 3 demonstrates the home page of the physical examination report. In Fig. 3 left, the first module summarizes the key attention items and gives the corresponding explanations. In Fig. 3 middle, the second module lists the general examination items; the third module lists the chemistry panel related items. In Fig. 3 right, at the bottom of the report, the customer can access his/her previous physical reports so as to compare to see whether the poor indicators of physical examination have been improved through the using of our personalized nutrition service.

Click each name of the physical examination item in Fig. 3, the second level page will be opened as described in Fig. 4. In Fig. 4 left, the first module gives the physical examination item name and its examination result (for example, the triglycerides is borderline high); based on the examination result, the second module gives some friendly health reminders; the third module explains in details about the examination item (for example, explains what are triglycerides and the relationship between triglycerides and health). In Fig. 4 right, the fourth module gives the matters that need to pay attention; the fifth module lists the diagnosis evidences for the physical examination item; the sixth module lists the reference scientific articles and clinical evidences.

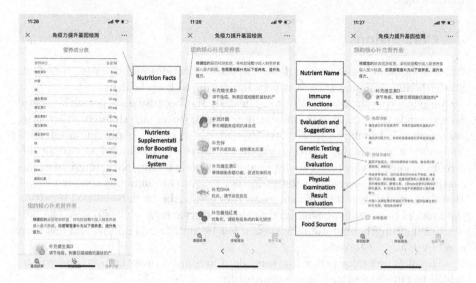

Fig. 5. The screen shots of the home page of the personalized nutrition report.

3.3 Dietary Assessment

As mentioned in Sect. 2, nutrition is a key factor for immune system, therefore, a balanced daily diet is very important for a healthy immune system. To acquire a customer's diet data, we rely on food frequency questionnaires [23, 24] to assess a customer's diet level.

3.4 Personalized Nutrition

Integrating the genetic testing data, physical examination data, as well as dietary assessment data, our data model calculates a personalized nutrition solution for each customer as described in Fig. 5.

In Fig. 5 left, the first module gives the personalized nutrition facts for each customer. In Fig. 5 middle, the second module lists personalized nutrients suggested for supplementation. Click the name of each nutrient, more detail information will be demonstrated as described in Fig. 5 right, for instance, the nutrition name part gives a brief summary about the relationship between the nutrient vitamin D and immune system; the immune function part explains more about how the nutrient vitamin D affects immune system; the evaluation and suggestions part, describes how the customer's immune capacity is evaluated based on genetic testing result, physical examination result, and dietary assessment result; the food sources part offers the foods containing a lot of the required nutrients.

Based on the personalized solution, customers can order a monthly customized nutrition box online, and our system will arrange a nutritional supplementation production factory to produce a customized nutrition box for each customer. The produced nutrition box will be posted to customer's home directly from factory.

4   Conclusions

Efficient immune response can defense against infections and diseases, therefore, strengthening immune system is very important to keep healthy.

Immune system is especially complicated, and because each person's genetic background, physical condition and nutritional status are different, therefore, each person's immune capacity is different, so in order to provide a effective immunity strengthening solution, we should provide personalized service for different persons. In this paper we integrate the genetic testing data, physical examination data, diet assessment data together to train an immune capacity evaluation data model, based on which, we further established a personalized nutrition data model to provide personalized nutrition service for each customer. The personalized strengthening immune system has been delivered online, and has been used by many customers.

The metabolomics (urine markers) data are under investigation, and will be added to our data model in the near future.

Acknowledgment. This research project is supported by Science Foundation of Beijing Language and Culture University (supported by "the Fundamental Research Funds for the Central Universities") (Approval number: 21YJ040002).

References

1. Guo, Q., et al.: The bioactive compounds and biological functions of Asparagus officinalis L - a review. J. Funct. Foods. **65**, 103727 (2020)
2. Aristizabal, B., Gonzalez, A.: Innate immune system. Autoimmunity: From Bench to Bedside [Internet]. In: Anaya, J.M., et al., (eds.), Bogota (Colombia). El Rosario University Press (2013). (Chapter 2)
3. Kennedy, M.A.: A brief review of the basics of immunology: the innate and adaptive response. Vet. Clin. North Am. Small Anim. Pract. **40**(3), 369–79 (2010)
4. Chaplin, D.D.: Overview of the immune response. J. Aller. Clin. Immunol. Author Manuscript **125**(2 Suppl. 2), S3-23 (2010)
5. Immune response. https://medlineplus.gov/ency/article/000821.htm. Accessed 22 July 2021

6. How to boost your immune system. https://www.health.harvard.edu/staying-healthy/how-to-boost-your-immune-system. Accessed 23 July 2021

7. Carr, A.C., Maggini, S.: Vitamin C and immune function. Nutrients **9**(11), 1211 (2017)

8. Hemila, H., Chalker, E.: Vitamin C for preventing and treating the common cold. Cochrane Database Syst. Rev. **2013**(1), CD000980 (2013)

9. Kongsbak, M., Levring, T.B., et al.: The vitamin D receptor and T cell function. Front Immunol. **4**, 148 (2013)

10. Martineau, A.R., et al.: Vitamin D supplementation to prevent acute respiratory tract infections: systematic review and meta-analysis of individual participant data. BMJ **356**, i6583 (2017)

11. Gammoh, N.Z., Rink, L.: Zinc in infection and inflammation. Nutrients **9**(6), 624 (2017)

12. Hemila, H., et al.: Zinc acetate lozenges may improve the recovery rate of common cold patients: an individual patient data meta-analysis. Open. Forum. Infect. Dis. **4**(2), ofx059 (2017)

13. Rerksuppaphol, S., Rerksuppaphol, L.: A randomized controlled trial of zinc supplementation in the treatment of acute respiratory tract infection in Thai children. Pediatr. Rep. **11**(2), 7954 (2019)

14. Reynolds, E.: Vitamin B12, folic acid, and the nervous system. Lancet Neurol. **5**(11), 949–60 (2006)

15. Lee, G.Y., Han, S.N.: The role of vitamin E in immunity. Nutrients **10**(11), 1614 (2018)

16. Garcia-Etxebarria, K., et al.: No major host genetic risk factor contributed to A(H1N1)2009 influenza severity. PLoS One. **10**(9), e0135983 (2015). [published correction appears in PLoS One. 2015;10(10):e0141661]

17. Kuparinen, T., Seppala, I., et al.: Genome-wide association study does not reveal major genetic determinants for anti-cytomegalovirus antibody response. Genes Immun. **13**(2), 184–90 (2012)

18. Tian, C., Hromatka, B.S., et al.: Genome-wide association and HLA region fine-mapping studies identify susceptibility LOCI for multiple common infections. Nat. Commun. **8**(1), 599 (2017)

19. Medici, M., et al.: Identification of novel genetic Loci associated with thyroid peroxidase antibodies and clinical thyroid disease. PLoS Genet. **10**(2), e1004123 (2014)

20. Cousminer, D.L., Ahlqvist, E., et al.: First genome-wide association study of latent autoimmune diabetes in adults reveals novel insights linking immune and metabolic diabetes. Diabetes Care. **41**(11), 2396–2403 (2018)

21. Childs, C.E., Calder, P.C., Miles, E.A.: Diet and immune function. Nutrients **11**(8), 1933 (2019)

22. Chandra, R.K.: Nutrition and the immune system: an introduction. Am. J. Clin. Nutr. **66**(2), 460S-463S (1997)

23. Johns, R., Kusuma, J., et al.: Validation of macro- and micro-nutrients including methyl donors in social ethnic diets using food frequency questionnaire and nutrition data system for research (USDA computerized program). SDRP J. Food Sci. Technol. **3**(4), 417–430 (2018)

24. Thompson, F.E., Subar, A.F.: Dietary Assessment Methodology. Nutrition in the Prevention and Treatment of Disease (Fourth Edition), Academic Press, ISBN 9780128029282 (2017). (Chapter 1)

Mining Outlying Aspects on Healthcare Data

Durgesh Samariya[✉] and Jiangang Ma

School of Engineering, Information Technology and Physical Sciences,
Federation University, Ballarat, Australia
{d.samariya,j.ma}@federation.edu.au

Abstract. Machine learning and artificial intelligence have a wide range of applications in medical domain, such as detecting anomalous reading, anomalous patient health condition, etc. Many algorithms have been developed to solve this problem. However, they fail to answer why those entries are considered as an outlier. This research gap leads to *outlying aspect mining* problem. The problem of outlying aspect mining aims to discover the set of features (a.k.a subspace) in which the given data point is dramatically different than others. In this paper, we present an interesting application of outlying aspect mining in the medical domain. This paper aims to effectively and efficiently identify outlying aspects using different outlying aspect mining algorithms and evaluate their performance on different real-world healthcare datasets. The experimental results show that the latest isolation-based outlying aspect mining measure, SiNNE, have outstanding performance on this task and have promising results.

Keywords: Outlier detection · Outlying aspect mining · Healthcare

1 Introduction

The application of machine learning (ML) and artificial intelligence (AI) algorithms in the healthcare industry helps to improve the health of patients more efficiently. These algorithms help in many ways, such as medical image diagnosis [13], disease detection/classification [9], detect anomalous reading, etc. Recently, researchers have been interested in detecting anomalous activity in healthcare industry. Anomaly or outlier[1] is defined as data instance which does not conform with the reminder of that set of data instances. The vast number of applications have been developed to detect outliers from medical data [8,10,14]. However, no study has been conducted to find out why these points are considered as outliers, i.e., on which set of features data point is dramatically different than others, as far as we know. The goal of outlying aspect mining is to identify the

---

[1] Anomaly and outlier are most commonly used terms in the literature. In this work, hereafter, we will use outlier term only.

© Springer Nature Switzerland AG 2021
S. Siuly et al. (Eds.): HIS 2021, LNCS 13079, pp. 160–170, 2021.
https://doi.org/10.1007/978-3-030-90885-0_15

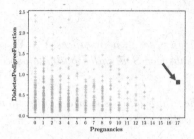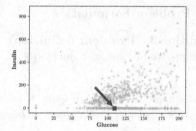

Fig. 1. Outlying aspects of patient A on different features. The red square point represents patient A. (Color figure online)

set of features where the given point (or a given outlier) is most inconsistent with the rest of the data.

In many healthcare applications, a medical officer wants to know, for a specific patient, the most outlying aspects compared to others. For example, you are a doctor having patients with Pima Indian diabetes disease. While treating a specific patient, you want to know, in which aspects this patient is different than others. For example, let's consider the Pima Indian diabetes disease data set[2]. For 'Patient A', the most outlying aspect will be having the highest number of pregnancies and low diabetes pedigree function (see Fig. 1), compared to other subspace.

Another example is, when a medical insurance analyst wants to know in which aspects the given insurance claim is most unusual. The above given applications are different than outlier detection. Instead of searching the whole data set for the outlier, in outlying aspect mining, we are specifically interested in a given data instance, and the goal is to find out outlying aspects where a given data instance stands out. Such data instance is called as a query q.

These interesting applications of outlying aspect mining in the medical domain motivated us to write this paper. In this paper, we introduce four outlying aspect mining methods and evaluate their performance on eight healthcare datasets. To the best of our knowledge, it is the first time when these algorithms are applied on healthcare data. Our results have verified their performance on outlying aspect mining task and found that isolation-based algorithm presents promising performance. It can detect more interesting subspace.

The rest of the paper is organized as follows. Section 2 summarizes the principle and working mechanism of four outlying aspect mining algorithms. The experimental setup and results are summarised in Sect. 3. Finally, we conclude the paper in Sect. 4.

2   Outlying Aspect Mining Algorithms

Before describing different outlying aspect mining algorithms, we first provide the problem formulation.

---

[2] The description of data set is provided in Table 1.

2.1 Problem Formulation

Definition 1 (Problem definition). *Given a set of n instances $\mathcal{X}$ ($|\mathcal{X}| = n$) in d dimensional space, a query $\mathbf{q} \in \mathcal{X}$, a subspace S is called outlying aspect of $\mathbf{q}$ if,*

- *outlyingness of $\mathbf{q}$ in subspace S is higher than other subspaces, and there is no other subspace with same or higher outlyingness.*

Outlying aspect mining algorithms, first requires a scoring measure to compute outlyingness of the query in subspace and search method to search for most outlying subspace. In the rest of this section, we review different scoring measures only. For search part, we will use Beam [15] search method because it is the latest search method and is used in different studies [11,15,16]. We re-produce the procedure of beam search in Algorithm 1.

Algorithm 1: $Beam(\mathbf{q}, \ell, \mathcal{X}, W, K, F)$

Input: $\mathcal{X}$ - a given data set, $\mathbf{q}$ - a query, ℓ - maximum dimension, W - beam width, K - number of top subspaces, F - a set of features

Output: set of outlying features of query $\mathbf{q}$

1 generate $2D$ subspaces ;
2 Add the top K subspaces to Ans;
3 **for** $\ell = 3$ *to* ℓ **do**
4   initialize $L_{(\ell)} = \Phi$;
5   **for** *each subspace* $S \in L_{(\ell-1)}$ **do**
6   **for** *each feature* F_i **do**
7   **if** $S \cup F_i$ *not considered yet* **then**
8   compute outlying score $\{S \cup F_i\}$;
9   **if** *the worst subspace score in S is worse than $\{S \cup F_i\}$* **then**
10   replace;
11   **end**
12   **if** $|L_{(\ell)}| < W$ **then**
13   append $\{S \cup F_i\}$ to $L_{(\ell)}$;
14   **end**
15   **else if** *the worst scored subspace in $L_{(\ell)}$ is worst than $\{S \cup F_i\}$* **then**
16   replace;
17   **end**
18   **end**
19   **end**
20   **end**
21 **end**
22 **return** *set of outlying features*

2.2 Density Rank

The scoring measure used in OAMiner [4] is based on kernel density estimation (KDE) [12].

Definition 2. *Given a query* **q***, the outlying degree based on KDE in subspace S is defined as follows.*

$$f_S(\mathbf{q}) = \frac{1}{n(2\pi)^{\frac{m}{2}} \prod_{i \in S} h_i} \sum_{x \in \mathcal{X}} e^{-\sum_{i \in S} \frac{(\mathbf{q}_i - x_i)^2}{2 h_i^2}} \tag{1}$$

where, $f_S(\mathbf{q})$ is a kernel density estimation of **q** *in subspace S ($|S| = m$), h_i is the kernel bandwidth in dimension i.*

Density is biased towards high dimension, therefore to eliminate effect of dimensionality biasedness, OAMiner [4] uses density rank as a measure of outlyingness.

2.3 Density Z-score

Recently, Vinh et al. (2016) [15] discussed the issue of using density rank as a measure of outlyingness and provided some examples where it can be counterproductive. They proposed to make density dimensionality unbiased with Z-score normalization.

Definition 3. *Given a query* **q***, the outlying degree based on Z-score normalization in subspace S is defined as follows.*

$$Z(f_S(\mathbf{q})) = \frac{f_S(\mathbf{q}) - \mu_{f_S}}{\sigma_{f_S}} \tag{2}$$

where μ_{f_S} and σ_{f_S} are the mean and standard deviation of densities of all data instances in subspace S, respectively.

2.4 SGrid

Wells and Ting (2019) [16] proposed sGrid density estimator, which is a smoothed variant of the traditional grid-based estimator (a.k.a histogram). Authors replaced the kernel density estimator to sGrid in the Beam [15] search. In experiments they shows that by just replacing kernel density estimator to sGrid density estimator, Beam search runs atleast two orders of faster than KDE. sGrid is dimensionally biased measure, thus it also required Z-score normalization to make the score dimensionality unbiased.

2.5   SiNNE

Very recently, Samariya et al.(2020) [11] proposed a **S**imple **I**solation score using **N**earest **N**eighbour **E**nsemble (SiNNE) measure originally inspired from Isolation using Nearest Neighbour Ensembles (iNNE) method for outlier detection [1]. SiNNE constructs t ensemble of models. Each model is constructed from randomly chosen sub-samples ($\mathcal{D}_i \subset \mathcal{X}, |\mathcal{D}_i| = \psi < n$). Each model have ψ hyperspheres, where radius of hypersphere is the euclidean distance between a ($a \in \mathcal{D}_i$) to its nearest neighbour in $\mathcal{D}_i$. The outlying score of $\mathbf{q}$ in model $\mathcal{M}_i$, $I(q|\mathcal{M}_i) = 0$ if $\mathbf{q}$ falls in any of the ball and 1 otherwise.

Definition 4. *The final outlying score of* $\mathbf{q}$ *using* t *models is :*

$$SiNNE(\mathbf{q}) = \frac{1}{t} \sum_{i=1}^{t} I(\mathbf{q}|\mathcal{M}_i) \tag{3}$$

where $I(\cdot)$ *is indicator function which gives output 0 if it is true otherwise 1.*

3   Evaluation and Discussion

In this section, we present the result of four scoring measures; Kernel Density Rank (RBeam), Density Z-score (Beam), sGrid Z-score (sBeam) and SiNNE (SiBeam) using Beam search on medical datasets. All experiments were run for 1 h and unfinished tasks were killed and presented as '‡'.

In this study, we used 8 publicly available benchmarking medical datasets for outlier detection; *BreastW* and *Pima* are from Keller et al. (2012) [7][3] and *Annthyroid, Cardiotocography, Heart disease, Hepatitis, WDBC* and *WPBC* are from Campos et al. (2016) [3][4]. The summary of each data set is provided in Table 1.

Table 1. An overview of the datasets used in this study.

Data set	# N	# d
Annthyroid	7129	21
BreastW	683	9
Cardiotocography	2114	21
Heart disease	270	13
Hepatitis	80	19
Pima	768	8
WDBC	367	30
WPBC	198	33

---

[3] Available at https://www.ipd.kit.edu/~muellere/HiCS/.

[4] Available at https://www.dbs.ifi.lmu.de/research/outlier-evaluation/DAMI/.

Table 2. Subspace discovered by RBeam, Beam, sBeam and SiBeam on real-world datasets. The top subspace for top five outlier queries are listed. **q-id** represent query point index and the numbers in a bracket are attribute index.

	q-id	RBeam	Beam	sBeam	SiBeam
Annthyroid	93	‡	‡	{5}	{2, 5, 16}
	952			{17}	{5, 13, 19}
	4921			{20}	{1, 18}
	5397			{7}	{7, 8, 18}
	6413			{19}	{2, 12, 19}
BreastW	8	{0, 8}	{6}	{8}	{2, 6, 8}
	36	{0, 4, 6}	{5, 6}	{0}	{1, 5, 6}
	70	{0, 6}	{0, 6}	{6}	{0, 5, 6}
	127	{0, 4}	{4}	{4}	{0, 2, 4}
	673	{6}	{6}	{8}	{0, 3, 8}
Cardioto.	140	{0, 14}	{0}	{15}	{15}
	379	{14, 16, 20}	{16}	{19}	{8, 16, 19}
	1477	{3, 16, 20}	{16}	{9}	{4, 9, 15}
	1585	{5, 12}	{5}	{5, 12}	{3, 5, 11}
	2074	{3}	{3}	{3}	{3, 6}
Heart disease	1	{0, 4}	{4, 10}	{4}	{3, 4}
	87	{2, 3, 9}	{10}	{10}	{2, 3, 9}
	159	{3, 11, 12}	{1, 12}	{1, 12}	{1, 3, 12}
	175	{6, 11, 12}	{6, 7}	{5, 6}	{7, 11, 12}
	235	{0, 9}	{10}	{10}	{0, 4, 7}
Hepatitis	28	{0, 15}	{4, 15}	{15}	{10, 15}
	38	{0, 13}	{13}	{8, 12}	{13, 18}
	57	{0, 15}	{3, 4, 15}	{2, 12}	{11, 13, 15}
	66	{5, 16, 18}	{13}	{13}	{5, 13, 17}
	78	{5, 8, 10}	{2, 4, 5}	{2, 12}	{1, 12, 16}
Pima	14	{0, 5}	{5}	{5}	{2, 5}
	36	{4, 6}	{6}	{4}	{2, 4, 6}
	213	{6}	{3}	{4}	{4, 6}
	304	{0, 3}	{3}	{3}	{0, 3}
	624	{0, 1, 3}	{1}	{1}	{0, 1, 7}
WDBC	6	{0}	{3}	{23}	{1, 19, 22}
	9	{1, 25}	{3}	{23}	{20, 28}
	28	{0, 6}	{28}	{16}	{0, 26, 28}
	79	{0, 17}	{8}	{16}	{0, 17}
	176	{1, 18}	{11}	{18}	{18, 22, 27}
WPBC	3	{0, 6}	{10}	{10}	{5, 10, 15}
	9	{0, 30}	{10}	{30}	{22, 28, 30}
	58	{0, 5}	{5}	{15}	{6, 8, 15}
	119	{1, 31}	{31}	{31}	{3, 22, 27}
	181	{7, 18}	{18}	{18}	{15, 17, 18}

We used default parameters of each algorithms as suggested in respective papers unless specified otherwise.

- Density rank and Density Z-score : KDE use Gaussian kernel with default bandwidth as suggested by [6];
- sGrid : block size parameter $w = 64$;
- SiNNE : subsample size $\psi = 8$, and ensemble size $t = 100$; and
- Beam search : beam width $W = 100$, and maximum dimensionality of subspace $\ell = 3$.

In terms of implementation, we used Java implementation of sGrid and SiNNE which is made available by the authors [16] and [11], respectively. We implemented RBeam and Beam in Java using WEKA [5]. All experiments were conducted on a machine with Intel 8-core i9 CPU and 16 GB main memory, running on macOS Big Sur version 11.1.

For each data set, we first use the state-of-the-art outlier detector called LOF [2] to detect the top five outliers; and then they are used as queries. Each scoring measure identifies outlying aspects for each queries.

Table 2 shows the subspace found by four scoring measures on real-world medical datasets. Note that, we do not have the ground truth on real-world data set to verify the quality of discovered subspaces. Thus, we visually present the discovered subspaces by different scoring measures of two queries[5] from each datasets.

Table 3, 4, 5, 6, 7, 8, 9 and 10 provides the visualization of discovered subspaces by different scoring measure on *Annthyroid, BreastW, Cardiotocography, Heart disease, Hepatitis, Pima, WDBC* and *WPBC*, respectively. Note that, each one dimensional subspace is plotted using histogram with 10 equal width bins. In

Table 3. Visualization of discovered subspaces on *Annthyroid* data set.

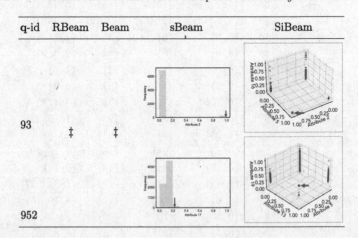

q-id	RBeam	Beam	sBeam	SiBeam
93	‡	‡		
952				

---

[5] Due to space limitation, we only present discovered subspaces of two queries. We choose queries where discovered subspaces are different for each scoring measure.

Table 4. Visualization of discovered subspaces on *BreastW* data set.

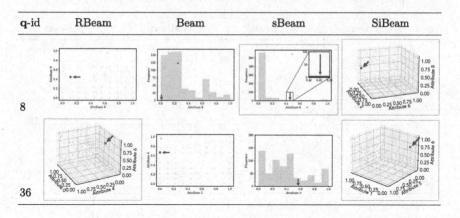

Table 5. Visualization of discovered subspaces on *Cardiotocography* data set.

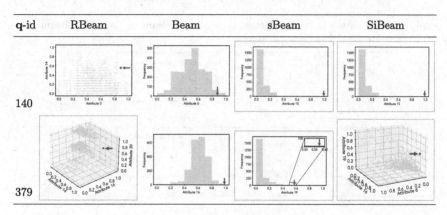

Table 6. Visualization of discovered subspaces on *Heart disease* data set.

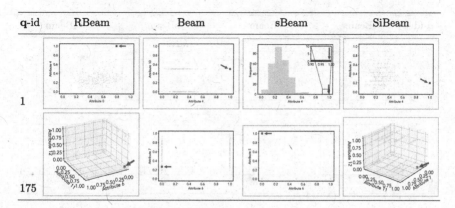

Table 7. Visualization of discovered subspaces on *Hepatitis* data set.

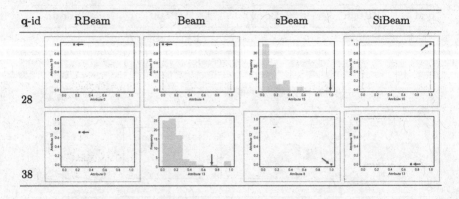

Table 8. Visualization of discovered subspaces on *Pima* data set.

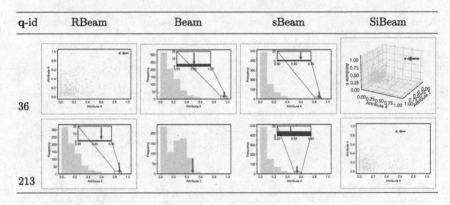

Table 9. Visualization of discovered subspaces on *WDBC* data set.

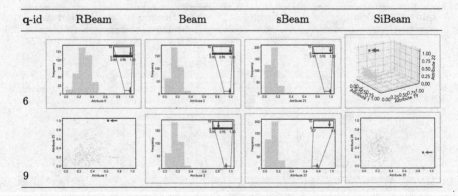

Table 10. Visualization of discovered subspaces on *WPBC* data set.

q-id	RBeam	Beam	sBeam	SiBeam
9				
58				

absence of better evaluation measure, we visually compared each discovered subspaces. The query is presented as red square and better subspace is highlighted in green color.

By looking at visualization of each discovered subspaces, we can say that, out of 16 queries (2 queries from eight datasets), SiBeam have comparatively better subspace in each query. While sBeam have better subspace in 11 queries out of 16. RBeam and Beam have better subspace in 11 and 5 queries out of 14[6], respectively. SiBeam is the only method which have better outlying subspace, as far as we can say from visualization.

4   Conclusion

In this paper, we present an interesting application of outlying aspect mining in healthcare domain. We first introduce four outlying aspect mining scoring measures which includes density rank, density Z-score, sGrid Z-score and SiNNE. Later, these algorithms are evaluated systematically on healthcare datasets. Our results on eight datasets shows that recently developed methods SiNNE and sGrid perform better than kernel density based measure. Apart from that, in medical domain it is important to have faster algorithm, thus, in this domain, kernel density based measures are not suitable if data set is huge in terms of data size and dimensionality.

Acknowledgement. This work is supported by Federation University Research Priority Area (RPA) scholarship, awarded to Durgesh Samariya. We are thankful to the anonymous reviewers for their critical comments to improve the quality of the paper.

---

[6] RBeam and Beam are unable to finish the process in 1 h for *Annthyroid* data set.

References

1. Bandaragoda, T.R., Ting, K.M., Albrecht, D., Liu, F.T., Wells, J.R.: Efficient anomaly detection by isolation using nearest neighbour ensemble. In: 2014 IEEE International Conference on Data Mining Workshop, pp. 698–705 (2014). https://doi.org/10.1109/ICDMW.2014.70
2. Breunig, M.M., Kriegel, H.P., Ng, R.T., Sander, J.: Lof: identifying density-based local outliers. In: Proceedings of the 2000 ACM SIGMOD International Conference on Management of Data, pp. 93–104. SIGMOD 2000, Association for Computing Machinery, New York, NY, USA (2000). https://doi.org/10.1145/342009.335388
3. Campos, G.O., et al.: On the evaluation of unsupervised outlier detection: measures, datasets, and an empirical study. Data Mining Knowl. Disc. 30(4), 891–927 (2016). https://doi.org/10.1007/s10618-015-0444-8
4. Duan, L., Tang, G., Pei, J., Bailey, J., Campbell, A., Tang, C.: Mining outlying aspects on numeric data. Data Mining Knowl. Disc. 29(5), 1116–1151 (2015). https://doi.org/10.1007/s10618-014-0398-2
5. Hall, M., Frank, E., Holmes, G., Pfahringer, B., Reutemann, P., Witten, I.H.: The WEKA data mining software: an update. SIGKDD Explor. Newsl. 11(1), 10–18 (2009). https://doi.org/10.1145/1656274.1656278
6. Härdle, W.: Smoothing techniques: with implementation in S. Springer Science & Business Media, New York (2012)
7. Keller, F., Muller, E., Bohm, K.: Hics: high contrast subspaces for density-based outlier ranking. In: 2012 IEEE 28th International Conference on Data Engineering, pp. 1037–1048 (2012). https://doi.org/10.1109/ICDE.2012.88
8. Laurikkala, J., Juhola, M., Kentala, E., Lavrac, N., Miksch, S., Kavsek, B.: Informal identification of outliers in medical data. In: Fifth International Workshop on Intelligent Data Analysis in Medicine and Pharmacology, Vol. 1, pp. 20–24 (2000)
9. Pham, T.D.: Classification of COVID-19 chest x-rays with deep learning: new models or fine tuning? Health Inf. Sci. Syst. 9(1), 1–11 (2021)
10. Prastawa, M., Bullitt, E., Ho, S., Gerig, G.: A brain tumor segmentation framework based on outlier detection. Med. Image Anal. 8(3), 275–283 (2004). https://doi.org/10.1016/j.media.2004.06.007
11. Samariya, D., Aryal, S., Ting, K.M., Ma, J.: A new effective and efficient measure for outlying aspect mining. In: Huang, Z., Beek, W., Wang, H., Zhou, R., Zhang, Y. (eds.) WISE 2020. LNCS, vol. 12343, pp. 463–474. Springer, Cham (2020). https://doi.org/10.1007/978-3-030-62008-0_32
12. Scott, D.W.: Multivariate Density Estimation: Theory, Practice, and Visualization. John Wiley & Sons, Hoboken (2015)
13. Tachmazidis, I., Chen, T., Adamou, M., Antoniou, G.: A hybrid AI approach for supporting clinical diagnosis of attention deficit hyperactivity disorder (ADHD) in adults. Health Inf. Syst. 9(1), 1–8 (2021)
14. van Capelleveen, G., Poel, M., Mueller, R.M., Thornton, D., van Hillegersberg, J.: Outlier detection in healthcare fraud: a case study in the Medicaid dental domain. Int. J. Acc. Inf. Syst. 21, 18–31 (2016). https://doi.org/10.1016/j.accinf.2016.04.001
15. Vinh, N.X., Chan, J., Romano, S., Bailey, J., Leckie, C., Ramamohanarao, K., Pei, J.: Discovering outlying aspects in large datasets. Data Mining Knowl. Disc. 30(6), 1520–1555 (2016). https://doi.org/10.1007/s10618-016-0453-2
16. Wells, J.R., Ting, K.M.: A new simple and efficient density estimator that enables fast systematic search. Pattern Recogn. Lett. 122, 92–98 (2019). https://doi.org/10.1016/j.patrec.2018.12.020

Multi-label Anomaly Classification Based on Electrocardiogram

Chenyang Li⬤ and Le Sun(✉)⬤

Engineering Research Center of Digital Forensics, Ministry of Education, and the Department of Jiangsu Collaborative Innovation Center of Atmospheric Environment and Equipment Technology (CICAEET), Nanjing University of Information Science and Technology, Nanjing 210044, China
{20201249417,LeSun1}@nuist.edu.cn

Abstract. Under the background of 5G and AI, it is particularly important to use cloud computing, Internet of things and big data technology to analyze massive physiological signals of patients in real time. Arrhythmia can cause some major diseases, such as heart failure, atrial fibrillation and so on. It's difficult to analysis them quickly. In this paper, a deep learning model of multi-label classification based on optimized temporal convolution network is proposed to detect abnormal electrocardiogram. The experimental results show that the accuracy of the model is 0.960, and the Micro F1 score is 0.87.

Keywords: Multi-label classification · Electrocardiogram · Classification of arrhythmia

1 Introduction

The statistics of World Health Organization show that every year around 17.5 million people died because of heart diseases. Detecting the early symptoms of heart diseases can help doctors to quickly make treatment decisions. Electrocardiogram (ECG) is the most commonly used tool to check heart diseases. People usually wear smart bracelets or professional detection equipments to collect ECG signals [10]. Internet of things and cloud computing technology are good helpers for human data collection and storage. However, due to the increasing number of patients, ECG data is also increasing rapidly. It is difficult to continue to diagnose diseases in such big data environment by only human experts. Therefore, it has become a significant research topic to automatically classify ECG records based on artificial intelligence techniques [2].

There are some researches on heartbeat classification. It is mainly the traditional machine learning method based on expert features and the most advanced deep learning method. Machine learning methods generally need to go through

Supported in part by the National Natural Science Foundation of China (Grants No 61702274) and PAPD.

three processes: data preprocessing, feature extraction and classification. Acquisition of ECG signal is easily affected by environment, such as body movement, breathing, electromagnetic interference of the surrounding environment. Therefore, the original ECG signal contains a variety of noises, which affect the signal classification. Preprocessing is an important measure of noise removal. Feature extraction techniques include: wavelet transform [23], principal component analysis [12], independent component analysis [7]. Many machine learning classification algorithms have been proved to be suitable for these features such as MLPNN [4] and SVM [1].

Due to the problems of data quality, expert experience and work efficiency, the limitations of traditional methods are highlighted. In recent years, deep learning has gradually been favored by scholars. Deep learning is an end-to-end process. Engineers using deep learning models do not need to extract features manually. The common classifiers are convolutional neural network [9] and recurrent neural network [5]. For multi-label classification, it is often necessary to design some more complex structural models to meet the needs of the task.

In this work, we proposed an improved temporal convolution network (TCN). In this improved TCN, we replace the weight normalization layer with the batch normalization layer. And we use the layer skip connection between every four basic blocks to reduce the time complexity. The rest of this paper is set as follows: Sect. 2 introduces the related work. Section 3 gives the details of our methods. In Sect. 4, we compared with other methods. Section 5 makes conclusion and presents future research directions.

2   RELATED WORK

2.1   Deep Neural Network

Zhu et al. [26] used residual neural network (ResNet) and squeeze-and-excitation blocks to learn ECG segment. Cai et al. [13] proposed a model named Multi-ECGNet which combines the advantages of ResNet and Xception. Feng et al. [6] used a model which combines ResNet and attention mechanism for ECG classification. Yang et al. [24] proposed an improved ResNet structure and introduced attention blocks as well. Nan et al. [5] presented a framework that detects ECG images by fine-grained mechanism. Ran et al. [16] proposed a EASTNet which extract the characteristics of abnormal heart and correlation between heartbeats via a deep network. Rong et al. [17] proposed a network based on ResNet and gated recurrent unit(GRU) to classify ECG data. Li et al. [14] proposed a multi-label ECG feature selection method based on sparse constraints. The method studies the correlation between abnormal cardiac. Yu et al. [25] proposed a light weight model which uses criterion and extended convolution to extract feature information. Natarajan et al. [15] developed a transformer network which combines manual ECG features. Li et al. [11] developed a system called DeepECG which combined convolutional neural network and transfer learning. Torres et al. [27] proposed to convert the original signal into TFR images and choose VGG-16 network for abnormal heart disease recognition. He et al. [29] designed a model structure including ResNet, bidirectional GRU and attention mechanism to identify arrhythmias.

2.2 Other Methods

Alexander et al. [22] developed a auto encoder to make an ECG embedding for classification. Wang et al. [20] proposed a method which combines Spark's cluster system to study the ECG big data. Wang et al. [21] proposed a method for Extreme Learning Machine which based on Adaptive algorithm. Baydoun et al. [3] proposed a method that converts the ECG into digitized data to trian by machine learning. Salem et al. [18] transferred the method from some image fields to ECG fields for classification. Satija et al. [19] developed a auto classification method for diagnosis in unsupervised conditions.

3 The Proposed Improved TCN

3.1 Data Preprocessing

For this work, we select five databases and they are CPSC Database [27], the PTB Diagnostic ECG Database [27], Georgia database [27], St Petersburg INCART 12-lead Arrhythmia Database [27] and the PTB-XL Database [27]. We choose wavelet transform to remove noise. Besides, we uniformly resample the datasets with different sampling rates 500 Hz. Considering the different record length, we only take a 10 s segments for each record, and selectively discard the segments less than 10 s.

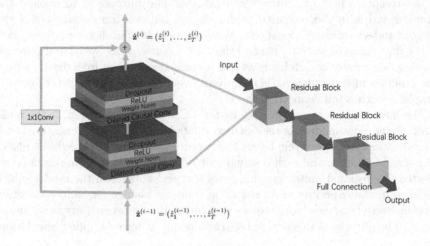

Fig. 1. TCN structure

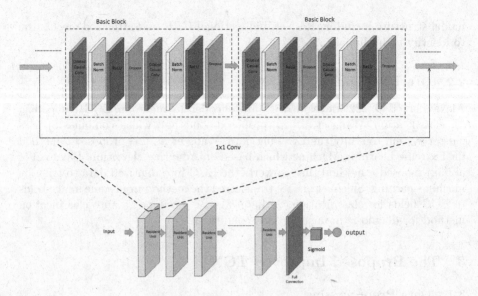

Fig. 2. Optimized TCN structure

3.2 Model

TCN model mainly consists of dilated convolution layer, weight normalization layer, relu activation layer and dropout layer. As shown in Fig. 1, one base block is stacked in the above order, and two base blocks form a residual block. Each residual block uses a skip connection. Dilated convolution adds a dilation rate to the receptive field of ordinary convolution. The purpose is to expand the sampling stripe in the receptive field area and balance the parameters of the network and the computational cost. Weights normalization is the normalization on the dimension of weights. It can bring faster convergence speed and stronger learning rate robustness. ReLU is used to prevent the gradient from disappearing. The function of dropout layer is to prevent over fitting of the model. Finally, it completes with a full connection layer.

We have made some optimizations for TCN. As shown in Fig. 2, the basic block of the new model consists of two dilated convolution layers, two batch normalization layers, two relu layers and two dropout layers. Double basic blocks form a residual unit, and each residual unit take a skip connection. Actually, we selected five residual units. This improves the performance of the model, which is shown in the experiment. At the same time, we change one skip connection between every two basic blocks to one skip connection between every two residual blocks. The purpose of this is to reduce the amount of down sampling calculation.

4   Experiment

4.1   Experiment Setup

Firstly, we read each ECG record and cut them into 10s segments. The dataset is divided as: 90% and 10% for training and testing, respectively. The parameter settings of the improved TCN model is as follows: the learning rate is 0.0001, the number of sample training batches is 100, the number of iterations is 500, the dropout rate is 0.1, the activation function is sigmoid and the initial value of dilation rate is 1. It is doubled every two Residual units. The optimizer uses Adma. The loss function is binary_crossentropy. Finally, We use the following metrics for evaluation: overall accuracy (ACC), mean Average Precision (mAP) and f1 score(F1). Besides, we introduce Hamming Loss (H-Loss) [30], Ranking Loss [30] and Coverage Error [31] to evaluate our experiment. Hamming Loss statistics related tags do not appear in the predicted tag set or irrelevant tags appear in the predicted tag set. The smaller it is, the better system performance is. Ranking Loss compare the related label set with the unrelated label set, and then count the times that the prediction possibility of the related label is less than that of the unrelated label. The smaller the value, the better the performance. Coverage error calculate We need to cover the distance of all true labels by ranking score. The best value is the average number of label per true label set. Formula 1 to formula 5 are their calculation methods.

$$ACC = \frac{TP + TN}{TP + TN + FP + FN} \tag{1}$$

$$PRE = \frac{TP}{TP + FP}, REC = \frac{TP}{TP + FN}, F1 = \frac{2 * PRE * REC}{PRE + REC} \tag{2}$$

$$H - Loss = \frac{1}{N}\Sigma_{i=1}^{N}\frac{XOR(Y_{i,j}, P_{i,j})}{L} \tag{3}$$

$$Coverage = \Sigma_{i=1}^{N}\frac{max(M_{l_1}, M_{l_2}, \ldots, M_{l_n})}{N} \tag{4}$$

$$Rankingloss = \frac{\Sigma_{j \in \mathbb{L}_i}\Sigma_{k \in \overline{\mathbb{L}}_i}I(P_{ij} \leqslant P_{ik})}{|\mathbb{L}_i| * |\overline{\mathbb{L}}_i|} \tag{5}$$

In formulae 1 and 2, TP means true positive. FP means false positive. TN means true negative. FN means false negative. N in formula 3 is the number of samples. L is the number of labels, $Y_{i,j}$ is the true value of the jth component in the ith prediction result, $P_{i,j}$ is the predicted value of the jth component in the ith prediction result. For coverage error, the N is the number of samples, $M_{l_i}(i \in 1, 2, 3, \ldots, n)$ is the label l_n is ranked from large to small according to all prediction probabilities. In formula 5, $\mathbb{L}_i$ is the positive label set and the $\overline{\mathbb{L}}_i$ is the negative label set which is possibility higher than the positive label set.

4.2   Result and Comparision

In Table 1, we make a comparison with the related work of multi-label classification. Our experiment is more complete and the evaluating metrics is more sufficient. Our F1-score 0.045 higher than Torres et al. [27] and 0.205 higher than the original TCN model. Besides, we also compare with the original TCN model in other metrics. According to the experiment results, our optimized model get lower H-Loss, lower coverage error, lower ranking loss and higher accuracy and mean Average Precision. It proves that our optimized model performs better.

Table 1. Compare with TCN and other works.

Model	F1 score	H-Loss	Coverage	mAP	Ranking loss	Accuracy
Optimized TCN	**0.870**	**0.03**	**2.21**	**0.79**	**0.123**	**0.960**
TCN	0.675	0.10	3.63	0.42	0.317	0.901
ResNet-50	0.764	-	-	-	-	-
VGG-19	0.813	-	-	-	-	-
Smisek et al.(2020) [28]	0.462	-	-	-	-	-
Torres et al.(2020) [27]	0.825	-	-	-	-	-

5   Conclusion

In this paper, we make some optimization to temporal convolution network and achieved good results. We use multiple metrics to evaluate our optimized model. Transplanting the model to wearable detection devices can significantly reduce labor costs and medical resource costs. In the future, we will use the Generative Adversarial Network (GAN) to enhance the data to balance dataset, so as to achieve better classification effect.

References

1. Almalchy, M.T., ALGayar, S.M.S., Popescu, N.: Atrial fibrillation automatic diagnosis based on ECG signal using pretrained deep convolution neural network and SVM multiclass model. In: 2020 13th International Conference on Communications (COMM), pp. 197–202 (2020)
2. Sun, L., Wang, Y., He, J., Li, H., Peng, D., Wang, Y.: A stacked LSTM for atrial fibrillation prediction based on multivariate ECGS. Health Inf. Sci. Syst. **8**(1), 1–7 (2020)
3. Baydoun, M., Safatly, L., Abou Hassan, O.K., Ghaziri, H., El Hajj, A., Ismaeel, H.: High precision digitization of paper-based ECG records: a step toward machine learning. IEEE J. Transl. Eng. Health Med. **7**, 1–8 (2019)
4. Bulbul, H.I., Usta, N., Yildiz, M.: Classification of ECG arrhythmia with machine learning techniques. In: 2017 16th IEEE International Conference on Machine Learning and Applications (ICMLA), pp. 546–549 (2017)

5. Nan, D., et al.: FM-ECG: A fine-grained multi-label framework for ECG image classification. Inf. Sci. **549**, 164–177 (2021)
6. Feng, Y., Vigmond, E.: Deep multi-label multi-instance classification on 12-lead ECG. In: 2020 Computing in Cardiology, pp. 1–4 (2020)
7. Islam, M.R., Bhuiyan, R.A., Ahmed, N., Islam, M.R.: PCA and ICA based hybrid dimension reduction model for cardiac arrhythmia disease diagnosis. In: 2018 IEEE 10th International Conference on Humanoid, Nanotechnology, Information Technology, Communication and Control, Environment and Management (HNICEM), pp. 1–7 (2018)
8. Jambukia, S.H., Dabhi, V.K., Prajapati, H.B.: Classification of ECG signals using machine learning techniques: a survey. In: 2015 International Conference on Advances in Computer Engineering and Applications, pp. 714–721. IEEE (2015)
9. Demir, F., Şengür, A., Bajaj, V., Polat, K.: Towards the classification of heart sounds based on convolutional deep neural network. Health Inf. Sci. Syst. **7**(1), 1–9 (2019). https://doi.org/10.1007/s13755-019-0078-0
10. Sadek, I., Biswas, J., Abdulrazak, B.: Ballistocardiogram signal processing: a review. Health Inf. Sci. Syst. **7**(1), 1–23 (2019). https://doi.org/10.1007/s13755-019-0071-7
11. Li, C., Zhao, H., Wei, L., Leng, X., Wang, L., Lin, X., Pan, Y., Jiang, W., Jiang, J., Sun, Y., Wang, J., Xiang, J.: DEEPECG: image-based electrocardiogram interpretation with deep convolutional neural networks. Biomed. Sig. Process. Control **69**, 102824 (2021)
12. Li, R., et al.: Arrhythmia multiple categories recognition based on PCA-KNN clustering model. In: 2019 8th International Symposium on Next Generation Electronics (ISNE), pp. 1–3 (2019)
13. Cai, J., Sun, W., Guan, J., You, I.: Multi-ECGNET for ECG arrhythmia multi-label classification. IEEE Access **8**, 110848–110858 (2020)
14. Li, Y., Zhang, Z., Zhou, F., Xing, Y., Li, J., Liu, C.: Multi-label classification of arrhythmia for long-term electrocardiogram signals with feature learning. IEEE Trans. Instrumen. Measure. **70**, 1–11 (2021)
15. Natarajan, A., et al.: A wide and deep transformer neural network for 12-lead ECG classification. In: 2020 Computing in Cardiology, pp. 1–4 (2020)
16. Ran, A., Ruan, D., Zheng, Y., Liu, H.: Multi-label classification of abnormalities in 12-lead ECG using deep learning. In: 2020 Computing in Cardiology, pp. 1–4 (2020)
17. Rong, P., Luo, T., Li, J., Li, K.: Multi-label disease diagnosis based on unbalanced ECG data. In: 2020 IEEE 9th Data Driven Control and Learning Systems Conference (DDCLS), pp. 253–259 (2020)
18. Salem, M., Taheri, S., Yuan, J.-S.: ECG arrhythmia classification using transfer learning from 2- dimensional deep CNN features. In: 2018 IEEE Biomedical Circuits and Systems Conference (BioCAS), pp. 1–4 (2018)
19. Satija, U., Ramkumar, B., Manikandan, M.S.: A new automated signal quality-aware ECG beat classification method for unsupervised ECG diagnosis environments. IEEE Sensors J. **19**(1), 277–286 (2019)
20. Wang, D., Ge, J., Wu, L., Song, X.: Mining frequent patterns for ECG multi-label data by FP-growth algorithm based on spark. In: 2019 7th International Conference on Information, Communication and Networks (ICICN), pp. 171–174 (2019)
21. Wang, S.-H., Li, H.-T., Wu, A.-Y.A.: Error-resilient reconfigurable boosting extreme learning machine for ECG telemonitoring systems. In: 2018 IEEE International Symposium on Circuits and Systems (ISCAS), pp. 1–5 (2018)

22. Wong, A.W., Salimi, A., Hindle, A., Kalmady, S.V., Kaul, P.: Multilabel 12-lead electrocardiogram classification using beat to sequence autoencoders. In: ICASSP 2021–2021 IEEE International Conference on Acoustics, Speech and Signal Processing (ICASSP), pp. 1270–1274 (2021)

23. Wu, Z., Feng, X., Yang, C.: A deep learning method to detect atrial fibrillation based on continuous wavelet transform. In: 2019 41st Annual International Conference of the IEEE Engineering in Medicine and Biology Society (EMBC), pp. 1908–1912 (2019)

24. Yang, S., Xiang, H., Kong, Q., Wang, C.: Multi-label classification of electrocardiogram with modified residual networks. In: 2020 Computing in Cardiology, pp. 1–4 (2020)

25. Yu, Y., Yang, Z., Li, P., Yang, Z., You, Y.: A real-time ECG classification scheme using anti-aliased blocks with low sampling rate. In: 2020 Computing in Cardiology, pp. 1–4 (2020)

26. Zhu, Z., et al.: Classification of cardiac abnormalities from ECG signals using SE-RESNET. In: 2020 Computing in Cardiology, pp. 1–4 (2020)

27. Torres, J.R., De Los Ríos, K., Padilla, M.A.: Cardiac arrhythmias identification by parallel CNNS and ECG time-frequency representation. In: 2020 Computing in Cardiology, pp. 1–4. IEEE (2020)

28. Smisek, R., Nemcova, A., Marsanova, L., Smital, L., Vitek, M., Kozumplik, J.: Cardiac pathologies detection and classification in 12-lead ECG. In: 2020 Computing in Cardiology, pp. 1–4. IEEE (2020)

29. He, R., et al.: Automatic classification of arrhythmias by residual network and bigru with attention mechanism. In: 2020 Computing in Cardiology, pp. 1–4. IEEE (2020)

30. Wei, G., Zhou, Z.H.: On the consistency of multi-label learning. Artif. Intell. **199**, 22–44 (2013)

31. Wu, X.Z., Zhou, Z.H.: A unified view of multi-label performance measures (2016)

Medical Data Mining (II)

Effective Tensor Based PCA Machine Learning Techniques for Glaucoma Detection and ASPP – EffUnet Classification

K. Venkatachalam[1]($\boxtimes$), Nebojsa Bacanin[2], Enamul Kabir[3], and P. Prabu[4]

[1] Department of Applied Cybernetics, Faculty of Science, University of Hradec Králové,
50003 Hradec Králové, Czech Republic
[2] Department of Computer Science, Singidunum University, 160622 Belgrade, Serbia
[3] School of Sciences, University of Southern Queensland, Toowoomba,
Darling Heights 4350, Australia
[4] Department of Computer Science, CHRIST (Deemed to be University),
Bangalore 560074, India

Abstract. Main problem in current research area focused on generating automatic AI technique to detect bio medical images by slimming the dataset. Reducing the original dataset with actual unwanted noises can accelerate new data which helps to detect diseases with high accuracy. Highest level of accuracy can be achieved only by ensuring accuracy at each level of processing steps. Dataset slimming or reduction is NP hard problems due its resembling variants. In this research work we ensure high accuracy in two phases. In phase one feature selection using Normalized Tensor Tubal PCA (NTT-PCA) method is used. This method is based on tensor with single value decomposition (SVD) for accurate dimensionality reduction problems. The dimensionality reduced output from phase one is further processed for accurate classification in phase two. The classification of affected images is detected using ASPP – EffUnet. The atrous spatial pyramid pooling (ASPP) with efficient convolutional block in Unet is combined to provide ASPP – EffUnet CNN architecture for accurate classification. This two phase model is designed and implemented on benchmark datasets of glaucoma detection. It is processed efficiently by exploiting fundus image in the dataset. We propose novel AI techniques for segmenting the eye discs using EffUnet and perform classification using ASPP-EffUnet techniques. Highest accuracy is achieved by NTT-PCA dimensionality reduction process and ASPP-EffUnet based classification which detects the boundaries of eye cup and optical discs very curiously. Our resulting algorithm "NTT-PCA with ASPP-EffUnet "for dimensionality reduction and classification process which is optimized for reducing computational complexity with existing detection algorithms like PCA-LA-SVM,PCA-ResNet ASPP –Unet. We choose benchmark datasets ORIGA for our experimental analysis. The crucial areas in clinical setup are examined and implemented successfully. The prediction and classification accuracy of proposed technique is achieved nearly 100%.

Keywords: Glaucoma detection · Tensor tubal PCA · ASPP · EffUnet · Convolutional neural network

© Springer Nature Switzerland AG 2021
S. Siuly et al. (Eds.): HIS 2021, LNCS 13079, pp. 181–192, 2021.
https://doi.org/10.1007/978-3-030-90885-0_17

1   Introduction

Intelligent technique for processing large database, observations, biomedical image processing, signal processing, and data mining, hyper spectral image analysis is a big challenge in large information processing era. Today all application requires large volume of data which cannot be processed by matrix techniques, with addition factorizing tensors become important role in extracting latent information. Principal component analysis (PCA) is most widely used approach in image matching and prediction. Even though there are lot of factorization techniques available in image processing, recently tensor based framework as tensor SVD, c-products, third order tensors receives good prediction results in recent image matching research work [1].

Optical neurodegenerative disease called Glaucoma which damages the optic nerves and results in loss of visualization is a dangerous disease in old age. The detection of diseases at early can prevent blindness [1]. Figure 1 shows the significant parts of eyes in optical fundus image. There are more machine learning techniques for processing medical image. But still sensitive portion of diseases are not feasibly identified. This motivates our research on detecting glaucoma in eye very effectively.

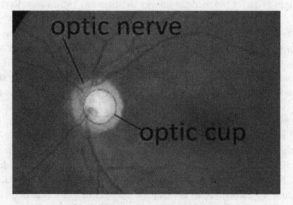

Fig. 1. Optic disc, cup and nerves

Some times miss classification of patients become big issue for prescribing medications. Clinical equipments and expert physicians are limited to access by all over the hospitals. Automatic glaucoma detection will become a low cost solution [2–6]. Screening the rural diseases with traditional complex algorithms results more false positive detections. Quality of the detection is based on the quality of training data. More training data always estimate less quality in outcome. Therefore it is need of automatic detection system with minimum computational power by less training images.

Normalized tensor based PCA is designed [1] with tensor 3 model for accurately matching and detecting the input fundus image which is affected or not. There may be 0.1% error which can be solved with further classification models. Atrous Spatial pyramid polling is a image segmentation module which perform semantic operation during segmentation process. ASPP generates the multiple rate of features layers for resampling. Before convolution process, features at multiple rates are resampled. ASPP uses multiple filters on original images which results in effective feature view. The traditional neural networks resample actual input features, but proposed ASSP perform mapping at multiple atrous convolution layer in parallel at various sampling rate.

The main contribution of the research work is,

- We design ASPP based EffUnet model for biomedical image classification. The main step is segmentation of optic disc and cup. The cup to disc ratio is calculated in image used for classification.
- Finally N-Parameter spatial generative statistical model is designed with EffUnet model for effective disc segmentation and classification.

1.1 Background

As to date hospitals use to diagnose glaucoma with clinical practice. There is a great demand for automatic detection of glaucoma from fundus photos. It is a challenging task in producing accurate detection results. Automatic identification of glaucoma uses two phases [2]: irregularity detection in cup and disc boundaries, second one is using deep learning techniques of artificial intelligence. The second technique has more benefits in achieving good results. Some data is used to train the deep learning model. Then the trained model identifies the input image is affected by glaucoma or not [3]. Though there is satisfied result, still image processing is a big issue in glaucoma detection. A current research concentrates on both dimensionality reductions and deep learning classifier. First dimensionality reduction reduces the features or noises. it slims the data for deep learning process. Secondly innovative deep learning algorithm is used to detect the glaucoma in the input image.

Rest of the article is arranged as follows: Sect. 2 has description about literature survey. Section 3 describes proposed algorithms and techniques. Section 3.2 analyses the results and experimental setup. Section 4 concludes the section with future scope.

2 Related Works

Biomedical images are processed originally using U shaped neural network called U-Net architecture [7]. This architecture has encoder, decoder, up sampling, down sampling, ReLU for activation purposes. Two convolution layers are present in encoder and decoder. Feature maps are splitted and processed in encoder. Later it was concatenated in decoder side. One of adapted version of Unet is Mnet [8]. It is a convolution neural network which process by multi-scaling input layer and output layers. VGG [9] based Ternaus Net in which VGG is used in encoder of Unet model. LinkNet uses ResNet-18 in its encoder section [10]. Instead of concatenation in decoding, it uses residual net -18 for concatenation. ResNet-34 [11] pre-trained as encoder. Main draw back in this model is computationally complex and expensive.

Recently there are many attempts in deep learning for segmenting optic discs and cup. Unet [12] and latest new Mnet uses same segmentation techniques with convolutional network based LSTM. This process executes in bidirectional way [13–15]. Some models provides low memory requirements for segmentation process. In [16–18] novel method of augmentation is used in Unet with variation in contrast. CDED net [19] is used neural network with less expensive framework were feature are reused in encoder and decoder.

The normal eye pressure in human is 12 to 22 mm in mercury component [20]. Due damage of optical fiber, pressure varies in eye [21]. There exists numerous techniques to detect glaucoma [22]. All manual technique are very expensive and require knowledge expertise to detect the diseases. The only preferred solution is automated techniques. Most widely used techniques are, Higher Order Spectra, Principal Component Analysis, Gabor Transform, Discrete Wavelet Transforms etc. [23]. Spectral power feature used to analyze glaucoma with coefficients and machine learning. PCA, Spectral is used to retrieve HOS based parameters and descriptors. Wavelet transform is used by representing its energy as frequency for local region analysis. The short time analyses of fourier transform is gabor transform which uses average, variance etc. for extracting the coefficients. EWT is decomposition techniques based on signal dependent in which spectrum of signal use to detect glaucoma. A feature extraction technique is used for similarity measuring of any two points and selects the color, shape and texture. In the article [24–26] the brain tumor detection is performed by using a dimensionality reduction and convolutional neural network [27–31, 32–34]. This technique achieves better results than the traditional techniques.

3   Proposed NTT-PCA with ASPP-EffUnet Classification and Detection Model

Our supervised automatic glaucoma classification model aims to provide accurate solution for wide spread usage among more bio medical image classification. It performs simple measurement technology for new datasets. Our working methodology is described in this section.

3.1   Proposed Framework

We introduce new AI algorithms in a two stage process as shown in Fig. 2. First the input images are processed using normalized tensor tubal based PCA algorithm (NTT-PCA) for dimensionality reduction of large dataset. This step finds very closest image in training database by matching with test data. Dimensionality reduction step removes all other irrelevant eye images that are not affected by glaucoma. It partially removes noises and unwanted data from input dataset. Now reduced data is fed as input to ASPP-EffUnet model for detecting diseases and classifying the affected image accurately. Finally cup to disc ratio is calculated and it helps to analyze glaucoma image is larger than normal eye image. Cup to disc ratio is calculated using boundaries of cup and disc. Here we

Input 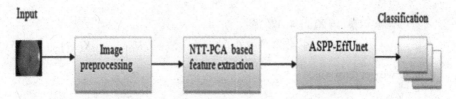 Classification

Fig. 2. Proposed NTT-PCA with ASPP-EffUnet architecture

notice CDR value for 36 direction at 10° differences up to 360°. EffUnet uses this value, so that massive training images does not required in this experiment.

Normalized Tensor Tubal –PCA (NTT-PCA)
Dimensionality reduction process in the image processing widely uses PCA for the feature classification. Some images are converted from color to grey scale for reducing cost of training process. It's not possible to convert all biomedical images, some images require colored for detecting the image. So we choose tensor based approach to process the colored images. In our dataset, glaucoma is detected based on eye color and disc appearance. So color image processing and acquiring high accuracy in classification is big challenge in our research work. Tensor based PCA allows to process improved databases of biomedical images. Important factor to consider here is high computational cost is required for processing massive database. For our image we use tensor product with discrete cosine transformation (DCT) [1].

Let tensor $P \in R^{n1,n2,n3}$ and $S \geq 1$ will be an integer. The tensor golub kahan bidiagonalzation [1] is defined as following computations. Let $A_k = K \times K$ upper matrix of diagonal which is given as,

$$\begin{bmatrix} \alpha_1 & \beta_1 & & & \\ & \alpha_2 & \beta_2 & & \\ & & \ddots & \ddots & \\ & & & \alpha_{k-1} & \beta_{k-1} \\ & & & & \alpha_k \end{bmatrix} \tag{1}$$

Let X_k and $P \times cX_K$ is executed as $(n_2 \times s \times g)$ and $(n_1 \times s \times n_3)$ front slices tensors of input image tensors $X_1 \dots\dots\dots\dots\dots X_k$ and $P \times cX_1 \dots\dots P \times cX_k$ respectively. Further U_k and $P^A \times cU_K$ will be computed from $(n_1 \times s \times n_3)$ and $(n_2 \times s \times n_3)$ for frontal slices of tensors $U_1 \dots\dots\dots\dots\dots U_k$ and $P^A \times cU_1 \dots\dots P^A \times cU_k$. Finally we express,

$$X_k := [X_1 \dots\dots X_k] \text{ and } P \times cX_K := [P \times cX_1 \dots\dots P \times cX_k] \tag{2}$$

$$U_k := [U_1 \dots\dots U_k] \text{ and } P^A \times cU_K := \left[P^A \times cU_1 \dots\dots P^A \times cU_k\right] \tag{3}$$

Final tensor gulab khan strategy gives,

$$P \times cX_K = U_k \circledast A_k \tag{4}$$

$$P^A \times cU_K = X_{k+1} \circledast A_k^{tensors}$$
$$= X_k \circledast A_k^{tensors} + \beta_k \left(H_{n \times s \times g} \ldots \ldots, H_{n1 \times s \times n3}, X_{k+1} \right) \qquad (5)$$

Finally we get tensor as,

$$U_k \circledast A_k = \left[U_k \circledast A_k^1 \ldots \ldots, U_k \circledast A_k^i \right] \qquad (6)$$

Where A_k^i is i^{th} column of A_k matrix.

Algorithm 1: Tensor global golub kahan algorithm for glaucoma prediction

Input: Images

Output: Tensor frontal slices

Step 1: Select tensor $X_1 \in R^{n2, s, n3}$, take modulo 1 for X_1 and set β_0

Step 2: for i=0 to k;

Compute:

a. $U_i = P \times cX_i - \beta_{i-1} U_{i-1}$

b. α_i is modulo 1 of X_1

c. Divide U_i with α_i update as U_i

d. $X_{i+1} = P^A \times cU_i - \times \alpha_i X_i$

e. β_i is modulo 1 of X_{i+1}

f. divide X_{i+1} with β_i update as X_{i+1}

Step 3: End for loop.

From the above tensor, non zero tensors are decomposed using normalization techniques as follows,

Algorithm 2: Normalization

Input: $P \in R^{n1, n2, n3}$ and tolerance TE=0

Output: tensor $\tilde{R}$ and tube fiber f

Step1: set tensor $\tilde{R}$ by computing discrete cosine transform (dct) for modulo 3 in P.

i.e. dct (P,[],3)

Step 2: for j= 1 to n3

$f_j = \| \tilde{R} \|$ of modulo 1;

If $f_j >$ TE, then $\tilde{R}(j) = \tilde{R}(j)/f(j)$

Else generate random tenors from n1, n2 and assign the random number to $\tilde{R}(j)$

F(j) = modulo 1 of $\tilde{R}(j)$;

$\tilde{R}(j) = \tilde{R}(j)/f(j)$;

$f_j = 0$;
End if;

R= dct ($\tilde{R}$,[],3), f= idct(f,[],3)   //decomposition

End for;

This normalization is executed in algorithm 1 for normalizing U_i and X_{i+1}. Based on this Algorithms 1 and 2, they are used for normalized tensor tubal –PCA algorithm and defined in below section.

NTT-PCA

Here we discuss about normalized tensor based PCA method in tensors order of 3 which can used in tough color image recognition like face [1], glaucoma, lungs etc. In matrix, set of Z is considered as number of training images where each pixel encoded in matrix as $n1*n2*n3$ for real tensor RT_i, where $1 < i < Z$. In our case for eye image with RGB, each layer at the frontal slices with encoding $n3 = 3$. Here we have to insert additional features, so contemplate $n3 > 3$ for additional process.

Let us assume one input test image (I_{in}) for training. In image, frontal slices of n3 as I_{in}^j is compressed to single column vectors of $vec\left(I_{in}^j\right)$, which forms length $LN = n1 \times n2$. The tensors are formed as $LN \times 1 \times n3$ with image X_{in} in matrix defined as $X_{in}(-; , -; , j) = vec\left(I_{in}^j\right)$. This procedure is executed by every input training image and obtains T tensors I_{in} with captive size of $LN \times 1 \times n3$. The average tensors of images is defined by, $\tilde{X} = \frac{1}{N}(\sum_{i=1}^{n} X_i)$ [1]. The training tensor $LN \times N \times n3$ is defined as $X = (\widetilde{X_1}, \ldots \ldots \widetilde{X_N})$, where $\widetilde{X_i} = X_i - \tilde{X}$. Next we need to consider SVD decomposition [1] for final tensor size $LN \times N \times n3$. Finally we consider matrix ideology, which uses singular suffice values used to capture the main features in image. This ideology is applied to RGB separately at three color layers. At end, generated values of RGB are approximated using minimum tubal rank tensor. Let us assume tensor for image is $B \in R^{n1 \times n2 \times n3}$ and SVD decomposition result $B = U \times cB \times cV^{tensor}$. Select the integer 'i' such that $i \leq \min(n1, n2)$. Value of B is approximated using i tubal rank tensor. Refer [1] for more details. By reducing singular value, image is truncated and its quality is increased by decreasing singular value rapidly. Based on these idea [1] used truncated tensor directly in c-SVD instead of using whole tensors in c-SVD.

3.2   ASPP-EffUnet Model for Glaucoma Detection

ASPP Model

The ASPP process input images by multi scaling based feature extraction. This high level extraction process impressed to propose Atrous convolutional neural network for glaucoma detection diseases. Glaucoma detection is a tedious job because we need process it with colored image. Due to lack of technology, manual detection is performed and it's more time consuming process. Our proposed ASPP with EffUnet model classify the affected image with high accuracy. In image processing, atrous convolution is defined as shown in Eq. (7)

$$M[i,j] = \sum_{n=1}^{n} k[i + pm.ln, j + pm.ln]x[pm], \tag{7}$$

where M[i, j] is output for the atrous convolution, k[i, j] is input signal, x represents of convolution kernel (filter) with length of ln, and pm represents parameter corresponding to stride with input sample. If we have rate (a) $= 1$, then standard atrous convolution is processed. Figure 2 gives example kernel image of 3 * 3 atrous. target pixel Rate is defined as a $= 1$, 2 and 4. If the eye have mild glaucoma, then rate of sampling will be lower to be 1. If eyes is heavily affected by glaucoma, sampling rate increases and size of atrous also increases.

Finally multi scaling ability are used to generate a feature map [30].

EffUnet Model

Efficient Unet (EffUnet) model is well generated AI technique with two stage architecture as shown in Fig. 2. As implemented in [2], first optic cup and disc segmentation is automatically processed using EffUnet by extracting actual boundaries in optic cup and disc as shown in Fig. 3 (optic disc). Algorithm called SpaGen [2] which is modified with N number of parameters for noise variance (instead of using one or two parameters) with cup-to-disc area ratio (CDAR).

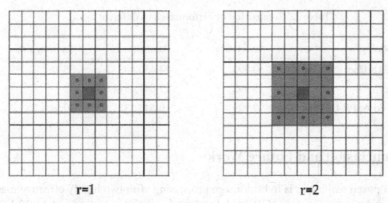

r=1   r=2

Fig. 3. Atrous convolution process in 2D images at rate = 1 and 2. Here, red pixels used to represent the target pixels and the red-dotted Pixels represent the pixels used in convolution. (Color figure online)

ASPP- EffUnet for Segmentation of Optic Disc and Cup

As designed in [2], EffUnet is developed as U shaped convolutional neural network by using encoder as pre-trained efficient net-B1. We joint ASPP model in U net structure which is our new ASPP-EffUnet deep learning network for our proposed work.

The main building blocks used in EfficientNet is mobile inverted based bottleneck convolution MBConv [2]. Additionally optimization with squeeze with excitation step is processed inside the U Net architecture.

In EffNet – B1, decoders blocks are arranged in upsampling network whereas each decoder has upsampling of 2 * 2 2D convolution of previous output with stride 2. The feature map from encoder section is concatenated. After concatenation, output tensor is passed to 2 convolution layer. These layers have exponential linear unit (ExLU) activation function which reduces gradient problems and computational complexity in deep learning networks. ExLU is expressed as,

$$f(p) = \begin{cases} p & (p > 0), \\ p(\exp(x) - 1) & (p < 0) \end{cases} \qquad (8)$$

Feature map is normalized with batch normalization and processed in ExLU. The outcome is fed as input to next decoder block. At end of architecture we have softmax layer to produce output image as similar to input image.

The optic disc and cup segmentation is processed to whole image by removing the black boundaries and resizing image as 512 * 512. The proposed ASPP-EffUnet model computes only less parameter which is lesser than 1.8 times of other models. Also it computes the image very faster than other models. Some comparison model is shown in below Table 1.

Table 1. Comparison of performance of different models

Methodology	Accuracy	Parameters	Training time
ResNet18-Unet	0.996	24,456,443	55
EffUnet	0.998	12,641,411	42
Proposed ASPP-EffUnet	0.999	9,543,233	30

4 Conclusion and Future Work

Our proposed technique is hybrid image processing with two highly effective machine learning algorithms such as NTT-PCA for dimensionality reduction and ASPP-EffUnet for classification model. The slimming the dataset is very challenging issue due its similarity features. Sometime we require intelligent analyzing techniques to adjudge the bio medical images with high accuracy. This algorithm computes good result and performance for ORIGA dataset for detecting glaucoma diseases using CDR and ACDR values of the eye. Fundus image is considered as more flexible and computationally simple for clinical diagnosis. We use this fundus image of detecting glaucoma with two stage architecture. NTT-PCA is first time applied in glaucoma image prediction by dimensionality reduction process. For the best classification we further use automated segmenting with statistical learning approach. The segmented images by proposed AI technique detect shapes of disc and cup and learn eye view with aspect ratio using N-parameter spatial generative algorithm. Every new segmentation pattern is trained in classification model so that accuracy of the classification is 99.99% which higher than other detection algorithm. In future efficient AI model can be identified for reducing the toughness in classification framework.

References

1. Hached, M., Jbilou, K., Koukouvinos, C., Mitrouli, M.: A multidimensional principal component analysis via the C-Product Golub–Kahan–SVD for classification and face recognition. Mathematics. **9**(11), 1249 (2021)
2. Krishna Adithya, V., et al.: EffUnet-SpaGen: an efficient and spatial generative approach to glaucoma detection. J. Imaging **7**(6), 92 (2021)
3. Divya, L., Jacob, J.: Performance analysis of glaucoma detection approaches from fundus images. Procedia Comput. Sci. **143**, 544–551 (2018)
4. Christopher, M., et al.: Retinal nerve fiber layer features identified by unsupervised machine learning on optical coherence tomography scans predict glaucoma progression. Invest. Ophthalmol. Vis. Sci. **59**(7), 2748–2756 (2018)
5. Wang, Z.-Y., Xia, Q.-M., Yan, J.-W., Xuan, S.-Q., Su, J.-H., Yang, C.-F.: Hyperspectral image classification based on spectral and spatial information using multi-scale ResNet. Appl. Sci. **9**(22), 4890 (2019)
6. Rossetti, L., et al.: Blindness and glaucoma: a multicenter data review from 7 academic eye clinics. PloS one **10**(8), e0136632 (2015)
7. Balyen, L., Peto, T.: Promising artificial intelligence-machine learning-deep learning algorithms in ophthalmology. Asia-Pac. J. Ophthalmol. **8**(3), 264–272 (2019)

8. Li, Z., He, Y., Keel, S., Meng, W., Chang, R.T., He, M.: Efficacy of a deep learning system for detecting glaucomatous optic neuropathy based on color fundus photographs. Ophthalmology **125**(8), 1199–1206 (2018)

9. Li, L., Xu, M., Liu, H., Li, Y., Wang, X., Jiang, L., et al.: A large-scale database and a CNN model for attention-based glaucoma detection. IEEE Trans. Med. Imaging **39**(2), 413–424 (2019)

10. MacCormick, I.J., et al.: Accurate, fast, data efficient and interpretable glaucoma diagnosis with automated spatial analysis of the whole cup to disc profile. PloS one **14**(1), e0209409 (2019)

11. Schmidt-Erfurth, U., Sadeghipour, A., Gerendas, B.S., Waldstein, S.M., Bogunović, H.: Artificial intelligence in retina. Prog. Retin. Eye Res. **67**, 1–29 (2018)

12. Ronneberger, O., Fischer, P., Brox, T.: U-net: convolutional networks for biomedical image segmentation. In: Navab, N., Hornegger, J., Wells, W., Frangi, A. (eds.) MICCAI 2015. LNCS, vol 9351, pp 234-241. Springer, Cham. https://doi.org/10.1007/978-3-319-24574-4_28

13. Fu, H., Cheng, J., Xu, Y., Wong, D.W.K., Liu, J., Cao, X.: Joint optic disc and cup segmentation based on multi-label deep network and polar transformation. IEEE Trans. Med. Imaging **37**(7), 1597–1605 (2018)

14. Iglovikov, V., Shvets, A.: TernausNet: U-net with VGG11 encoder pre-trained on imagenet for image segmentation. arXiv prerint. arXiv preprint arXiv:180105746 (2018)

15. Chaurasia, A., Culurciello, E.: LinkNet: exploiting encoder representations for efficient semantic segmentation. In: 2017 IEEE Visual Communications and Image Processing (VCIP). IEEE (2017)

16. Kumar, E.S., Bindu, C.S.: Two-stage framework for optic disc segmentation and estimation of cup-to-disc ratio using deep learning technique. J. Ambient Intell. Humaniz. Comput. 1–13 (2021)

17. Khan, M.K., Anwar, S.M. (eds.): M-Net with bidirectional ConvLSTM for cup and disc segmentation in fundus images. In: 2020 IEEE-EMBS Conference on Biomedical Engineering and Sciences (IECBES). IEEE (2021)

18. Imtiaz, R., Khan, T.M., Naqvi, S.S., Arsalan, M., Nawaz, S.J.: Screening of Glaucoma disease from retinal vessel images using semantic segmentation. Comput. Electr. Eng. **91**, 107036 (2021)

19. Tabassum, M., et al.: CDED-Net: joint segmentation of optic disc and optic cup for glaucoma screening. IEEE Access. **8**, 102733–102747 (2020)

20. Shen, S.Y., et al.: The prevalence and types of glaucoma in Malay people: the Singapore Malay eye study. Invest. Ophthalmol. Vis. Sci. **49**(9), 3846–3851 (2008)

21. Nyúl, L.G. (ed.): Retinal image analysis for automated glaucoma risk evaluation. In: Medical Imaging, Parallel Processing of Images, and Optimization Techniques, MIPPR 2009. International Society for Optics and Photonics (2009)

22. Borgalli, R.A., Gautam, H.P., Parayil, W.G.: Automated glaucoma detection techniques using fundus image. Int. J. Technol. Enhanc. Emerg. Eng. Res. **3**(12), 1–8 (2015)

23. Kolář, R., Jan, J.: Detection of glaucomatous eye via color fundus images using fractal dimensions. Radioengineering. **17**(3), 109–114 (2008)

24. Sadiq, M.T., Yu, X., Yuan, Z.: Exploiting dimensionality reduction and neural network techniques for the development of expert brain–computer interfaces. Expert Syst. Appl. **164**, 114031 (2021)

25. Sadiq, M.T., Yu, X., Yuan, Z., Aziz, M.Z., Siuly, S., Ding, W.: A matrix determinant feature extraction approach for decoding motor and mental imagery EEG in subject specific tasks. IEEE Trans. Cogn. Dev. Syst. (2020)

26. Sarki, R., Ahmed, K., Wang, H., Zhang, Y.: Automated detection of mild and multi-class diabetic eye diseases using deep learning. Health Inf. Sci. Syst. **8**(1), 1–9 (2020). https://doi.org/10.1007/s13755-020-00125-5

27. Supriya, S., Siuly, S., Wang, H., Zhang, Y.: Automated epilepsy detection techniques from electroencephalogram signals: a review study. Health Inf. Sci. Syst. **8** (1), 1–15 (2020)

28. Du, J., Michalska, S., Subramani, S., Wang, H., Zhang, Y.: Neural attention with character embeddings for hay fever detection from Twitter. Health Inf. Sci. Syst. **7**(1), 1–7 (2019). https://doi.org/10.1007/s13755-019-0084-2

29. He, J., Rong, J., Sun, L., Wang, H., Zhang, Y., Ma, J.: A framework for cardiac arrhythmia detection from IoT-based ECGs. World Wide Web **23**(5), 2835–2850 (2020). https://doi.org/10.1007/s11280-019-00776-9

30. Jiang, H., Zhou, R., Zhang, L., Wang, H., Zhang, Y.: Sentence level topic models for associated topics extraction. World Wide Web **22**(6), 2545–2560 (2019)

31. Li, H., Wang, Y., Wang, H., Zhou, B.: Multi-window based ensemble learning for classification of imbalanced streaming data. World Wide Web **20**(6), 1507–1525 (2017). https://doi.org/10.1007/s11280-017-0449-x

DEPRA: An Early Depression Detection Analysis Chatbot

Payam Kaywan$^{(\boxtimes)}$, Khandakar Ahmed, Yuan Miao, Ayman Ibaida, and Bruce Gu

Intelligent Technology Innovation Lab (ITIL), Institute for Sustainable Industries and Liveable Cities (ISILC), Victoria University, Melbourne, Australia
{payam.kaywan,Khandakar.ahmed,yuan.miao,ayman.ibaida,bruce.gu}@vu.edu.au

Abstract. The application of Artificial Intelligence (AI) in the assessment and treatment of mental health has gained momentum in recent years due to the evidential development of chatbots. There are promising outcomes from recent attempts such as facilitation to detect the depression level in patients' profiles, which have improved the aspiration of finding a solution to assist medical professionals in detecting depression. However, experts believe the promise is still far from the expectations since most of the chatbots found in literature has conscious decision from selectable answer. In addition, the participants are required to have longer period of the interactions with the chatbot which suffer great losses of the participation. Furthermore, the user privacy and scientific evaluations of early depression detection are not guaranteed due to the customized chatbot platforms. Motivated by these, we proposed and developed DEPRA based on contemporary bot platforms with early depression detection to tackle the mental health symptoms. DEPRA is built on Dialogflow as a conversation interface and uses personalized utterances collected from a focused group to train it. Moreover, the interaction time was reduced remarkably by the setup of DEPRA. A structured early detection depression interview guide for the Hamilton Depression Scale (SIGH-D) and Inventory of Depressive Symptomatology (IDS-C) underpins the formation. DEPRA can act as the proxy between the health professional and the patient. Moreover, the DEPRA integrated with social network platform which provide convenience of the attractions for the participants. More than 40 participants interact with DEPRA and the analysis of their response establishes the promise of its use in mass screening for early detection of depression. User experience survey demonstrates that the overall user satisfaction level is approbatory.

Keywords: Chatbot · Conversational system · Depression analysis · User experience

1 Introduction

In this research, we establish the trend on early detection of depression to target the best momentum to tackle the issue. Suicidal trends are significantly increas-

S. Siuly et al. (Eds.): HIS 2021, LNCS 13079, pp. 193–204, 2021.
https://doi.org/10.1007/978-3-030-90885-0_18

ing among young and aged women in countries with low and middle salaries and these statistics have reached approximately 800,000 cases annually [8]. Intentional self-harm remains one of the top five leading causes of death among Australians aged between 15 and 44, with the lowest median age of death at 43.9 [2]. Therefore, the early depression detection analysis has compulsory beneficial with early warnings for the behaviours such as suicidal thoughts, self-harm and mental health. The chatbots are recently receiving remarkable consideration by the societies as they bring three major advantages to the medical world: a) reducing the gap between the available resources compared to the number of people, b) mitigating the risk caused by the social stigma, and c) addressing the fear of being judged by others. As the concept of Artificial Intelligence (AI) and the technology beneath it are in its initial formation it is considered that more studies are required to prove the possibility of applying these technologies. So far, revealing personal and health details have not been reported but there are concerns that chatbots might be a breaching hole.

A systematic literature review identifies ten studies conducted over the last half decade [18]. Most of the chatbots cited in the literature focus on delivering cognitive behavioural therapy (CBT), tracking the adherence of physical activity and medication, and healthy lifestyle recommendations. By AI early depression detection participants can benefit from medical treatments. With DEPRA, the requirement of early depression detection is at the focus of this research. We are aware that if the depression is detected at early stages there are hopes to cure the patients. Besides, it removes the reliance on a short set of multiple choice responses and includes open-ended responses for the participants. Moreover, DEPRA chatbot study duration is approximately 30 min for each participant. Another aspect of DERPRA is that it is benefiting from scoring systems. SIGH-D [23] and IDS-C [2] are based on medical psychiatrist achievements where a set of questions are shared with the patients to rate the severity of their depression. As a result, DEPRA can detect depression levels by probing mood, feelings of guilt, suicide ideation, insomnia, agitation or retardation, anxiety, weight change, and somatic symptoms. The contribution of this paper can be summarized as below:

- DEPRA is capable of assisting participants to find out about their mental health and medical professionals to realize their role in achieving the cure for the patients who are suffering from depression.
- Implementing a conversation flow based on the structured interview guide for SIGH-D and IDS-C which is derived from the experience of a group of psychiatrists. This makes DEPRA chatbot a unique chatbot that shares the same stem of clinically proved questions.
- The validity of the questions used in the DEPRA chatbot has been measured by applying closed group participation. This is arranged by designing open-ended questions for the participants. Regarding social media, DEPRA is benefiting from integration with Facebook Messenger. So, the participants can interact with the chatbot through social media to share their responses.
- DEPRA takes approximately 30 min to complete. As the results suggested there are high satisfaction rates reported by the participants in relevance to

the responses. The questions were easy to comprehend and respond to, not as time consuming as a real psychiatrist session, text messaging via social media platforms has a higher degree of preference compared to talking in a consultation session.

The rest of the paper is organized as follows. In Sect. 2, the Related Work will be discussed. In Sect. 3, Methodology will be briefly presented. In Sect. 4, Experiment and Results are elaborated. Finally, Sect. 5 will discuss the Conclusion and Future Works.

2   Related Work

Contemporary mental health bots built using conversational agents over the last half decade aims to a) provide psychosocial intervention in improving mental health, life-style or work efficiency and b) identify depression and its level in patients. The experiment duration time is considered a feature for any chatbots when it is less than one week. The reason behind this feature is that the participants would not be monitored for long durations and this can create a hassle to track the participants when they should have self-control over the research which in some cases it would be impossible to track the trend and it results in inaccurate consequences.

2.1   Psychosocial Intervention

In this section, we will discuss different intervention types and the chatbots. Regarding the work that has been conducted in this area so far, Ly et al. [4] conducted research to measure the effectiveness of smartphone apps in the CBT interventions. Shim chatbot considered 28 participants including males and females and it was based on a text-only method of collecting data. The same as Woebot [6] which offers the CBT, Sharma et al. [12] designed a chatbot for CBT. The focus of this chatbot is on the depression level of the participants. Gardiner et al. [7] studied urban women to consider the possibility of applying Embodied Conversational Agent (ECA) to implement changes in their lifestyle. By using 3D Gabby chatbot, the participants, mainly women, were divided into 2 categories: a) an ECA which included mindfulness, stress management, physical activities during the day and eating habits. b) The same as the first group but with the mediation to be considered daily for one month. By the end of the research, some women reduced the average level of drinking alcohol in order to control their stress level and they managed to consume more fruits in their daily diet.

Within another research by Bickmore et al. [3], the Laura chatbot was designed to use a 3D environment for a patient's hospital discharge plan. The goal was to how hospitalized patients would react to a chatbot when they were at the stage of being discharged from the hospital. The patients declared a high rate of satisfaction regarding the easiness of using the chatbot, fluency of receiving discharge information from the agent compared to the medical staff. Besides, Podrazhansky et al. [11] design a chatbot mobile app for mental health. It is meant to collect data from the users in natural ways such as text, voice, or video. Machine learning algorithms along with NLP applied to locate a mental disorder and offer prevention methods. Besides, Sharma et al. [13] reveals a chatbot designed to predict and manage stress. Continued stress can be the main cause of some serious illnesses such as headaches, heart attacks and depression. In another study, Tielman et al. [16] promoted a therapy system 3MR2 that includes a digital diary and a 3D WorldBuilder where patients can recreate their traumatic memories intending to treat posttraumatic stress disorder (PTSD). All of the participants had previous PTSD follow up therapies. The digital agent unlike a therapist has limitations to steer a conversation and bring patients back on track during a therapy session.

Lucas et al. [9] mention two studies with the same 3D chatbot. This chatbot is used as a consultant to deal with military veterans with PTSD symptoms. Another study by Tielman et al. [6] revealed the fact that whether verbal or text-based psychoeducation is more effective for improving adherence where text-based agents result in higher adherence than voice-based agents. Moreover, Shinozaki et al. [14] considered IT employees in a study to analyse anxiety and emotional problems that they face as the consequence of the low success rate of development projects. A study by Kharel et al. [14] considered early detection of depression with the aid of machine learning (ML) that was performed on patients' MRI images. Due to limitations in the small dataset, the experiment, the use of ML algorithms and features were restricted.

2.2 Early Depression Detection

As recommended by Akbari et al. [1] late depression detection can lead to suicidal trends in the patients. A computer-aided mechanism should be applied for early depression detection. Another phase of the Tielman et al. [17] research focuses on depression detection. Participants were advised to describe one of their unpleasant memories and explain their experiences on that memory in a digital note after being assisted with verbal or textual psychoeducation guidance. As a result, it was concluded that the presentation of psychoeducation via text provided more adherence rather than verbal presentation. More research has been conducted by Bickmore et al. [4] with the aid of Laura 3D chatbot. Antipsychotic medicine adherence and change in lifestyle of patients suffering from schizophrenia was examined. Regarding Philip et al. [10], research was conducted with 179 participants for a period of one day participation. A 3D chatbot was used to benefit from Embodied Conversational Agents (ECAs) which are software with high potential but they have not been used more often in the studies of mental disorders. There were two goals for this study: a) testing efficiency of diagnostic system related to major depressive disorders (MDD). b) evaluation of acceptability on ECA. As the conclusion of this study, it is derived that ECAs have a high potential to be utilized for standard and wellperformed applications in the interviews [5].

According to the related work, most of the chatbots are designed for therapeutic purposes and there is not sufficient work related to early depression detection. DEPRA is considered a unique chatbot that has been specifically designed for fulfilling the goal of early depression detection. In this research, we focus on the features of DEPRA and its capabilities as an early depression detection chatbot. With the aid of Dialogflow, we have designed and implemented a chatbot that can assist the participants to reflect their emotions into the chatbot. As mentioned before, it is critical to detect depression at early stages to create hopes to cure the mental disorder when it comes to medical professionals attention. This research and its achievements such as open-ended questions, closed group participation, experiment duration and following structured interview guide generate a basis to collect the data from participants to make sure they are supported by medical professionals when it is required. If the participants are diagnosed with the symptoms there would be consultation sessions as well as medical support to overcome the clinical symptoms [15].

3   Methodology

In this section, we have designed the DEPRA as an agent under Dialogflow. The participant has access to its smartphone, laptop, desktop or other devices. Facebook Messenger is a connection between the participant and the agent. In order to establish the connectivity, the agent, in this case DEPRA, which has been designed in Dialogflow under Google Cloud and Node.js receives a record from the participant by Facebook Messenger. At the backend, the agent will save the data into AWS database. In order to create and modify the tables in database, we have applied MySQL Workbench client. The AWS Educate is the core database which saves all the records when the interaction takes place between the agent and the participant. Figure 1 summarizes the general trend of the process:

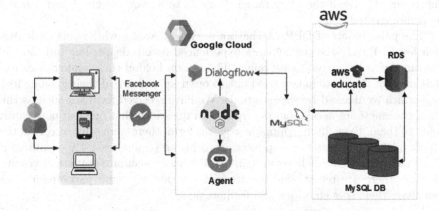

Fig. 1. DEPRA chatbot design and implementation schema

3.1   Conversation Design

DEPRA has been implemented on the Dialogflow platform as a conversational environment for communication and interaction between the bot and the participants. The analysis of the responses from the potential patients and the participants, in general, makes it possible to have a review of the participants and derive the symptoms rating scale out of the set of responses. In order to design the conversation, we developed a conceptual model with 27 psychometric questions. One of the key features of the DEPRA chatbot is the time duration in which the participants should allocate to fulfil the experiment. DEPRA chatbot study duration is approximately 30 min interaction with the participants. The DEPRA chatbot is based on scoring systems. Two scoring systems are applied to the results of the DEPRA chatbot; Inventory of Depressive Symptomatology Self-Rated (IDS-SR) and Quick Inventory of Depressive Symptomatology Self-Rated (QIDS-SR). One of the major features of this chatbot is the open-ended responses. Then, their responses are manually scored. Moreover, it is possible to pass the parameters from one intent to another intent. Input and output contexts are tools in DEPRA so the parameters are passed internally.

The flowchart in Fig. 2 illustrates the design of conversational flow and how the sequence of questions deal with the depression symptoms such as mood, reactivity of mood, outlook and so forth. The sequence commences with a question: "How have you been feeling since last week?". Then, according to the response, a value between 0 to 3 allocates to the score of this specific question. The range of the scores are graded according to 0 for unlikely and 3 for very severe. The score would be saved in a parameter and the trend continues to the next questions. The same scoring method will be applied from 0 to 3 range. When all the 27 questions are answered by the participant for each symptom, the overall score will be calculated. If the overall score is less than 13, there would be no depression for the participant. If the score is between 13 and 25 mild depression result will be generated. The range between 25 and 38 demonstrates moderate depression. Moreover, the score range between 38 and 48 generates severe depression. Lastly, if the score ranges from 48 to 84 very severe depression will be demonstrated.

The participants of DEPRA chatbot survey showed a wide range of depression levels. Rarely the participants experienced severe depression and most of the range was in the moderate range. The reason behind these statistics can be that most of the participants tried not to open up and reveal their genuine feelings which were asked by the questions. We have received feedback such as this chatbot sometimes asks about very personal questions that one can not readily reply to them. Even after signing the consent form, there were some uncertainties about privacy and how the responses are going to be analyzed. By encouraging more participants we believe we can achieve more accurate statistical results. Besides, there are remarkable opportunities to attract more participants who can share their true emotions and feelings.

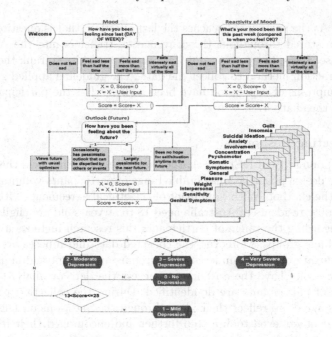

Fig. 2. Design of the chatbot conversational flow

3.2 Implementation and Integration

As the first step in the implementation phase of building the virtual agent, the concept of intent in the Dialogflow platform was addressed. For each question, we required an intent to be defined. Intents consist of training phrases, actions, parameters, responses, contexts and events. Dialogflow contexts are similar to natural language contexts. In our case, input and output contexts were used to manage the flow of conversation and to pass the value of parameters in the code. We use inline editor to develop and deploy the code and the service within Dialogflow platform. Furthermore, one of the significant features of the DEPRA chatbot is the open-ended way of responding to the questions. With the input and output contexts, we can receive or pass the parameters to the other intents respectively. This can be crucial in the design phase as we should be able to have control over the parameters.

Following the implementation and deployment, we have configured a Facebook messaging app and integrated Facebook Messenger with Dialogflow. To complete the integration the Facebook Messenger Platform was used to create a messaging app and to configure the integration between the Facebook app and the Dialogflow to send messages to the end-user through the Facebook Messenger API. Facebook Messenger was chosen as the proxy due to its popularity around the world and benefiting from most population of active users compared to other platforms such as WhatsApp, We Chat and so forth. When a participant interacts with DEPRA by sending a message on Facebook, a mutual conversation takes place. As the participant reaches the last question, that is question number 27, the data stored throughout the conversation transfers into the AWS Educate database. Then, the participants have the opportunity to rank the DEPRA and its interaction method to collect the data. The guideline applied guarantees that the symptoms of depression have been addressed as the participants make progress on the chatbot.

3.3 Collecting Responses

Due to the popularity of DEPRA chatbot and its user friendliness that was the result of the design phase, a considerable range of participants voluntarily interacted with the chatbot. With fulfillment of the ethical agreements with Victoria University, only residents of Australia aged 18 to 80 years old are eligible to participate. Regarding the range of participants this research includes a variety of genders and age groups. Moreover, the collected data and reposes are stored in an AWS Educate database under secure circumstances. Only administrator of the research group have the authority to access the data or analyze the data. The details of participants are de-identified. During the collection phases, the participants agreed to reflect their ideas through the questions on DEPRA and the several contacts even took a step further and encouraged their friends and family who were eligible to be a part of the experiment. As per the initial plan, a closed group was considered. As the participants follow the questions and they answer through by reaching the final question they will receive a greeting message as well as a link to the evaluation form where they have the opportunity to fulfil the user experience survey.

3.4 Database

Regarding the database for this study, we benefit from Amazon Web Services (AWS) Educate database. To connect to this database we are using MySQL Workbench as an integrated development environment to manage the database using a structured query language (SQL). As per the ethics policy of the research, the participants' information was de-identified and stored in separate tables. Regarding ranking, the manual scores were analysed based on two methods: IDS-SR and QIDS-SR. In the IDS-SR method, we evaluate each response on a scale of 0 to 3 by following SIGH-D and IDS-C. Then, the total score for each participant was calculated. For the QIDS-SR method, a summation of different categories is added upon a scale of 0 to 3. However, for three psychometric themes related to sleep symptoms (4 items), weight symptoms (4 items) and psychomotor symptoms (2 items), only the highest and maximum score on each theme should be used for calculation.

4   Experiment and Results

In this section, we discuss the experimental results that were generated throughout the research progress. Further explanations are provided regarding participants and user satisfaction.

4.1 Participants

The prerequisites for the participants to be a part of this study are to be a resident of Australia, at the time of taking the responses, and to age between 18 to 80 years old. Moreover, Fig. 3 proves both the IDS-SR method and QIDS-SR method will result in the same level of accuracy for the analysis. The difference in the score range is based on the fact that IDS-SR and QIDS-SR are applying different ranges to consider the level of depression to discover the severity of the depression in any participants groups.

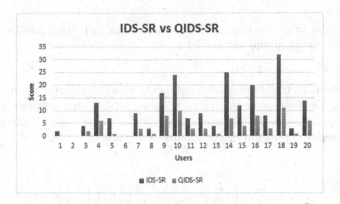

Fig. 3. Comparison of severity for IDS-SR and QIDS-SR.

4.2 User Satisfaction Analysis

A ranking form has been designed and it was included as a link to the data collection phase. After participants finalized their interaction with the chatbot, this ranking form link was offered to them. A range of 5 questions as well as an open-ended question was shared with the participants. Question 1 concerned if the set of questions in DEPRA chatbot are easy to comprehend and respond. Question 2 demonstrates the time spent on the survey compared to a real psychiatrist session. Question 3 discussed if the participants feel more comfortable answering the questions and use text messaging compared to talking to a psychiatrist. Question 4 mentioned if the sequence of questions directs them to share the severity of their health specifically the level of depression. Question 5 checked with the participants if they recommend this survey participation to their friends, colleague or acquaintances. As mentioned earlier, question 6 was an open-ended question concerning any more comments from the participants.

Comparison between IDS-SR and QIDS-SR along with the severity of depression according to age group and gender of the participants are displayed. Despite the severity of 2, moderate, for males in their 20 s, in most of the other age groups and genders, the ratio remained as 1, mild, for the rest of the groups. As a result,

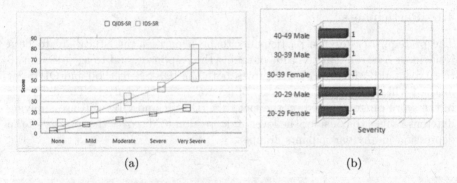

(a)   (b)

Fig. 4. Severity of depression: (a) Total score ranges in IDS-SR and QIDS-SR; (b) Total number in age groups and gender.

males between 20 to 29 are considered as the most vulnerable group that more researchers for depression should be targeted within this sensitive age group. Figure 4 (a) compares the two methods of scoring and Fig. 4 (b) summarizes the severity level of depression in age groups and genders.

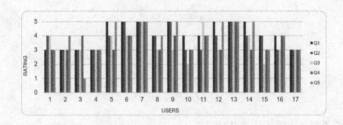

Fig. 5. Participants rating.

Access to electronic healthcare systems looks to be a necessity, so this paper is contributing to fulfilling this gap and provides a platform that anyone can interact with a chatbot. DEPRA chatbot has been designed to complete this task. In addition, one of the participants recommended that a reply after every answer would provide a more human element interaction when dealing with the DEPRA chatbot. In Fig. 5 the summary of rating by the participants are shown.

5   Conclusion and Future Works

As the role of DEPRA chatbot and its ability to collect data from participants were examined, it is concluded that chatbots can be applied to collect data and assist medical science with the application of early detection of depression. By collecting data from participants they can share their symptoms with a chatbot and as per the initial analysis the severity of depression, if it exists, will be determined. The suggestions to contact a psychiatrist and pursing further medical consultations will be shared with the participants. The next step would be to locate more participants to enrich our dataset with more responses and more relevant expressions to be supplied by the participants. We have 25 participants and we are seeking more people to participate.

As we generated our dataset by using the DEPRA chatbot, the future work will be to expand the number of participants and create a more robust dataset with various responses from the participants. Our future works will focus on automatic scoring methods based on Natural Language Processing (NLP) and sentiment analysis. A more precise and comprehensive open-ended conversational chatbot will be developed.

References

1. Akbari, H., Sadiq, M.T., Payan, M., Esmaili, S.S., Baghri, H., Bagheri, H.: Depression detection based on geometrical features extracted from SODP shape of EEG signals and binary PSO. Traitement du Signal **38**(1), 13–26 (2021). https://doi.org/10.18280/ts.380102
2. Australia, Y.B.: Australian bureau of statistics. Canberra, Australia 161 (2008)
3. Bickmore, T.W., Mitchell, S.E., Jack, B.W., Paasche-Orlow, M.K., Pfeifer, L.M., ODonnell, J.: Response to a relational agent by hospital patients with depressive symptoms. Interact. Comput. **22**(4), 289–298 (2010). https://doi.org/10.1016/j.intcom.2009.12.001
4. Bickmore, T.W., Puskar, K., Schlenk, E.A., Pfeifer, L.M., Sereika, S.M.: Maintaining reality: Relational agents for antipsychotic medication adherence. Interact. Comput. **22**(4), 276–288 (2010). https://doi.org/10.1016/j.intcom.2010.02.001
5. Cacheda, F., Fernandez, D., Novoa, F.J., Carneiro, V., et al.: Early detection of depression: social network analysis and random forest techniques. J. Med. Internet Res. **21**(6), e12554 (2019). https://doi.org/10.2196/12554
6. Fitzpatrick, K.K., Darcy, A., Vierhile, M.: Delivering cognitive behavior therapy to young adults with symptoms of depression and anxiety using a fully automated conversational agent (WOEBOT): a randomized controlled trial. JMIR Ment. Health **4**(2), e19 (2017)
7. Gardiner, P.M., et al.: Engaging women with an embodied conversational agent to deliver mindfulness and lifestyle recommendations: a feasibility randomized control trial. Patient Educ. Counseling **100**(9), 1720–1729 (2017). https://doi.org/10.1016/j.pec.2017.04.015
8. INITIATIVE, S., TARGET, W.G.: Universal health coverage for mental health
9. Lucas, G.M., et al.: Reporting mental health symptoms: Breaking down barriers to care with virtual human interviewers. Front. Robot. AI **4**, 51 (2017)
10. Philip, P., et al.: Virtual human as a new diagnostic tool, a proof of concept study in the field of major depressive disorders. Sci. Rep. **7**(1), 1–7 (2017)
11. Podrazhansky, A., Zhang, H., Han, M., He, S.: A chatbot-based mobile application to predict and early-prevent human mental illness. In: Proceedings of the 2020 ACM Southeast Conference, pp. 311–312. ACM SE 2020, Association for Computing Machinery, New York, NY, USA (2020). https://doi.org/10.1145/3374135.3385319

12. Sharma, B., Puri, H., Rawat, D.: Digital psychiatry-curbing depression using therapy chatbot and depression analysis. In: 2018 Second International Conference on Inventive Communication and Computational Technologies (ICICCT), pp. 627–631. IEEE (2018)
13. Sharma, T., Parihar, J., Singh, S.: Intelligent chatbot for prediction and management of stress. In: 2021 11th International Conference on Cloud Computing, Data Science Engineering (Confluence), pp. 937–941 (2021). https://doi.org/10.1109/Confluence51648.2021.9377091
14. Shinozaki, T., Yamamoto, Y., Tsuruta, S.: Context-based counselor agent for software development ecosystem. Computing **97**(1), 3–28 (2015)
15. Stankevich, M., Latyshev, A., Kuminskaya, E., Smirnov, I., Grigoriev, O.: Depression detection from social media texts. In: Data Analytics and Management in Data Intensive Domains: I International Conference DADID/RCDL 2019, pp. 352–496 (2019)
16. Tielman, M.L., Neerincx, M.A., Bidarra, R., Kybartas, B., Brinkman, W.P.: A therapy system for post-traumatic stress disorder using a virtual agent and virtual storytelling to reconstruct traumatic memories. J. Med. Syst. **41**(8), 1–10 (2017). https://doi.org/10.1007/s10916-017-0771-y
17. Tielman, M.L., Neerincx, M.A., van Meggelen, M., Franken, I., Brinkman, W.P.: How should a virtual agent present psychoeducation? Influence of verbal and textual presentation on adherence. Technol. Health Care Official J. Eur. Soc. Eng. Med. **25**(6), 1081–1096 (2017)
18. Vaidyam, A.N., Wisniewski, H., Halamka, J.D., Kashavan, M.S., Torous, J.B.: Chatbots and conversational agents in mental health: a review of the psychiatric landscape. Canadian J. Psych. Revue. canadienne de psychiatrie **64**(7), 456–464 (2019). https://doi.org/10.1177/0706743719828977

Machine Learning Algorithm for Analysing Infant Mortality in Bangladesh

Atikur Rahman[1]([✉])(iD), Zakir Hossain[2](iD), Enamul Kabir[3](iD),
and Rumana Rois[1](iD)

[1] Department of Statistics, Jahangirnagar University, Dhaka, Bangladesh
{arahman,rois}@juniv.edu
[2] Department of Statistics, University of Dhaka, Dhaka, Bangladesh
zakir.hossain@du.ac.bd
[3] School of Sciences, University of Southern Queensland, Toowoomba, Australia
Enamul.Kabir@usq.edu.au

Abstract. The study aims to investigate the potential predictors associated with infant mortality in Bangladesh through machine learning (ML) algorithm. Data on infant mortality of 26145 children were extracted from the latest Bangladesh Demographic and Health Survey 2017–18. The Boruta algorithm was used to extract important features of infant mortality. We adapted decision tree, random forest, support vector machine and logistic regression approaches to explore predictors of infant mortality. Performances of these techniques were evaluated via parameters of confusion matrix and receiver operating characteristics curve. The proportion of infant mortality was 9.7% (2523 out of 26145). Age at first marriage, age at first birth, birth interval, place of residence, administrative division, religion, education of parents, body mass index, gender of child, children ever born, exposure of media, wealth index, birth order, occupation of mother, toilet facility and cooking fuel were selected as significant features of predicting infant mortality. Overall, the random forest (accuracy = 0.893, precision = 0.715, sensitivity = 0.339, specificity = 0.979, F1-score = 0.460, area under the curve: AUC = 0.6613) perfectly and authentically predicted the infant mortality compared with other ML techniques, including individual and interaction effects of predictors. The significant predictors may help the policy-makers, stakeholders and mothers to take initiatives against infant mortality by improving awareness, community-based educational programs and public health interventions.

Keyword: Machine learning, boruta algorithm, random forest, auc.

1 Introduction

Infant mortality is defined as the death of infants during the first year of their life [1]. Infant mortality is a key health indicator to assess the progress of child

© Springer Nature Switzerland AG 2021
S. Siuly et al. (Eds.): HIS 2021, LNCS 13079, pp. 205–219, 2021.
https://doi.org/10.1007/978-3-030-90885-0_19

health and the development of a country. One of the important millennium development goals (MDGs) is to reduce child mortality, particularly infant mortality, all over the world [2]. Globally, 4.0 million infants died within the first year of life in 2018 which accounts for 75% of all under-five deaths. The infant mortality rate has reduced worldwide to 29 deaths in 2018 from 65 per 1000 live births in 1990 [3].

In Bangladesh, the infant mortality rate has decreased to 38 in the year 2014 from 87 in 1993 [4]. The reduction in infant mortality by two-thirds of a country indicating the progress towards achieves the MDG-4 [5]. To meet the sustainable development goals (SDGs), reducing the infant mortality rate will make a significant contribution to improving children's health. Bangladesh is far away from achieving the target to get down infant mortality by 5 deaths per 1000 live births [4, 6].

A number of studies examined the causes and investigated the potential factors affecting infant mortality. It was reported that the factors related to mothers like her education had a significant positive impact on infant mortality [7,8]. It was also noted that the infant mortality was significantly higher in mothers who did not attend antenatal care follow up during pregnancy [9,10]. A short birth interval between two pregnancies was a highly significant determinant for infant mortality [11]. Moreover, maternal age, multiple births, domestic violence, place of residence, preterm, and having metabolic disorders were identified as statistically significant determinants associated with infant mortality [12–16].

Infant mortality is the consequence of various socio-economic and demographic factors, including factors related to infants themselves. Low birth weight of infants was one of the most important determinants of infant mortality [9,17,18]. Infant mortality was significantly higher among mothers from low income families than those who belong to middle and rich families [11]. In Bangladesh, infant mortality was significantly higher among mothers who give their births at home instead of health centre and also belong to the class of lower income groups [4,19]. Antenatal care during pregnancy, wealth status, birth size at the time of delivery, and gender of child were potential risk factors for higher rate of infant mortality [4]. A recent study reported that the higher educational attainments of mothers were the protective factors of infant mortality in Bangladesh [18].

Most mortality-related studies analyzed the data by the logistic regression (LR) model, particularly for binary responses. The LR model requires to fulfil all the underlying unavoidable assumptions, predictors are independent of each other and having a significant association with the outcome variable, for estimating the parameters. Therefore, this commonly used prognostic modelling approach is sometimes challenging for estimating the model parameters correctly and also the incorrect estimation algorithm provides misleading information. Recently, the machine learning (ML) and data mining approaches are the further improvement of modelling health data that incorporate artificial intelligence and explore more hidden information from a large volume of data [20–24]. In the area of health research, ML generally aims to predict several clinical outcomes based on multiple predictors [25,26].

In this study, we adapted four different well-known ML techniques: decision tree (DT), random forest (RF), support vector machine (SVM), and LR for the classification and prediction of the significant factors associated with infant mortality in Bangladesh. Moreover, systematic performances of these ML approaches are investigated by comparing accuracy, sensitivity, specificity and precision values.

2   Methods and Materials

2.1   Data and Variables

Infant mortality data were extracted from the latest country-wise representative survey, Bangladesh Demographic and Health Survey (BDHS) 2017–18 [27]. A two-stage stratified random sampling design was used for collecting data in this survey and the detailed information is available at https://dhsprogram. com/data/available-datasets.cfm. The data related to infant mortality were collected from reproductive mothers and 26145 infants were included in this study after excluding missing cases. The binary outcome variable: infant death (death of a live birth before the age of one year) is considered in this study. Infant mortality is the consequence of a variety of multiple factors. The various maternal, socio-economic, demographic and environmental factors were considered as exposure variables such as maternal age at first marriage, maternal age at first birth, mother's body mass index, birth interval between two subsequent pregnancies, antenatal care service during pregnancy, receiving a tetanus toxoid (TT) injection during pregnancy, administrative regions, place of residence, religion, educational attainment of both mother's and father's, occupational status of mother's, women empowerment, exposure of media, total children ever born, child sex, birth order number, sources of drinking water, type of toilet facilities and type of cooking fuel.

2.2   Models

This study aimed to assess the potential predictors associated with infant mortality and to predict infant mortality in Bangladesh using different ML classification models: DT, RF, SVM and LR. Our methodology involves accordingly data pre-processing, feature (the risk factors) selection using Boruta algorithm, splitting the entire data set into training and test data sets applying ML models in the training data set and evaluate the performance of these models on the test data set, and finally predicting infant mortality based on the entire data set using the best performed model. The performances were evaluated using five performance parameters (accuracy, sensitivity, specificity, precision, and F1-score) obtained from the confusion matrix, and the area under the receiver operating characteristics (ROC) curve (AUC). All ML models were performed using the scikit-learn module in Python programming language version 3.7.3. Only the Boruta algorithm was implemented to select the risk factors using the Boruta package in the R programming language [28].

2.3 Boruta Algorithm

Boruta algorithm was performed to extract the relevant risk factors for infant mortality in Bangladesh. This is a wrapper build algorithm around the RF classifier to find out the relevance and important features with respect to the outcome variable [29].

2.4 Decision Tree (DT)

The DT is one of the most simple and intuitive techniques in ML, based on the divide and conquer paradigm [30]. In a DT technique, tests (on input patterns) and categories (of patterns) are used as inner and leaf nodes, respectively. This technique also assigns a class number to an input array by filtering the array down via the tests in the tree [31].

2.5 Random Forest (RF)

The RF algorithm consists of taking hyper-parameters identifying the number of trees and the maximum depth of each tree [32]. The RF is an ensemble learning approach for classification using a large collection of decorrelated DT [33]. In this experiment, we have used 501 DT and Gini for impurity index to implement the RF algorithm in Python.

2.6 Support Vector Machine (SVM)

The SVM is a supervised ML technique used for analyzing data and recognizing patterns [34,35]. A model or classification function is constructed in the SVM training algorithm in order to assign new values into one class on either side of a hyper plane, building it a non-probabilistic binary linear classifier for the two-class learning task. The kernel trick is used in a SVM technique to map the data into a high-dimensional space prior solving the ML task as a convex optimization problem [33–36]. New values are then predicted belonging to a group on the basis of the side of the partition in which these values fall. The nearest data points to the hyper plane that divides the classes are considered as support vectors [33]. We examined SVM models using the sigmoid kernel (the best performed kernel for BDHS 2017–18 infant mortality data set) for this analysis.

2.7 Logistic Regression (LR)

The LR, a probabilistic model, is used for classification problem and predicting the likelihood of the incidence of an event [33]. The association between a categorical response variable and a dichotomous categorical outcome or feature is modelled by the LR. It is used as a binary (multiple) model to predict binary (multiple) responses, the outcome of a categorical response variable, based on one or more exposure variables [30].

2.8 Confusion Matrix Performance Parameters

The graphical representation of real versus predicted class accuracies is obtained by a confusion matrix [33]. To visualize the performance of the classification algorithm, the confusion matrix is used for the comparison of predicted versus real classifications in the form of true positive, false positive, true negative and false negative [33]. Therefore, the performance parameters: accuracy (number of data points correctly classified by the classifier), sensitivity (how well a classification algorithm classifies data points in the positive class), specificity (how well a classification algorithm classifies data points in the negative class) and precision (number of data points correctly classified from the positive class) are measured [33].

2.9 Receiver Operating Characteristic (ROC) Curve

The ROC curve is an alternative and useful visualization technique for classifiers operating on datasets. Fawcett [37] provided a complete and informative introduction about the ROC analysis, emphasising usual misconceptions. The ROC curve reveals the sensitivity of the classifier considering the true positives and false positives rates. When the classifier is outstanding, the true positive rate will increase, and area under the ROC curve (AUC) will be close to 1 [30].

3 Statistical Results: Univariate and Bivariate Analysis

The frequency and percentage distributions of exposure variables, and the prevalence of infant mortality are presented in Table 1. As shown in the table, more than three quarters of mothers (82.6%) married before their legal recommended age of first marriage (at least 18 years) in Bangladesh. The enormous percentage of mothers (88.0%) had their first birth at 20 years or below. Approximately one-third (32.8%) of the mothers were overweight or obese, over half (55.3%) were normal and 11.9% were thin. The birth interval between two subsequent pregnancies for the majority (76.1%) of live births were more than two years. Only 0.4% and 0.3% of the mothers received ANC services and TT-injection, respectively during their pregnancy period. In this study, 70.0% of children were selected from rural and 30.0% from urban areas. The vast majority of participants were Muslim (92.1%), while only 7.9% of children were non-Muslim. With regards to mothers education, 27.0% had no education and only 4.8% of the mothers had higher education. Besides, 32.5% of fathers were illiterate, and 9.4% had higher education.

Table 1 shows that more than fifty percent (58.1%) of the mothers were employed, while 41.9% were unemployed. The proportion of children from low-income families was higher (45.9%) than rich (34.1%) and middle class (20.0%) families. The majority (82.4%) of respondents' mothers were not empowered, while the rest (17.6%) were fund to be empowered. Almost fifty percent (44.9%) of the children's mothers had mass-media exposure in Bangladesh. Half of the children were male and half were female. 46.7% of the children were the first ranked children, 27.7% were the second ranked children and the rest were third or higher ranked children. More than three quarters (80.6%) of mothers had 3 or more number of children, 42.4% of the mothers used to defecate in the unhygienic places, only 13.5% children were from households with less polluted cooking fuel and only 7.1% had no facilities of safe drinking water.

The prevalence of infant mortality was higher among mothers who were married before their legal age of 18 years and had their first child before 20 years (Table 1), although age at first marriage and age at first birth were found to be statistically insignificant factors for infant mortality. The percentage of infant mortality was higher for mothers who were underweight (12.2%) and had less than 2 years preceding birth interval (19.7%) in comparison with their counterparts. Mothers BMI (p<0.001) and birth interval (p<0.001) were found to be significantly associated with infant mortality in Bangladesh. The variables antenatal care and TT injection during pregnancy were also found to be statistically insignificant determinants with infant mortality. The administrative divisions showed significant association (p<0.001) with infant mortality and the prevalence varied from 8.0% (Chittagong) to 11.1% (Mymensingh). Infant mortality was comparatively lower in urban areas (9.2%) than rural areas (9.8%), though the place of residence was statistically insignificant (p = 0.144). Infant mortality was found to be significantly higher among non-Muslim (11.4%) as compared with Muslim (9.5%) and the religion was strongly associated with (p<0.001) infant mortality.

The educational attainment of both mothers (p<0.001) and fathers (p<0.001) showed a significant association with infant mortality. The decreasing trend of infant mortality was observed with mothers and fathers increasing levels of education. However, the proportion of infant mortality was found to be higher among working (10.2%) mothers in comparison to non-working (8.9%) mothers. The occupational status of mothers (p<0.001) was also significantly associated with infant mortality. The proportion of infant mortality was decreasing significantly with the increasing levels of wealth index (p<0.001). Mass-media exposure of mothers was found to be statistically significant (p = 0.002) for their infant mortality and this mortality was lower (9.0%) among mothers who were exposed to mass media than their counterparts (10.2%). The percentage of infant mortality was higher for the male children (10.9%), first order birth (10.3%), and mothers having 3 or more children (11.1%). All these variables: child of sex (p<0.001), birth order (p = 0.002), total children ever born (p<0.001) were significantly associated with infant mortality. Households with unhygienic toilet facility (10.5%) and polluted (9.9%) cooking fuel showed a significant (p<0.001) higher prevalence of infant mortality than those with hygienic toilet facility and less polluted cooking fuel.

Table 1. Background characteristics and chi-square (χ^2) test statistic associated with corresponding p-value.

Variables	n(%)	Infant death n = 2523 (9.7%)	χ^2-value	p-value
Age at first marriage			6.155	0.013
<18	21586 (82.6)	2128 (9.9)		
18 and above	4559 (17.4)	395 (8.7)		
Age at first birth			2.951	0.086
≤20	22998 (88.0)	2246 (9.8)		
>20	3147 (12.0)	277 (8.8)		
Mother's BMI			52.295	<0.001*
Normal	14471 (55.3)	1456 (10.1)		
Underweight	3101 (11.9)	379 (12.2)		
Overweight and obesity	8573 (32.8)	688 (8.0)		
Birth interval			957.434	<0.001*
≤2 years	6256 (23.9)	1234 (19.7)		
>2 years	19889 (76.1)	1289 (6.5)		
Antenatal care during pregnancy			0.106	0.745
No	26051 (99.6)	2513 (9.6)		
Yes	94 (0.4)	10 (10.6)		
TT-Injection during pregnancy			0.914	0.339
No	26076 (99.7)	2514 (9.6)		
Yes	69 (0.3)	9 (13.0)		
Region			27.940	<0.001*
Dhaka	3276 (12.5)	316 (9.6)		
Barisal	2936 (11.2)	265 (9.0)		
Chittagong	4244 (16.2)	341 (8.0)		
Khulna	2826 (10.8)	259 (9.2)		
Mymensingh	3122 (11.9)	345 (11.1)		
Rajshahi	2859 (10.9)	311 (10.9)		
Rangpur	3273 (12.5)	334 (10.2)		
Sylhet	3609 (13.8)	352 (9.8)		
Place of residence			2.139	0.144
Urban	7855 (30.0)	726 (9.2)		
Rural	18290 (70.0)	1797 (9.8)		
Religion			7.723	0.005*
Non-Muslim	2074 (7.9)	236 (11.4)		
Muslim	24071 (92.1)	2287 (935)		
Maternal education			82.227	<0.001
No education	7055 (27.0)	831 (11.8)		
Primary	10534 (40.3)	1030 (9.8)		
Secondary	7292 (27.9)	594 (8.1)		
Higher	1264 (4.8)	68 (5.4)		
paternal education			63.747	<0.001*
No education	8496 (32.5)	929 (10.9)		
Primary	9162 (35.0)	942 (10.3)		
Secondary	6031 (23.1)	493 (8.2)		
Higher	2456 (9.4)	159 (6.5)		
Mother's occupation			10.889	<0.001
Not working	10961 (41.9)	980 (8.9)		
Working	15184 (58.1)	1543 (10.2)		
Wealth index			25.853	<0.001
Poor	11994 (45.9)	1265 (10.5)		
Middle	5226 (20.0)	504 (9.6)		
Rich	8925 (34.1)	754 (8.4)		
Women empowerment			0.077	0.781
No	21533 (82.4)	2013 (9.7)		
Yes	4612 (17.6)	440 (9.5)		
Exposure of media			9.662	0.002*
Non-exposure	14406 (55.1)	1464 (10.2)		
Exposure	11739 (44.9)	1059 (9.0)		
Child sex			46.344	<0.001
Female	13083 (50.0)	1100 (8.4)		
Male	13062 (50.0)	1423 (10.9)		
Birth order			12.302	0.002*
One	12215 (46.7)	1262 (10.3)		
Two	7094 (27.1)	637 (9.0)		
Three and more	6836 (26.1)	624 (9.1)		
Total children ever born			252.454	<0.001*
1 or 2	5071 (19.4)	190 (3.7)		
3 and more	21074 (80.6)	2333 (11.1)		
Toilet facility			14.479	<0.001*
Hygienic	15065 (57.6)	1364 (9.1)		
Unhygienic	11080 (42.4)	1159 (10.5)		
Cokking fuel			8.757	<0.001*
Less polluted	3526 (13.5)	292 (8.3)		
Polluted	22619 (86.5)	2231 (9.9)		
Drinking water			0.496	0.481
Safe water	24294 (92.9)	2353 (9.7)		
Unsafe water	1851 (7.1)	170 (9.2)		

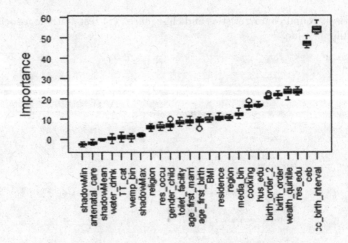

Fig. 1. Features selection using the Boruta algorithm

3.1 Machine Learning (ML) Results

3.1.1 Features Selection

Figure 1 reveals that with the aid of the Boruta algorithm, seventeen variables i.e., age at first marriage, age at first birth, birth interval, place of residence, administrative division, religion, education of parents, BMI, gender of child, children ever born, exposure of media, wealth index, birth order, occupation of mother, toilet facility and cooking fuel were selected among all surveyed variables as the risk factors to predict infant mortality in Bangladesh. Hereafter, these seventeen variables were used to evaluate the performance of ML algorithms.

3.1.2 Machine Learning (ML) Models Evaluation

The performance of different ML models were evaluated using five performance parameters of the confusion matrix (Table 3) and the realized confusion matrices of different ML models using a single run (Table 2), and the area under the ROC curve (Fig. 2). Considering 70% observations as the training data and 30% observation as the test data with the random seed 1119, using the scikit-learn module, we estimated accuracy, sensitivity, specificity, precision, and F1-score of DT, RF, SVM, and LR algorithms to predict infant mortality in Bangladesh and the results are illustrated in Table 2 and 3.

Table 2 illustrates various realized confusion matrices of different ML models using random seed 1119. The confusion matrix compares the actual target positive 761 and negative 7083 cases with those predicted by the different ML models. The DT model has True Positive (TP) = 125, True Negative (TN) = 6440, False Positive (FP) = 643, and False Negative (FN) = 636, i.e., 125 positive and 6440 negative classes data points were correctly classified by the DT, and 643 negative and 636 positive classes data points were incorrectly classified by the DT model. The maximum 371 positive and 6935 negative classes data

Table 2. Realized confusion matrices of different machine learning models

Label	Actual	DT (predicted)		RF (predicted)		SVM (predicted)		LR (predicted)	
		+ve	−ve	+ve	−ve	+ve	−ve	+ve	−ve
Positive	761	125	636	371	390	78	683	0	761
Negative	7083	643	6440	148	6935	707	6376	0	7083

+ve = Positive label, −ve = Negative label

Table 3. Accuracy, sensitivity, specificity, precision, and F1-score of different machine learning models

Models	Accuracy	Sensitivity	Specificity	Precision	F1-score
DT	0.837	0.164	0.909	0.163	0.164
RF	0.893	0.339	0.979	0.715	0.460
SVM (sigmoid kernel)	0.823	0.103	0.900	0.099	0.101
LR	0.903	0.000	1.000	NA	0.00

NA: Not applicable

points were correctly classified by the RF model, whereas the LR model failed to correctly classify any positive class data points though classified correctly all negative class data points.

Table 3 shows that the RF model was the efficient one to predict infant mortality based on the higher value of the performance parameters in all cases. For instance, the RF model provided 89.3% of accurate predictions (accuracy = 0.893), 33.9% of positive cases that were predicted as positive (sensitivity = 0.339), 97.9% of negative cases that were predicted as negative (specificity = 0.979), 71.5% of positive predictions that were correct (precision = 0.715), and 46.0% of F1-score indicating moderate precision and recall (F1-score = 0.460). Though, commonly used LR model provides the highest accuracy score (accuracy = 0.903) and specificity score (specificity = 1.00), but completely failed to estimate the precision of the test. Furthermore, the sensitivity and F1-score were also zero in that case. Figure 2 illustrates the estimated AUC of DT, RF, SVM, and LR models, which were run using the scikit-learn module in Python 3.7.3 by considering 70% observations as training data and 30% observation as test data with the random seed 1119. To predict infant mortality in Bangladesh the estimated AUC scores were 0.5416, 0.6613, 0.5443, and 0.7123 for the ML models DT, RF, SVM with the sigmoid kernel, and LR, respectively. Although the LR algorithm showed the maximum AUC among all examined ML models, however it completely failed to classify the positive cases. Therefore, performance of the RF model is comparatively better among all situations. Consequently, to predict infant mortality, the RF algorithm performed better based on the precision, sensitivity, specificity and accuracy measures, and the ROC approaches.

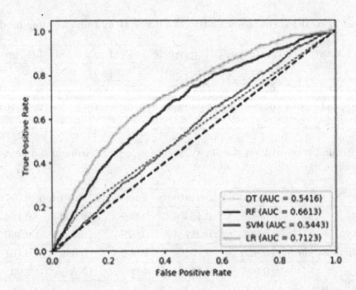

Fig. 2. The ROC curves to predict infant mortality in Bangladesh using DT, RF, SVM, and LR models

3.2 Random Forest (RF) Model for Predicting Infant Mortality

For the entire dataset, therefore, the best performed ML model, the RF model, was fitted to predict infant mortality in Bangladesh using the selected risk factors: age at first marriage, age at first birth, birth interval, place of residence, administrative division, religion, education of parents, BMI, gender of child, children ever born, exposure of media, wealth index, birth order, occupation of mother, toilet facility and cooking fuel, and the top one tree from the forest is visualized in Fig. 3. All the nodes have five parts (feature's question, gini, samples, value and class) with a question based on a value of a feature, except the terminal leaf nodes have four parts (gini, samples, value and class) [38]. The part 'gini' indicates the Gini Impurity of the node, which is the average weighted Gini Impurity decreases as the path move down the tree, 'samples' is the number of observations in the node, 'value' is the number of samples in each class, and 'class' indicates the majority classification for points in the node ('class' is the prediction for all samples in the leaf node) [38].

Each feature's question has either a True (left nodes) or a False (right nodes) answer that splits the node. Based on the answer to the question, a data point moves down the tree and reaches a leaf node (the final decision). Moreover, the blue-type colored leaf indicates a prediction of infant mortality and the orange-type colored leaf indicates a prediction of not infant mortality as shown in Fig. 3. To predict any given respondent's data, simply move down the tree in Fig. 3, using the answer to the feature's question until arriving at a leaf node where the class is the prediction.

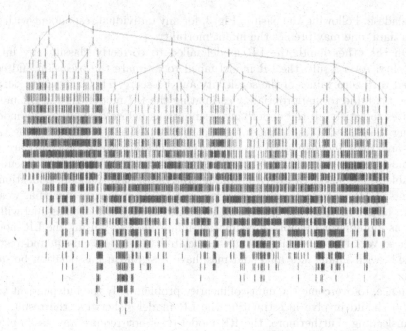

Fig. 3. Top one tree from the fitted RF model to infant mortality in Bangladesh

4 Discussion and Conclusion

Infant mortality is one of the most important public health problems universally; the problem is even more devastating in densely populated countries like Bangladesh. Motivated by such a noticeable public health concern, this research was conducted to find the significant factors and prediction of infant mortality in Bangladesh using different ML algorithms.

The study results reveal that age at first marriage, age at first birth, birth interval, place of residence, administrative division, religion, education of parents, BMI, gender of child, children ever born, exposure of media, wealth index, birth order, occupation of mother, toilet facility and cooking fuel were the major significant factors for predicting infant mortality using the ML features selection algorithm-Boruta. However, birth interval, administrative division, religion, education of parents, BMI, gender of child, children ever born, exposure of media, wealth index, birth order, occupation of mother, toilet facility and cooking fuel were only the significant factors for infant mortality using the conventional chi-squared test.

We evaluated the performance of different ML models: DT, RF, SVM and LR to predict infant mortality in Bangladesh using the performance parameters of the confusion matrix and the AUC. The RF model performed better to predict infant mortality in Bangladesh. The RF model considered the individual and interaction effects of all the selected factors to predict infant mortality in

Bangladesh. Following the path in Fig. 3, for any individual respondent with the given data, one may predict the infant mortality.

On the other hand, the LR model failed to correctly classify any infant mortality. As a result, the LR model failed to estimate the precision and concluded with zero values of the sensitivity and F1-score. This incomplete output is observed due to inappropriately estimating the LR model. As the LR model requires to satisfy all the underlying assumptions before estimating the model, among them predictors having a significant association with the outcome variable and their independence (to avoid the multicollinearity problem) are the foremost assumptions that need to satisfy. In this analysis, only the independent variable(s) among birth interval, administrative division, religion, education of parents, BMI, gender of child, children ever born, exposure of media, wealth index, birth order, occupation of mother, toilet facility and cooking fuel will be used as a predictor variable in estimating infant mortality using the LR model, as these variables were significantly associated (using the chi-squared test in Table 1) with infant mortality and may have a significant association between them.

Hence, to overcome the multicollinearity problem only the independent variable(s) should involve in estimating the LR model, otherwise, the results will be misleading. Furthermore, the RF model does not require any assumptions in estimating the model. Therefore, considering the better performance, the RF model will be better and authentic (in terms of fulfilling the assumptions) to predict infant mortality in Bangladesh in this study.

Conventional chi-square test identified only fourteen variables as significant factors, whereas the ML framework identified seventeen variables as significant factors for predicting infant mortality in this analysis. Needless to say, this study introduces the application of different ML models in the prediction of infant mortality, for instance, DT and RF, which do not require any assumptions and very easy (available) to implement in any standard software. Furthermore, the RF model included all these seventeen significant variables to predict infant mortality using their individual and interaction effects. Considering the high accuracy in prediction, better performance, and assumptions-free feature, the RF model is found to be more authentic and informative to predict infant mortality in Bangladesh.

Acknowledgements. The authors are thankful to the authority of Bangladesh Demographic and Health Survey (BDHS) for making their data available for free. Authors would also like to express their gratitude to Department of Statistics, Jahangirnagar University, Savar, Dhaka, Bangladesh; Department of Statistics, University of Dhaka, Bangladesh; and Faculty of Health, Engineering and Sciences (HES) of University of Southern Queensland, Australia for the technical support.

Funding Information. There is no funding for this work.

Data Availibility Statement. We used secondary data from the Demographic and Health Surveys (DHS) Program. The data are available online at https://dhsprogram. com/data/available-datasets.cfm.

Conflicts of interest. No conflict of interest exits among the authors.

Patient Consent for Publication. Not applicable.

Ethics Statement. This article does not include any data of human participants conducted by any of the authors. The Bangladesh Demographic and Health Survey (BDHS) was approved by ICF Macro Institutional Review Board and the National Research Ethics Committee of the Bangladesh Medical Research Council. Written consent was given by participants in relation to this survey before the interview. All identification of the survey participants was dis-identified before publishing the data. In this study, we used the secondary data that are freely available on the DHS website: https://dhsprogram.com/data/available-datasets. cfm.

References

1. CDC: Infant Mortality. Centers for Disease Control and Prevention (2018). https://www.cdc.gov/reproductivehealth/MaternalInfantHealth/InfantMortality. htm. Accessed 14 July 2021
2. World Health Organization (WHO). Millennium development goals (MDGs) (2018). http://www.who.int/topics/millennium-development-goals/about/en. Accessed 14 July 2021
3. World Health Organization (WHO). The global health observatory (2018). https://www.who.int/data/gho/data/themes/topics/indicator-groups/indicator-group-details/GHO/infant-mortality. Accessed 14 July 2021
4. Vijay, J., Patel, K.K.: Risk factors of infant mortality in Bangladesh. Clin. Epidemiol. Global Health **8**, 211–214 (2020)
5. Hajizadeh, M., Nandi, A., Heymann, J.: Social inequality in infant mortality: what explains variation across low and middle income countries? Soc. Sci. Med. **101**, 36–46 (2014)
6. World Health Organization (WHO). Success factor for women's and child's health: Bangladesh (2015). www.who.int
7. Quansah, E., Ohene, L.A., Norman, L., Mireku, M.O., Karikari, T.K.: Social factors influencing child health in Ghana. PLoS One **11**(1), 1–10 (2016)
8. Kiross, G.T., Chojenta, C., Barker, D., Tiruye, T.Y., Loxton, D.: The effect of maternal education on infant mortality in Ethiopia: a systematic review and meta-analysis. PLoS One **14**(7), e0220076 (2019)
9. Dube, L., Taha, M., Asefa, H.: Determinants of infant mortality in community of Gilgel gibe field research center, Southwest Ethiopia: a matched case control study. BMC Public Health **13**, 401 (2013)
10. Leal, M.D., Bittencourt, S.D., Torres, R.M., Niquini, R.P., Souza, P.R., Jr.: Determinants of infant mortality in the Jequitinhonha valley and in the north and northeast regions of Brazil. Rev Saude Publica **51**(12), 1–9 (2017)

11. Khadka, K.B., Lieberman, L.S., Giedraitis, V., Bhatta, L., Pandey, G.: The socio-economic determinants of infant mortality in Nepal: analysis of Nepal demographic health survey. BMC Pediatr. **15**(152), 1 (2015)

12. Santos, S.L., Santos, L.B., Campelo, V., Silva, A.R.: Factors associated with infant mortality in a northeastern Brazilian capital. Rev. Bras. Ginecol. Obstet. **38**(10), 482–491 (2016)

13. Baraki, A.G., et al.: Factors affecting infant mortality in the general population: evidence from the 2016 Ethiopian demographic and health survey (EDHS); a multilevel analysis. BMC Pregnancy Childbirth **20**, 299 (2020)

14. Varghese, S., Prasad, J.H., Jacob, K.S.: Domestic violence as a risk factor for infant and child mortality: a community-based case-control study from southern India. Natl. Med. J. India **26**(3), 142–146 (2013)

15. Mohamoud, Y.A., Kirby, R.S., Ehrenthal, D.B.: Poverty, urban-rural classification and term infant mortality: a population-based multilevel analysis. BMC Pregnancy Childbirth **19**, 40 (2019)

16. de Bitencourt, F.H., Schwartz, I.V.D., Vianna, F.S.L.: Infant mortality in Brazil attributable to inborn errors of metabolism associated with sudden death: a time-series study (2002–2014). BMC Pediatr. **19**, 52 (2019)

17. Vilanova, C.S., et al.: The relationship between the different low birth weight strata of newborns with infant mortality and the influence of the main health determinants in the extreme south of Brazil. Popul. Health Metrics **15**, 1–10 (2019)

18. Hajipour, M., et al.: Predictive factors of infant mortality using data mining in Iran. J. Comprehen. Pediatr. **12**(1), 1–8 (2021)

19. Dancer, D., Rammohan, A., Smith, M.D.: Infant mortality and child nutrition in Bangladesh. Health Econ. **17**(9), 1015–1035 (2008)

20. Alghamdi, M., Al-Mallah, M., Keteyian, S., Brawner, C., Ehrman, J., Sakr, S.: Predicting diabetes mellitus using SMOTE and ensemble machine learning approach: the Henry Ford Exercise Testing (FIT) project. PLoS One **12**, 1 (2017)

21. Supriya, S., Siuly, S., Wang, H., Zhang, Y.: Automated epilepsy detection techniques from electroencephalogram signals: a review study. Health Inf. Sci. Syst. **8**(1), 1–15 (2020). https://doi.org/10.1007/s13755-020-00129-1

22. Pandey, Y.Z.D., Yin, X., Wang, H.: Accurate vessel segmentation using maximum entropy incorporating line detection and phase-preserving denoising. Comput. Vision Image Underst. **155**, 162–172 (2017)

23. Sarki, R., Ahmed, K., Wang, H., Zhang, Y.: Image Preprocessing in Classification and Identification of Diabetic Eye Diseases. Data Sci. Eng. 1–17 (2021)

24. Supriya, S., Siuly, S., Wang, H., Zhang, Y.: EEG sleep stages analysis and classification based on weighed complex network features. IEEE Trans. Emerg. Topics Comput. Intell. **5**, 236–246 (2018)

25. Sarki, R., Ahmed, K., Wang, H., Zhang, Y.: Automated detection of mild and multi-class diabetic eye diseases using deep learning. Health Inf. Sci. Syst. **8**(1), 1–9 (2020). https://doi.org/10.1007/s13755-020-00125-5

26. Mateen, B.A., Liley, J., Denniston, A.K., Holmes, C.C., Vollmer, S.J.: Improving the quality of machine learning in health applications and clinical research. Nat. Mach. Intell. **2**(10), 554–556 (2020)

27. National institute of population research and training (NIPROT), Bangladesh demographic and health survey 2017–2018. Mitra and Associates, Dhaka, Bangladesh and ICF International, Calverton, Maryland, USA (2019)

28. R Core Team: a language and environment for statistical computing. Vienna: R Foundation for Statistical Computing. http://www.R-project.org

29. Kursa, M.B., Rudnicki, W.R.: Feature selection with the Boruta package. J. Statist. Softw. **36**(11), 1–13 (2010)
30. Igual, L., Seguí, S.: Introduction to Data Science. Springer, Cham (2017)
31. Nilsson, N.L.: Introduction to Machine Learning. Stanford University, Stanford, CA (1997)
32. Breiman, L.: Random forests. Mach. Learn. **45**(1), 5–32 (2001)
33. Awad, M., Khanna, R.: Efficient Learning Machines. A press, Berkeley, CA (2015)
34. Burges, C.J.: A tutorial on support vector machines for pattern recognition. Data Mining Knowl. Disc. **2**(2), 121–167 (1998)
35. Müller, K.R., Mika, S., Rätsch, G., Tsuda, K., Schölkopf, B.: An introduction to kernel-based learning algorithms. IEEE Trans. Neural Netw. **12**(2), 181–201 (2001)
36. Vapnik, V.N.: The Nature of Statistical Learning Theory. Springer-Verlag, New York (1995)
37. Fawcett, T.: Introduction to ROC analysis. Pattern Recogn. Lett. **27**, 861–874 (2006)
38. Koehrsen, W.: An implementation and explanation of the random forest in Python. Towards Data Sci. **31**, 1 (2018)

Medical Data Processing

Applications and Challenges of Deep Learning in Computer Vision

Chetanpal Singh[✉]

Holmes Institute, Melbourne, Australia
Csingh@holmes.edu.au

Abstract. Deep learning has gained a lot of prominence in the past few years, with it even taking precedence over other learning techniques quite significantly. The use of computer vision is a very good example of its widespread application. As the amount of data generated becomes more, the complexity of the analysis also increases. This is the ideal application of the Deep Learning Method and it is known to outperform other traditional Machine Learning algorithms by quite some margins as the latter has issues in dealing with high-volume data. The specialty of deep learning is that it is applicable for texts as well as image data alike. Two important algorithms of deep learning that have multiple utilities are Convolutional Neural Network and Deep Belief Network. By using a Convolutional Neural Network, one can extract information from images by detection and recognition. It can be used in the medical science field by locating out tumors accurately and identifying its type and using robots for navigation by locating the hurdles. The main aim of this review paper is to provide a brief about the deep learning methods used. It includes a description of their structure, functioning, and limitation and also includes their utility in computer vision like for object identification, human face, and activity recognition etcetera. In the end, a brief description of the future usage of it and how the newer challenges can be dealt with is shared here.

Index Terms: Deep learning · Computer vision · Convolutional Neural Network · Deep belief network · Recurrent Neural Network · Restricted Boltzmann machine · Autoencoders · Machine learning · Artificial intelligence

1 Introduction

Nowadays, the generation of huge data is leading to complex data analysis which is well-managed by the use of a Deep Learning system. Traditional algorithms are unable to deal with these data packets and solve all the associated problems and Deep Learning becomes more useful in such a situation. It can deal with texts and images and other forms of data alike. The process of application of Deep Learning involves using multiple layers and since the computational data is more profound, it replaces the traditional

© Springer Nature Switzerland AG 2021
S. Siuly et al. (Eds.): HIS 2021, LNCS 13079, pp. 223–233, 2021.
https://doi.org/10.1007/978-3-030-90885-0_20

algorithm (Shetty and Siddiqa 2019). Another important aspect to keep in mind is that machine learning algorithms that have a traditional approach have certain limitations to their processing ability which is not the case with the Deep Learning algorithm. The performance is enhanced when the amount and complexity of the data are more. For example, a neural network like ANN has multiple layers hidden between the layers for input and output.

The algorithm of Deep Learning software is such that it can be instructed and trained to work with a large dataset related to texts, sounds, images, and even videos and speeches in a time series model (Patel and Thakkar 2020). The approach is multi-layered which is ideal for deep neural networks. Some are even of the opinion that Deep Learning is a subset system of Machine Learning itself and it uses a lot of data for performing jobs like an acknowledgment of pictures and uncovering multiple layers of information using a multi-layered neural network.

The main reasons that have boosted the application of Deep Learning are the availability of datasets that are of the highest quality and publicly available and which have GPU computing abilities. Recently, there has been a shift from CPU to GPU-based utilities as well which has accelerated the Deep Learning algorithm significantly. Alleviating the problem of the vanishing gradient and the disengagement from saturation functions as well as the proposal of the new techniques of regularization along with TensorFlow and Mxnet ensures that the prototyping becomes all the more efficient and faster in functioning (Voulodimos et al. 2018).

There were quite a few problems related to computer vision that have been solved using Deep Learning models. These include the detection of objects, recognition of action, segmentation of the semantics, and estimation of different human poses. The purpose of this review is to give a proper idea of the architecture related to Deep Learning and other algorithms used in the application of computer vision. Convolutional Neural Network (CNN), Deep Belief Network (DBN), and Recurrent Neural Network (RNN) are a few of the algorithms being discussed here. The application of these algorithms depends on the type of data and its performance.

1.1 Research Objective

The main aim of the research is to help researchers in the field of multimedia analysis and people working with computer vision. It is also useful for general researchers of machine learning who want to delve into deep learning in finer details. The main tasks that are reviewed are recognition of face and activity, object and face detection etcetera.

1.2 Research Motivation

One of the main agendas of Artificial Intelligence is to create machines that have similar functionality and understanding abilities as humans. This has led to the formation of a subset of AI called computer vision that is mainly concerned with the processing of visual data. Computer vision has developed a lot in recent years using Artificial Networks and Deep Learning (Hassaballah and Awad 2020). It involves the taking of unstructured data in the form of images as well as videos and processing them into something good. These advances have even been instrumental in boosting the use of Computer Vision in the domains that already exist and the newer ones. It has become a part of everyday neural network computations in more ways than one.

1.3 Research Gap

Machine learning and deep learning techniques are one of the most promising technologies of modern times. It primarily deals with working with high-level data using hierarchical structures. Implementation of machine learning techniques helps in the advanced application of programming in low-cost computing hardware. It is being used across a wide range of devices and tools. At present, several attempts have been made to improve the advancement of deep learning algorithms. It is realized that deep learning approaches offer satisfactory results compared to the various top-of-the-line methods. Despite progress in this field, it remains to be a relatively new technology. This paper discusses the recent advancements in deep learning and its application across various domains of computer science.

2 Literature Review

The purpose of the Computer Vision System is to replicate the human vision system as accurately as possible. It takes images and videos and analyzes them to extract information from them as well as uses it to bring out important information and related decisions. DBN and CNN are two Deep Learning methods that have had the maximum application in this regard. The concept that CNN is based on is when a neuron has several parameters that are applied in patches, a translational kind of invariance is formed. (Hassaballah and Awad 2020) utilizes the Convolutional Neural Network to remove errors and get conducive results concerning tasks of pattern recognition.

The problem that arises commonly with CNN is that of overfitting. This mainly arises because many parameters are learned and used. Augmentation of data and stochastic pooling has been suggested to deal with it. Some of the parameters are also trained instead of taking random numbers. It is known as pretraining and it has been employed concurrently (Patel and Thakkar 2020). The idea behind it is to make the learning process faster and also improve the capacity of network generalization. Speaking from an overall perspective, CNN has been deemed to be much better than the traditional algorithms for computer vision and tasks related to the recognition of patterns. It is due to this reason CNN has become very popular in recent times among all.

2.1 Computer Vision Applications

The discussion is done concerning applications of CNN in computer vision aspects like object detection, face recognition, image captioning, robot navigation and medical image analysis, human pose estimation, and activity and action recognition.

- **Object Detection**

  The method of identifying from digital video and images the presence of semantic objects belonging to a specific class is called Object Detection. Using CNN features is the most general method for these object detection frameworks. It includes building a huge set of candidate windows present in the sequel classified with these features. For deriving object proposals, the process in (Kaushal et al. 2018) uses selective search. Furthermore, for every proposal, the CNN features are extracted, and then to select whether the object is in the windows or not, features are integrated into an SVM classifier. However, the preciseness in detecting the accurate position of an object is a miss, although the approximate positions can be found successfully. Generally, favorable results are achieved by these methods when they adhere to the joint object detection- semantic segmentation approach.

  For real-time object detection, the YOLO technique is required. Detection and localization of objects in an image are done by the CNN network used by YOLO (Vickyet al. 2017; Kaushal et al. 2018). Due to fast features, YOLO is integrated with real-time.

- **Medical Image Analysis**

  CNN mainly comprises medical image analysis. Useful processes such as detection of abnormality, segmentation, classification of disease are mainly analyzed with the help of Image analysis (Xu et al. 2018). Moreover, this process also helps to diagnose computer-aided MRIs or X-rays. CNN can also diagnose prostate cancer. Locating prostate cancer needs CAD or a Computer-Aided Diagnosis system (Reda et al. 2018).

  Semantic segmentation requires a helix network that is similar to the CNN, but the CNN does not have layers at the end of the network that is fully connected, therefore MRI brain image requires FCN for lesion segmentation. To dissect the 3D image that helps in learning the shape of an object, FCN plays a crucial role.

  There are two crucial drawbacks of FCN. This process fails to examine the depth of contusions. The second issue is that FCN fails to examine huge objects. Due to differentiation in class ratio, FCN fails to inspect (Xu et al. 2018). Therefore, to overcome the backlash, an appropriate methodology that includes 3D patching authentic images and then modifies the patches so that there is a minimum difference of class ratio.

- **Face Recognition**

  A significant performance in face detection has been done by a Convolutional DBN (Amritkar and Jabade 2018). Moreover, because of the enhanced transformation invariance and feature learning properties, change has also been brought about by CNNs.

  CNN's are also the base for DeepFace by Facebook (Zhao et al. 2019) and FaceNet by Google. In FaceNet, the training mechanism grasps the clustering of the face representation of a singular person. It also defines the representation function of triplet loss. On the contrary, in DeepFace, the system models any face in 3D and then aligns it to make it viewed as the frontal face. However, the interpretation of the presentation is not seamless in DeepFace despite its excellent performance rates. This is because, during the training process, the faces of a singular person are not usually clustered. Apart from these, the core of OpenFace also uses CNN. This open-source face recognition tool is good for mobile computing since it has a quick execution time and is small sizewise. However, the accuracy is not very high.

- **Robot Navigation**

  An automatic robot needs GPS and sensors to navigate. Convolutional neural networks are required to make the vision-based system that helps in the motion of a robot (Hassaballah and Awad 2020). Appropriate data and complex computation are required to implement this process. To identifying the lane, the object needs to be enforced.

- **Autonomous Vehicles**

  The AI community is persevering to develop vehicles that do not need human drivers to navigate roads. With the help of deep neural networks, a considerable amount of progress is made. To Code vehicles to sense their surroundings is the utmost hurdle for self-driving vehicles (Dargan et al. 2019). Several companies are taking many measures to handle the issue, but computer vision technology is the main sector every company has. GPS and image analysis techniques are incorporated to build autonomous vehicles (Vicky et al. 2017). It is possible only through deep learning algorithms as it helps to transmit data without extreme training as it helps to identify unfamiliar objects or by using an image processing method that helps in detecting the edge/lane for swift movement.

- **Image captioning**

  In CNN, the image captioning process is more effective. Integrating the RNN and CNN helps to generate text sentences, which makes the prime architecture of the image captioning process. Image captioning is the process that helps to identify the factors in an image and autonomously code a description in a text sentence.

  CNN and RNN can also be used to extract features and generate text that helps to describe the image can be a solution of image captioning (Amritkar and Jabade 2018). To encode and decode the caption, LSTM is required (Amritkar and Jabade 2018). The image captioning application of CNN also helps in answering the visual question if extended. To formulate textual sentences, unique RNN or LSTM can be used (Wu et al 2018). There are two issues regarding this process, firstly the images paint helps to identify the image, and secondly, the language aspect helps to textualize the image in proper English. The result section includes a summary of different proposals that use CNN regarding this issue.

2.2 Current Challenges

The main assay of Deep Learning is to support the theoretical reasoning of individuals that helps to utilize machinery. But there are some drawbacks.

- **Managing Constant Input Data:** The inspection of facts involved in the training process of DL. Notwithstanding, the fact that it is a swift process that does not provide enough time to render accurate data, therefore, the professional needs to modify the algorithm.
- **Ensured Conclusion Transparency:** There are no sectors left to enhance DL as it is already modified to the brim. The overall algorithm needs to be modified again for a single phenomenon that is to point out the issues.
- **Resource-Demanding Technology:** DL is a resource-demanding technology. As this technology requires high storage and hi-tech GPU to render a model, ML requires much less time than DL to acknowledge. Despite these drawbacks, DL is still effective in learning corporations and provides advantages to analysts and educators.

2.3 Literature Gap

Issues such as motion detection, robotic, video processing, language processing, verification, and recognition are involved in computer vision, which can be corrected through DL. The sector of computer vision is enhancing rapidly with the help of CNN. The determination of pre-trained facts helps in adjusting, confirming, and utilizing through DL. The process of segmentation helps to provide a pixel clear image of an object whereas object detection only consists of drawing a rectangle box in the place of the object. DL is an essential means but raises somber problems as mentioned by (Patel and Thakkar 2020). As DL is not transparent, there are problems to acknowledge the rules working in the system. It is not easy to understand the algorithms of the vehicle using DL that can be the reason for the lack of information.

3 Methods and Materials

There are several similarities in the functioning of Neural Networks and Deep Learning. Supervised as well as unsupervised learning is being assisted by DL. Machine Learning is not efficient to rectify the problems of computer vision and therefore DL is appropriate. This combines two major proposals namely Training and Testing.

a) The training stages - it comprises explaining the homogeneous factors and labeling of a considerable amount of data. This helps in comparing the features and providing acute reasoning and conclusion for the training model when required. Here are some steps that are included in the DL training process.

1. Data labeling.
2. A set of binary questions which includes true or false is being delved into

3. Efficient responses are being directed for data classification.
4. Several values are being extracted from the data bar.

b) The testing stages - help to generate a conclusion by exposing the data with the help of the previous facts. The machine will be assembled with a new feature extraction process from fundamental data to develop ancient machine learning. The flaws can be corrected by the machine with the help of ML instruction that is generated by analysts.

In deep learning, excess training has a negative impact, but this process helps to redress it. The supervised learning includes examples as well as data training that helps in supporting the system to render appropriate decisions by the analyst for ML. Human assistance is required to solve a large number of tasks by a computer. This includes ancient machine learning.

However, there are some visible differences between Deep Learning and Machine Learning. It has been observed that Deep Learning needs hi-tech GPU and hardware which are not required by Machine Learning. While deep learning offers some unique features, Machine Learning requires professional analysts to extract such features; however, ML is transparent in comparison to DL. Deep Learning provides extensive knowledge to get end-to-end solutions but in the case of Machine Learning, the problem is segmented into beats and later combined to arrive at a solution. For effective results, DL requires a huge amount of data which is not the case in Machine Learning. The machine is ready to intake useful data and provides decisions until the data is credible. For concluding the process of deep learning, it confers the use of several leveled processes, which provides a positive factor.

4 Results and Discussion

Artificial intelligence has a segment known as Deep Learning which is a part of Artificial Neural Networks. Machine learning is efficient for solving small dataset algorithms but for a considerable amount of datasets, the Deep learning algorithm is optimum. With the help of topics such as captioning, object detection, and object recognition professionals can compare both models (Kaushal et al. 2018).

As CNN uses filters for computation therefore it does not require examining every bit of the image meticulously. The project mentions the applications of CNN in computer vision through medical image analysis that consists of digital medical images like MRI scan, ECG, X-ray, EEG to locate any signs of irregularities (Xu et al. 2018). There is no need for human assistance in vehicles and autonomous systems if the robot uses CNN for navigation. To acquire image captions RNN is integrated with CNN.

Technical failures such as time series problems, natural language processing, video processing, speed recognition, text recognition, and image recognition can be easily determined with the help of DL and NN.

The onerous deep learning is more effective and provides benefits than machine learning algorithms. If there is a need to render more effective and fast solutions, graphical processing support must be provided to Deep Neural Networks, as they are difficult to learn and train upon. The deep learning algorithm is used in several advanced technologies such as the face recognition system in Apple, Cortana personal assistant, SIRI, self-driven cars by Google and the latest introduction is the Amazon Go store (Vicky et al. 2017) (Table 1).

4.1 Analysis of Applications of Deep Learning Models in Computer Vision

Table 1. Applications of deep learning models in computer vision

Application	Methodology technique and description	References
Object detection	• Detection and localization of objects in an image are done by the CNN network used by YOLO	(Kaushal et al. 2018) (Vicky et al. 2017)
Medical image analysis	• MRI brain image with FCN for lesion segmentation • CNN can also diagnose prostate cancer	(Xu et al. 2018) (Reda et al. 2018)
Face recognition	• Face recognition is carried out through Convolutional DBN • CNN's are also the base for DeepFace by Facebook and FaceNet by Google	(Amritkar & Jabade, 2018) (Zhao, et al., 2019)
Robot navigation	• Convolutional neural networks are required for Robot Navigation	(Hassaballah and Awad 2020)
Autonomous vehicles	• GPS and image analysis techniques are used in operating autonomous vehicles	(Vicky et al. 2017)
Image captioning	• CNN and RNN can also be used to extract features and generate text in image captioning • LSTM is required for coding and decoding the caption • unique RNN or LSTM can be used to formulate textual sentences	(Amritkar and Jabade 2018) (Amritkar and Jabade 2018) (Wu et al. 2018)

5 Conclusion

In the past few years, deep learning has garnered the attention of many industries to a great extent as it has a promising future in the field of computer vision. CNN has been implemented in different tasks, from face recognition, object detection to activity recognition and human pose estimation. But there are benefits and disadvantages associated with such a technology. Feature learning is one of the unique advantages of CNNs. However, there is no possibility of transformation in CNN's technology which is regarded as a great support in most computer vision applications. But the disadvantage is that it depends on the availability of the label data.

The coverage that has been presented above cannot be called exhaustive. One will not get a brief description of recurrent neural networks by reading the above paper even though it has great importance in deep learning, but the review has not listed this category. The Recurrent neural network is implemented in problems like text classification, handwriting recognition, music recognition as well as machine translation. Still, it has got significantly less application in computer vision problems, and this is the reason why the recurrent neural network is not mentioned correctly in the paper.

Moreover, according to the paper, it can be concluded that to get potential output in serious learning problems, CNN plays a crucial role by providing proper image input. But one drawback of CNN is that the investment required is high, one needs a high category GPU, and if there is no GPU present in the process, it becomes prolonged as it involves a lot of Training data. However, there are solutions to overcome these kinds of drawbacks, and one of the best ways is to utilize models which can be fine-tuned according to the requirement.

Undoubtedly, deep learning is one of the fastest-growing technologies of recent times. The growing use of machine learning algorithms in various domains shows its dynamic nature and utility. Advancements in these fields have further improved its accuracy along with the integration of deep learning. It has become an integral part of several everyday processes. It will also become an essential tool for future advancements and research. The hierarchical structure of the layers is beneficial for supervision and learning purposes. It also plays a significant role in the successful integration of deep learning algorithms. At present, deep learning is being integrated into the development of security tools with the help of face recognition and speech recognition. Digital image processing is also making use of more advanced processing approaches. Deep learning has emerged as one of the most exciting and promising technologies for the more extensive implementation of artificial intelligence.

Therefore, it can be safely concluded that we will find a more optimized form of data and computation resources with the development in this field. Integration of deep learning techniques across various domains is gradually revolutionizing everyday operations. It is one of the most reliable and efficient technologies that is still in its initial stages. More applications of deep learning techniques will give it the much-needed boost for large-scale implementation. Deep learning technology will be helpful in fields like natural language processing, health care, remote sensing, and more.

5.1 Future Work

- Enhancing the capability of deep networks by integration of diversity between features
- Improving deep networks with the inclusion of non-static and sophisticated scenarios that can work with multiple noise types
- Development of neural networks that are compatible with an unsupervised learning environment
- Deep reinforcement learning will give future direction to this technology

- Deep networks will affect factors like efficiency inference and accuracy in the development
- Maintenance and processing of various data types
- Development of deep generative models with advanced and superior modeling abilities
- Automatic reception of ECG signal through deep learning
- Deep neural network for tracking videos and object detection

From the above discussion, it is clear that deep learning technologies will significantly impact all domains in the future. It will promote the development of conventional machine learning techniques for various applications. Deep learning technologies serve as the most effective supervisor and efficient approach to machine learning. Researchers will now be able to perform a quick evaluation of potential issues associated with application development. Deep learning will help in obtaining more accurate and productive results.

5.2   Open Research Questions

This paper mainly deals with the advancement of applications dependent on CNN as it is mainly used for images. Various recent research papers have stated that CNN strategies have exceeded the accuracy of human testers with their advancement. However, there is still a big scope in terms of the advancement made. The theoretical foundation of CNN strategies fails to show that under what conditions and when they will have an optimal structure and enhanced performance for specific tasks.

Despite being one of the most promising technologies of recent times, the results documented in the literature of the study show specific shortcomings. There are significant challenges in the large-scale integration of deep learning technology. Theoretical groundwork is necessary to explain the various aspects of the technology in real life. It would help in the optimal selection of the model type and structure that would help comprehend the reasons. For architectures and algorithms, there are several approaches for effective implementation. These are some of the significant issues that can affect the extensive scale integration of machine learning techniques. It will also continue to attract the attention of researchers in this field in the coming days.

References

Amritkar, C., Jabade, V.: Image caption generation using deep learning technique. Fourth Int. Conf. Comput. Commun. Control Autom. (ICCUBEA) **2018**, 1–4 (2018)

Dargan, S., Kumar, M., Ayyagari, M.R., Kumar, G.: A survey of deep learning and its applications: a new paradigm to machine learning. Arch. Comput. Methods Eng. **27**(4), 1071–1092 (2019). https://doi.org/10.1007/s11831-019-09344-w

Hassaballah, M., Awad, A.I.: Deep Learning in Computer Vision: Principles and Applications. CRC Press, Boca Raton (2020). https://doi.org/10.1201/9781351003827

Kaushal, M., Khehra, B., Sharma, A.: Soft computing based object detection and tracking approaches: state-of-the-art survey. Appl. Soft. Comput. **70**, 423–464 (2018)

Kautz, T., Groh, B., Hannink, J., Jensen, U., Strubberg, H., Eskofer, B.: Activity recognition in beach volleyball using a DEEp Convolutional Neural NETwork: leveraging the potential of DEEp Learning in sports. Data Min. Knowl. Disc. **31**(6), 1678–1705 (2018)

Patel, P., Thakkar, A.: The upsurge of deep learning for computer vision applications. Int. J. Electr. Comput. Eng. (IJECE) **10**(1), 538–548 (2020)

Reda, I., et al.: A new CNN-based system for early diagnosis of prostate cancer. In: 2018 IEEE 15th International Symposium on Biomedical Imaging (ISBI 2018)

Shetty, S.K., Siddiqa, A.: Deep learning algorithms and applications in computer vision. Int. J. Comput. Sci. Eng. **7**(7), 195–201 (2019)

Vicky, M., Aziz, G., Hindersah, H., Prihatmanto, A.: Implementation of vehicle detection algorithm for self-driving car on toll road cipularang using Python language. In: 2017 4th International Conference on Electric Vehicular Technology (ICEVT)

Voulodimos, A., Doulamis, N., Doulamis, A., Protopapadakis, E.: Deep learning for computer vision: a brief review. Comput. Intell. Neurosci. **2018**, 1–13 (2018). https://doi.org/10.1155/2018/7068349

Wu, Q., Shen, C., Wang, P., Dick, A., Hengel, A.: Image captioning and visual question answering based on attributes and external knowledge. IEEE Trans. Pattern Anal. Mach. Intell. **40**(6), 1367–1381 (2018)

Xu, B., et al.: Orchestral fully convolutional networks forsmall lesion segmentation in brain MRI. In: Proceeding of IEEE International Symposium on Biomedical Imaging, pp. 889–892 (2018)

Zhao, C., Chen, K., Wei, Z., Chen, Y., Miao, D., Wang, W.: Multilevel triplet deep learning model for person re-identification. Pattern Recogn. Lett. **117**, 161–168 (2019)

Generating Data Models to Manage Individual Information Related to Environmental Risk Factors and Social Determinants of Health

Miguel Atienza-Maderuelo[1]($\boxtimes$), Paloma Collado[1] (iD),
and Fernando Martin-Sanchez[2] (iD)

[1] National Distance Education University (UNED), Madrid, Spain
matienza74@alumno.uned.es
[2] Instituto de Salud Carlos III, Madrid, Spain

Abstract. In 2005, Wild coined the term Exposome and defined it as the totality of exposures individuals encounter from conception until death. Economy, behavior, social, cultural, and environmental matters, among others, influence and modify the health status of individuals along their life. Multiple diseases find their origin in the interaction between the Genome and the Exposome. Therefore, there is a need to integrate both data sources, considering human health from a holistic perspective.

There is still a scarcity of accepted standards to represent human exposure data, nonetheless. From a Biomedical Informatics' perspective, representing people's Exposome data constitutes a great challenge, considering that it is based on Big Data sources that changes very fast through time, and space. Overcoming this challenge is mandatory to consider human exposure in health assessment studies. This work tries to partially contribute to address the difficulty of representing these kinds of data, proposing interoperable and interchangeable data models, ready to be used to improve clinical decision making, patients proactivity in health care, biomedical research and health systems management and efficiency.

Keywords: Biomedical research · Exposome · Expotype · Archetype · Precision medicine

1 Introduction

Lately, health systems in developed countries have presented good results despite constant low levels of investment. However, COVID-19 pandemic [1] has set unprecedented pressure, revealing vulnerabilities when facing unexpected perturbations. With that in mind, considering just how biological systems function, or dominating the latest surgery advances is not sufficient anymore. Multiple complexities must be considered, such as those related to social, environmental, or economic factors, among others, delivering and making this knowledge available to patients, aiming for a patient centric perspective, jointly with the traditional clinical approach. Patients must be observed and considered

© Springer Nature Switzerland AG 2021
S. Siuly et al. (Eds.): HIS 2021, LNCS 13079, pp. 234–244, 2021.
https://doi.org/10.1007/978-3-030-90885-0_21

holistically, perceiving their context globally. This will enable better clinical decision making as well as more efficient health systems [2].

Social, economic, political factors, among others external matters taking part in people's life and context, must now be considered for an integral health care transformation. A relevant number of complex diseases such as cancer, cardiovascular and respiratory diseases, or diabetes, deemed as usual death causes in societies, find part of their provenance in non-genetic factors, such as the ones mentioned [3]. The full environmental exposure people experience throughout their lifespan from the prenatal period, comprises the main topic related to the present article, the Exposome [4].

The Exposome relates to all those non-genetic risk factors affecting people's health, jointly with their genetic endowment. It includes social, environmental, and cultural factors, among others [5]. The Exposome stands as a new concept, being complementary to the Genome. Jointly, the interactions between them shape people's health situation or sickness. This is how the individual Phenotype is generated, resulting from the interactions mentioned between the Genome, and the external or environmental elements to which an individual is exposed (expotype) [6].

2 Objective

In technical terms, the Exposome constitutes a source of Big Data that changes through time and space, and so its implementation poses a great challenge for biomedical informatics and health care systems. It requires considering individual data related to the different elements surrounding the individual, and how this data change over time. Having said that, nowadays, dynamic environmental and psychosocial data can be gathered on a real time basis, using wearable devices, smartphones, or social networks. Also, computing infrastructures now make it possible to process this amount of information for a better understanding of disease causes and development mechanisms. Notwithstanding, there are not yet enough accepted data standards to represent this kind of data in an interchangeable and interoperable manner.

This Exposome's complexity being mentioned requires certain investments and coordinated support. Deploying more capable methodologies to evaluate individual exposures is urgent. For this purpose, data sharing and collaboration is required through the different disciplines taking part in health care. To succeed, it is mandatory to enable the research community to easily access tools, data, and exposure measures. Creating databases and methodologies for representing data to evaluate exposure is fundamental. In these terms, an accessible inventory would enable knowledge sharing between different studies and research lines [7].

In this project, several Exposome data examples have been analyzed, developing the required data models to collect, integrate and store the related data for further investigation, in a context of precision medicine. To do so, information processing methods have been developed, aiming to generate partial aspects of an individual's Exposome (Expotypes), from diverse data sources related to environmental risk factors affecting health. For this purpose, different information flows have been analyzed and data structures have been defined, illustrating a method to generate Expotypes for further research. These Expotypes have been represented following ISO-EN13606, a standard focused on modelling health data, based on Archetypes. Through this process, a common criteria to gather, represent and managed Exposome's data is pursued, making it possible to generate data models aimed to enable integrated and holistic health research, including all risk factors affecting health and complex diseases' development, both genetic and non-genetic. Through these examples, we aim to generate standard data models to support biomedical research and public health policies. This will enable health systems to analyze people's individual real time data, considering diary evolution of measures such as weight, physical activity, or blood pressure, to suggest proactive recommendation to people, anticipating possible health issues.

Through analysis such as the one being described here; biomedical informatics adds value and improve data management of environmental data affecting health. Certain research areas could specifically benefit from advances in this field:

- Biomedical research, as the one focused on understanding causes and mechanisms responsible for complex diseases' evolution.
- Precision medicine, as the integrative approach to health that considers all those risk factors affecting people's health and taking part in disease's development, for a better disease understanding [8].
- Digital epidemiology, as the field focused on pandemic and disease tracking and evolution, using digital monitoring devices such as wearables or smartphones. Indicators such as heart rate or sleep patterns are related to certain disease symptoms and can be tracked and measured through this kind of devices [9] (for example, fever related to COVID-19).

3 Previous Definitions

Expotyping is a new term that refers to individual Expotypes generation, meaning generating partial aspects of an individual's Exposome [10]. This new term can be presented by analogy to the terms of Genotype and Phenotype.

The Genome includes all the genes of a human organism and represents its complete DNA [11]. Drilling down into this term, the Genotype refers to the genetic information belonging to a specific individual [12]. Besides, the concept of Phenome relates to all those features presented by a human organism in relation to its genetic and exposure record [13], and so the Phenotype is defined as the structural and/or functional characteristics that can be observed on an individual, generated by the interaction between its Genotype and its context [14]. Ultimately, the Expotype represents a specific set of exposures accumulated by an individual during a certain time/space window, responsible of a particular Phenotype. In this regard, to fully understand how diseases are developed, assessing how the environment interacts with the genomic information generating specific phenotypes is a crucial step.

In addition to the terms presented above, one more key concept must be presented, as it is especially relevant to represent the data on a standard basis, the Archetype. As introduced before, the Expotypes generated have been represented following ISO-EN13606 recommendations through Archetypes. This framework establishes a dual development environment for health information systems, consisting in separating the medical knowledge from the information being introduced in systems. By doing this, medical information systems are able to adapt and evolve as the medical knowledge does so.

Archetypes stand as a mechanism for clinical concepts formal representation, automatically actionable by information systems [15]. They allow medical knowledge to be represented in computational terms, enabling health information structures to be modelled. Archetypes make it possible to build Expotype data models, integrating them with data related to the Genotype and Phenotype, aiming for a holistic approach in health care.

4 Methodology

Given the context defined above, this study tackles the generation of three Expotypes especially relevant nowadays, COVID-19, pollution, and physical activity. For each of them, it is mandatory to firstly study how their most important factors behave, enabling afterwards their modelling through Archetypes.

4.1 Expotype Design and Modelling

As explained, previous to the Expotypes modelling through Archetypes, studying which are the primary factors involved in the Expotype is mandatory. To do so, a first analysis aimed to gather a high-level view around Expotypes' composition has been conducted, enabling a clearer guidance for their subsequent data modelling. This step is required to establish the basis for a most exhaustive Expotype characterization through Archetypes, matching the most important factors comprising them with the data available to be gathered through devices such as the mentioned wearables, smartphones, or even traditional questionnaires. The information gathered from these sources will constitute a partial view of an individual's Exposome. On a similar basis, information related to its Genotype or Phenotype could be extracted and modelled through Archetypes, aiming for a common data storage manner, enabling a holistic approach for biomedical research.

4.2 Archetype Development

Having established conceptual Expotype's models, meaning the relevant factors taking part on each of them, the study advances towards Archetypes' construction by using the "LinkEHR" platform [16]. "LinkEHR" brings the required tools to guarantee semantic interoperability in data, such as the possibility to create Archetypes from clinical information models, or transforming clinical information to certain standards like openEHR, HL7 CDA or ISO 13606. "LinkEHR" is a key tool in digital health, not only because of the Archetypes construction mechanism, but also because allows to create an interoperable semantic framework. Through this tool, the proposed Archetypes have been created, generating real interoperable data models.

5 Results

5.1 COVID-19 Expotype

Expotype design and modelling. In viral pathogens transmission, environmental factors such as humidity or temperature have been proven strongly relevant [17]. Viruses live longer periods of time on surfaces if the environment stays dry and cold, hence increasing transmission possibilities. In general, environmental conditions influence diseases' transmission through three different axis, social factors, microbiological factors, and physiological factors [18], in addition to physical factors such as humidity or solar radiation. Moreover, measuring the time spent outdoors and indoors stands as a critical factor for COVID-19's transmission, as well as ventilation levels and measures.

A relevant part of COVID-19's transmission has been proven to occur in places where people expose themselves to longer periods of contact, such as gyms or restaurants [19]. Furthermore, sociological factors such as protection measures utilization, and social distancing maintenance, are also relevant for SARS-Cov-2 transmission. Moreover, as temperature increase stands as a regular symptom for people infected with this virus, COVID-19 pandemic has enforced societies to implement certain measures such as temperature periodical controls, in addition to protection measures such as the use of

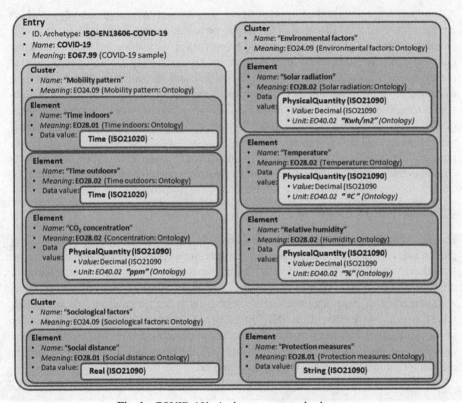

Fig. 1. COVID-19's Archetype proposal schema.

masks or hydroalcoholic gel. Considering these measures presented above may result extremely useful in terms of pandemic's evolution digital tracking, research, and patient's treatment. Hence, the following Archetype model is proposed (Fig. 1).

COVID-19's Archetype Construction. Having set the main factors considered for COVID-19's Expotype modelling, the Expotype model is developed. as explained before, the data model based on archetypes has been built by using the platform "LinkEHR". "LinkEHR" enables introducing the different factors studied, with the possibility to relate them to the adequate measure units and limits (Fig. 2).

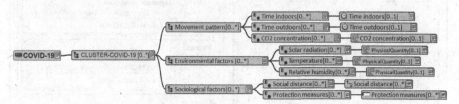

Fig. 2. COVID-19 Archetypes' data model designed using LinkEHR tool.

5.2 Pollution Expotype

Expotype Design and Modelling. Linking pollution with the previous study, air pollution and its exposure stand as a proven risk factor for COVID-19's transmission and symptoms, as it is related to heart and lung diseases. That being said, pollution could be related to 15% of COVID-19 deaths globally [20]. In general, pollution is considered as an international health issue, affected by several factors such as the social and the economic context, or lifestyle habits, among others. Anthropogenic pollution causes death to seven million people each year, globally [21]. The continuous exposure to pollution can be related to chronic diseases development such as asthma, lung deficiency, cardiovascular diseases, or diabetes [22].

In this sense, it is extremely relevant to be able to gather data around individual's exposure to pollution, bearing in mind its variation through time and space. Tracking individuals' situation, and matching their behavior to pollution data gathered from public air quality probes, can provide insight about individual's exposure to pollution rates, even differentiating between concentration from different particles, such as sulfur dioxide, ozone, cadmium, nitrogen dioxide, amongst others.

In this study, data from public air quality probes provided by Madrid's City Council have been used, matching their position with the measures provided over the different concentrations and particles. Having set the most relevant factors compounding the pollution Expotype, it has been modelled as follows (Fig. 3).

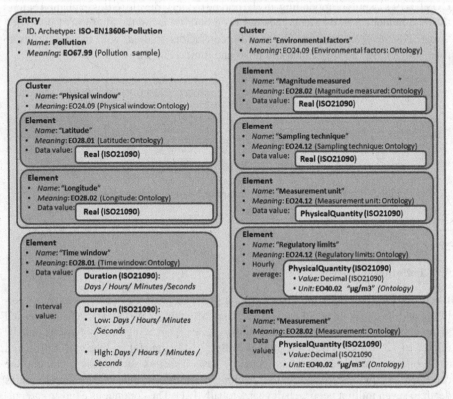

Fig. 3. Pollution's Archetype proposal schema.

Pollution's Archetype Construction. Once modelled the pollution's expotype, its construction through the use of archetypes is represented as follows. Once more, "LinkEHR" allows us to configure the units being measured, like the use of grades when establishing pollution's location through latitude and longitude (Fig. 4).

5.3 Physical Activity Expotype

Expotype design and modelling. Regular physical activity contributes to enhance muscular and respiratory capacity, bone health and functional capacity, reducing hypertension risk, cardiovascular diseases, and strokes, among others [19]. In addition, in general, people with more sedentary habits present shorter life expectancy than those individuals remaining active [23].

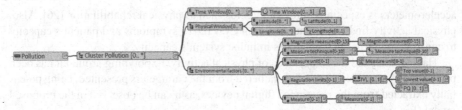

Fig. 4. Pollution Archetypes' data model designed using LinkEHR tool.

Being conscious of the benefits of physical activity and how it contributes to health, makes it mandatory to evaluate and measure it. Nowadays, physical activity is already being measured through devices such as smartphones or wearables, through the different sensors they incorporate. These devices have the capacity to measure relevant aspects related to people wellbeing, such as treatments efficacy, activity levels, sports performed and body reactions related to them, among others [24]. On this last point, monitoring certain parameters such as heart rate, blood pressure, respiratory rate, blood oxygen saturation, or body temperature is extremely interesting for health care [25]. Furthermore, being able to evaluate postural hygiene and body movement by using these devices'

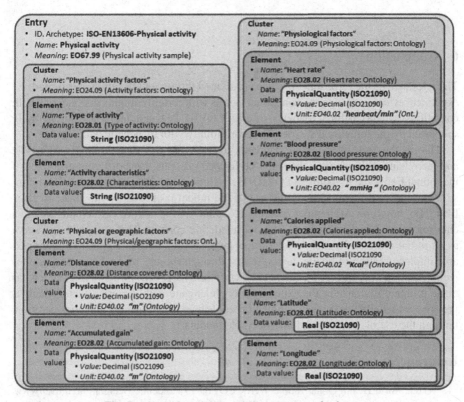

Fig. 5. Physical Activity's Archetype proposal schema.

accelerometers is especially relevant in fields such as physical rehabilitation [26]. Also, physical activity finds its connection with COVID-19 symptoms and patient's capacity to confront the virus, as it enhances immune system's capacity.

Having analyzed the importance of physical activity, Expotyping around it has been performed by considering the data gathered from the parameters presented, being potentially extracted from the mentioned digital devices, as it can be observed in the proposed model (Fig. 5).

Physical Activity's Archetype Construction. As with the previous examples, physical activity's archetype has been constructed as follows (Fig. 6).

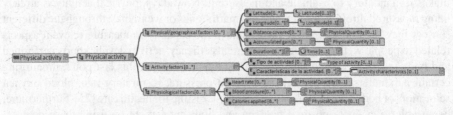

Fig. 6. Physical Activity Archetypes' data model designed using LinkEHR tool.

6   Conclusions

The relevance of the Exposome has been presented throughout the study performed. As explained, evidence relates environmental factors with certain complex diseases or health conditions, such as asthma, diabetes, or even COVID-19 pandemic. These are partially supported by the individual's exposure record jointly with its genetic endowment.

Due to the lack of accepted standards to represent this data in an interoperable and interchangeable manner, the study performed presents three different examples of individual Expotype modelling, COVID-19, pollution, and physical activity. Their construction has been supported by the use of the model proposed by the standard ISO-EN13606, based on Archetypes, making it available to gather, integrate and store this data for research purposes, in a precision medicine context. These models will serve as an initial point and example for further investigation, and an Exposome interoperable implementation in health care systems, through the use of Archetypes. Societies are nowadays experiencing a context characterized by COVID-19 pandemic, which has made it urgent to consider the exposures people engage with. External factors such as the ones modelled in the present study must contribute to a holistic health consideration, through the use of standard and interoperable models.

References

1. WHO: World Health Organization. WHO. COVID-19 Pandemic Declaration. https://www.who.int/director-general/speeches/detail/who-director-general-s-opening-remarks-at-the-media-briefing-on-covid-19---11-march-2020. Accessed 10 June 2021

2. Skochelak, S.E., et al.: Health Systems Science. 2nd Edn. (2020). https://www.elsevier.com/books/health-systems-science/skochelak/978-0-323-69462-9. Accessed 16 Feb 2021
3. Manolio, T.A., et al.: Finding the missing heritability of complex diseases. Nature **461**(7265), 747–753 (2009). https://doi.org/10.1038/nature08494
4. Wild, C.P.: Complementing the genome with an 'exposome': the outstanding challenge of environmental exposure measurement in molecular epidemiology. Cancer. Epidemiol. Biomark. Prev. **14**(8), 1847–1850 (2005). https://doi.org/10.1158/1055-9965.EPI-05-0456
5. Wild, C.P.: The Exposome: from concept to utility. Int. J. Epidemiol. **41**(1), 24–32 (2012). https://doi.org/10.1093/ije/dyr236
6. Martin-Sanchez, F., et al.: Use of informatics to characterise the Exposome of COVID-19. BMJ Health Care Inf. **28**, e100371 (2021). https://doi.org/10.1136/bmjhci-2021-100371J
7. Stingone, A., et al.: Toward greater Implementation of the Exposome research paradigm within environmental epidemiology. Annu. Rev. Public Health **38**, 315–327 (2017). https://doi.org/10.1146/annurev-publhealth-082516-012750
8. Collins, F.S., Varmus, H.: A new initiative on precision medicine. N. Engl. J. Med. **372**(9), 793–795 (2015). https://doi.org/10.1056/nejmp1500523
9. Sanchez, F.M., Gray, K., Bellazzi, R., Lopez-Campos, G.: Exposome informatics: considerations for the design of future biomedical research information systems. J. Am. Med. Inf. Assoc. **21**(3), 386–390 (2014). https://doi.org/10.1136/amiajnl-2013-001772
10. Martin-Sanchez, F.J., Lopez-Campos, G.H.: The new role of biomedical informatics in the age of digital medicine. Methods Inf. Med. **55**(5), 392–402 (2016)
11. Goldman, A.D., Landweber, L.F.: What is a genome? PLOS Genet. **12**(7), e1006181 (2016). https://doi.org/10.1371/journal.pgen.1006181
12. What is genotype? What is phenotype? – pgEd. https://pged.org/what-is-genotype-what-is-phenotype/. Accessed 14 Apr 2021
13. Mahner, M., Kary, M.: What exactly are genomes, genotypes and phenotypes? And what about phenomes? J. Theor. Biol. **186**(1), 55–63 (1997). https://doi.org/10.1006/jtbi.1996.0335
14. El sueño de lo posible: bioética y terapia génica - Lydia Feito Grande - Google Libros. https://books.google.es/books?id=LY1DwRobYbQC&lpg=PA35&dq=genotipo%20es&hl=es&pg=PA35#v=onepage&q=genotipo%20es&f=false. Accessed 14 Apr 2021
15. Maldonado, J.A., Moner, D., Tomas, D., Angulo, C., Robles, M., Fernandez, J.T.: Framework for Clinical Data Standardization Based on Archetypes, pp. 454–458 (2007)
16. VeraTech for Health: "LinkEHR" https://linkehr.veratech.es/. Accessed 10 June 2021
17. Barreca, A.I., Shimshack, J.P.: Absolute humidity, temperature, and influenza mortality: 30 years of county-level evidence from the United States. Am. J. Epidemiol. **176**(suppl_7), S114–S122 (2012). https://doi.org/10.1093/aje/kws259
18. González, P.: Es la COVID-19 una enfermedad estacional? https://theconversation.com/es-la-covid-19-una-enfermedad-estacional-148039. Accessed 10 June 2021
19. Chang, S., et al.: Mobility network models of COVID-19 explain inequities and inform reopening. Nature **589**(7840), 82–87 (2021). https://doi.org/10.1038/s41586-020-2923-3
20. Pozzer, A., Dominici, F., Haines, A., Witt, C., Münzel, T., Lelieveld, J.: Regional and global contributions of air pollution to risk of death from COVID-19. Cardiovasc. Res. **116**(14), 2247–2253 (2020). https://doi.org/10.1093/cvr/cvaa288
21. WHO: World Health Organization. Air pollution. https://www.who.int/health-topics/air-pollution#tab=tab_1. Accessed 10 June 2021
22. Eze, I.C., et al.: Long-term air pollution exposure and diabetes in a population-based Swiss cohort. Environ. Int. **70**, 95–105 (2014). https://doi.org/10.1016/j.envint.2014.05.014
23. Bauman, A.E.: Updating the evidence that physical activity is good for health: an epidemiological review 2000–2003. J. Sci. Med. Sport **7**(1), 6–19 (2004). https://doi.org/10.1016/S1440-2440(04)80273-1

24. Dinh-Le, C., Chuang, R., Chokshi, S., Mann, D.: Wearable health technology and electronic health record integration: Scoping review and future directions. JMIR mHealth uHealth **7**(9), e12861 (2019). https://doi.org/10.2196/12861

25. Dias, D., Cunha, J.P.S.: Wearable health devices—vital sign monitoring, systems and technologies. Sensors **18**(8), 2414 (2018). https://doi.org/10.3390/s18082414

26. Tokucoglu, F.: Monitoring physical activity with wearable technologies. Arch. Neuropsych. **55**(Suppl 1), S63 (2018). https://doi.org/10.29399/npa.23333

MKGB: A Medical Knowledge Graph Construction Framework Based on Data Lake and Active Learning

Peng Ren[1], Wei Hou[2(✉)], Ming Sheng[1], Xin Li[3], Chao Li[1], and Yong Zhang[1]

[1] BNRist, DCST, RIIT, Tsinghua University, Beijing 100084, China
{renpeng,shengming,li-chao,zhangyong05}@tsinghua.edu.cn
[2] Henan University, Kaifeng 475004, China
houwei@henu.edu.cn
[3] Beijing Tsinghua Changgung Hospital, School of Clinical Medicine, Tsinghua University, Beijing 102218, China
Horsebackdancing@sina.com

Abstract. Medical knowledge graph (MKG) provides ideal technical support for integrating multi-source heterogeneous data and enhancing graph-based services. These multi-source data are usually huge, heterogeneous, and difficult to manage. To ensure that the generated MKG has higher quality, the construction of MKG using these data requires a large number of medical experts to participate in the annotation based on their expertise. However, faced with such a large amount of data, manual annotation turns out to be a high labor cost task. In addition, the medical data are generated rapidly, which requires us to manage and annotate efficiently to keep up with the pace of data accumulation. Prior researches lacked efficient data management for massive medical data, and few studies focused on the construction of large-scale and high-quality MKG.

We propose a **M**edical **K**nowledge **G**raph **B**uilder (MKGB) based on Data Lake and active learning, which is used to solve the problems mentioned above. There are four modules in MKGB, data acquiring module, data management framework module based on Data Lake, active learning module for reducing labor cost and MKG construction module. With the efficient management for extensive medical data in data management framework based on Data Lake, MKGB uses active learning based on doctor-in-the-loop idea to reduce the labor cost of annotation process, while ensuring the quality of annotation and enabling the construction of large-scale and high-quality MKG. Based on the efficient data management, we demonstrate that our approach significantly reduces the cost of manual annotation and generates more reliable MKG.

Keywords: Data management · Data Lake · Active learning · Medical knowledge graph

1 Introduction

With the massive growth of data in medical domain, knowledge graph plays an increasingly important role. On the one hand, knowledge graph technology can effectively

S. Siuly et al. (Eds.): HIS 2021, LNCS 13079, pp. 245–253, 2021.
https://doi.org/10.1007/978-3-030-90885-0_22

organize huge amounts of medical multi-source heterogeneous data [1]. On the other hand, knowledge graph technology is effective in applications such as patient information extraction, personalized drug recommendation, and clinical decision making [2]. We broadly divide the construction process of medical knowledge graph (MKG) into three steps: data acquisition, data annotation and graph generation.

The researches of medical data management in the early stage adopted Database [3, 4] and Data Warehouse [5, 6]. More recently, confronted by the challenges brought by Database and Data Warehouse in medical data management, researchers began to pay attention to Data Lake technology.

For data annotation, many methods have been developed to achieve precise matching, such as template-based models [7], statistical-based methods [8], hybrid approaches [9], and deep-learning based approaches [10]. Although these methods achieve competitive performance in annotation tasks, the quality of the annotation results cannot be guaranteed in the face of new data without domain experts to provide judgment criteria. To address this issue, researchers focus on active learning [11]. Active learning is a technique for real-time labeling of data, which aims to optimize neural network learning by selecting the more informative data for labeling without exhaustive data labeling. Currently, most active learning methods combine sample selection strategies and deep learning models [12–14]. However, most of these methods annotate data automatically without the intervention of domain experts, the quality of annotation in real scenarios cannot be guaranteed.

Existing data management and annotation methods for building MKG have shortcomings in efficiency and quality control, respectively.

To solve the above problems, we propose a MKG construction platform based on Data Lake and active learning to manage medical multi-source heterogeneous data efficiently. Meanwhile, we achieve quality-assured medical data annotation to generate large-scale and high-quality MKG.

The rest of this paper is organized as follows. The review of related work is provided in Sect. 2. The platform architecture is described in Sect. 3. The modules are presented and analyzed in Sect. 4. The practical application is evaluated in Sect. 5. Finally, the conclusion is given in Sect. 6.

2 Related Work

In this section, we discuss three related topics, i.e. knowledge graph in medical domain, Data Lake in medical domain and active learning in medical domain.

Knowledge Graph in Medical Domain. To construct a medical related knowledge graph, previous work used different methods according to different data sources. An automatic approach for constructing a knowledge graph of knee osteoarthritis in Chinese was designed by Li et al. [15], and was used for knowledge retrieval from electronic medical records (EMRs). Chen et al. [16] utilized non-linear functions in building the knowledge graph to better understand existing model assumptions.

Although the MKGs mentioned above play a certain role for different data sources, few of them could manage the data in high performance. Unlike them, our proposed platform can efficiently manage medical data while building large-scale MKGs.

Data Lake in Medical Domain. The concept of Data Lake was first put forward by Dixon to deal with the challenges brought by Data Warehouse [17]. Due to the flexibility of Data Lake technology and the diversity of diseases, the existing researches work on Data Lake management framework in medical domain can be divided into two categories, namely, Data Lake technology research and disease analysis research.

With regard to Data Lake technology, Mesterhazy et al. [18] aimed at the cloud-based distributed computing technology to carry out rapid turnover of medical imaging, thus generating a medical image Data Lake processing framework. Bozena et al. [19] integrated fuzzy technology and declarative U-SQL language into data analysis, and developed a fuzzy search scheme for big Data Lake.

In terms of disease diversity research, Alhroob et al. [20] designed a data management framework based on Data Lake technology for semi-structured data of cardiovascular. Kachaoui et al. [21] came up with a Data Lake framework combining semantic web services and big data features in order to predict the case of COVID-19.

Different from these researches, we consider the real-time requirements of medical decision making and add distributed storage and processing modules to manage medical data efficiently.

Active Learning in Medical Domain. High-quality annotation of data through active learning techniques is a core part of achieving the construction of high-quality MKG.

In medical image processing, O-MedAL, an active learning method Smailagic et al. [12] proposed, which calculates the distance between unlabeled data and all training centers in the feature space, and then selects the unlabeled data with the maximum distance for labeling. Nath et al. [22] combined the U-net network model with the QBC and proposed a joint optimized QBC active learning method for image segmentation.

In medical natural language processing, Sheng et al. [13] combined CNN-CNN-LSTM and active learning algorithm, and proposed a framework called AHIAP that could extract quality entities and relations in EMRs. Carvallo et al. [14] proposed a combined logistic regression uncertainty sampling method based on four linguistic models, which was applied to the medical document screening task with better results.

Due to the sensitivity and importance of medical data, these active learning based methods for data annotation have a poor quality control module. Instead, we propose an active learning method with DITL idea.

3   The Framework of MKGB

3.1   The Framework of MKGB

As shown in Fig. 1, the platform architecture consists of four modules:

(1) Data acquiring module. It provides a large amount of medical data for the data management, such as EMRs, ECGs, CTs, etc.
(2) Data management module. It takes Data Lake technology as its core, and manages medical multi-source heterogeneous data in a unified and efficient way.

(3) Active learning module. It is composed of active learning and quality control, which jointly fulfill the task of high-quality data annotation.

(4) Output module. It generates large-scale and high-quality MKG according to the annotated medical data.

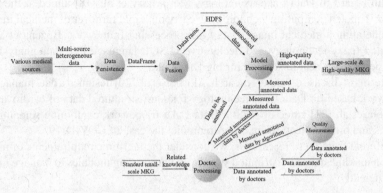

Fig. 1. The framework of MKGB

3.2 The Workflow of MKGB

Firstly, the platform imports the original medical data into the Data Lake in the form of data stream, which provides these data with storage interface, storage space and access permissions. Then, the data management module completes the unified and efficient management of data through its components such as conversion, cleaning, accelerated storage and analysis, thus preparing for data annotation.

In order to ensure the quality of data annotation and lower the cost of manual annotation, we adopt the active learning method with DITL. When the data is annotated, a small amount of data annotated by the model is first sent to the doctor, who makes the initial judgment on the data annotation. After that, the agent, which integrates the sample selection strategy, data enhancement and quality control components, conducts the second judgment on the data. Finally, the data and annotations at this time are input into the deep learning model to complete the iterative training of the model. When the model reaches a stable state or the data in the Data Lake is fully annotated, the process will be terminated.

When the process terminates, the remaining data can be automatically annotated directly by employing the model at this time if there is data left in the Data Lake, and all the final annotated data will be used as the basis for building the MKG.

4 Modules

4.1 Data Management Module

As shown in Fig. 2, at the bottom of the Data Lake platform, the distributed file system HDFS provides the basic storage, and the Spark provides the computing power.

Besides, the DataFrame and Delta Lake work together to fuse data for efficient and unified data storage. The core module is a number of data processing methods customized by Spark and Delta Lake, and these methods are released as RESTful APIs to support data exploration and analysis.

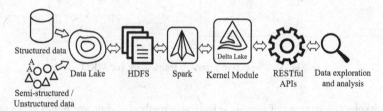

Fig. 2. The data management workflow

Data Overview. There are two forms of data sources according to the way of obtaining data. The first one is the transportation type. In transportation type, the interface designed by the Data Lake platform is used to upload the data files to the reserved space of the Data Lake using SFTP protocol, and then the data is carried to the data cluster inside the Data Lake. The second type is pipeline. Accessing the Database by protocol, this form of data itself will not be put inside the Data Lake to save, it will read the data into the memory for using, fusing or querying, and then calculate with other data in the memory. The calculation results are saved to HDFS.

Data Management. Due to the complexity and diversity of the medical data, we propose to convert heterogeneous data from different sources into one form. The data model DataFrame, which is the core of our data management, is a distributed collection of data organized in named columns. The idea of our data management is to first transform data in a discrete manner and then merge the transformed unified data. At the same time, in order to handle the problem of data flow pressure, the conversion among data is accelerated by Spark, which can significantly increase the conversion efficiency.

4.2 Active Learning Module

In this module, we adopt Zhang's work [23] and further add the DITL, thus forming a method that can be applied to knowledge graph construction, as shown in Fig. 3.

The Workflow of Active Learning. In the process of the module, the active learning algorithm iteratively selects the most informative data from the Data Lake and sends it to the doctor for annotating.

Star-up Procedure

In the initial stage of the module, the executors of the selection strategy are deemed as the agent to dynamically select the samples with the most information. At the beginning,

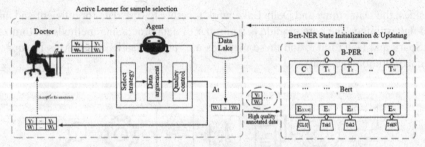

Fig. 3. The active learning framework for MKG

the agent selects a strategy of sample selection, a method of data argument and a method of quality control. In the meanwhile, the data that need to be annotated are prepared in the Data Lake. After the preparation, Bert-NER, the initialized sequence annotating model, is used to randomly select a part of medical data for annotating. The agent then selects the most informative data from the data verified by the doctor and transmits it to BERT-NER model, and updates the model.

Loop Procedure

After the initialization phase, BERT-NER model is warmed up, and at time t, the quality of medical data annotation by the model begins to improve. At this time, the model, combined with the agent, selects the data $(w_1, w_2, \ldots, w_k)$ from the Data Lake with the action A_t to annotate, and then transmits the annotated data to the doctor for judgment. After the doctor judges the data, the data is transmitted to the agent again. Then, the agent selects a part of the data and applies the method of data enhancement to generate new data consistent with the judged data label to accelerate the convergence of the model state. The quality control module of the agent screens the new data generated, removes the data with poor quality generated after data enhancement, and retains the data that conforms to the characteristics of medical data. In the end, the data $(w_i, \ldots)$ reviewed by the doctor and the agent are transmitted to BERT-NER model, which automatically learns features of new data, dynamically updates parameters.

Termination Procedure

Once the model reaches the required state or the data in the Data Lake is fully annotated, the doctor and agent will not continue the subsequent step.

If there is still data left in the Data Lake when the model reaches the required state, the data in the Data Lake can be completely annotated by directly annotating the remaining data with the model in this state.

Measurement Module. Medical data is unique and important, and errors can have irreparable consequences for doctor decisions and patient care. Therefore, it is important to ensure the quality of data annotation.

Methodology

We implement a double-layer annotation quality control method.

The first layer: the medical data annotated by the model is transmitted to the doctor for the first judgment, and the doctor decides whether to accept the data or annotate the data again.

The second layer: the medical data judged by the doctor is transmitted to the agent for the first time. The agent adopts the strategy of sample selection to select the sample with the highest information content to be transmitted to the data argument module. Then, the data argument algorithm is used to amplify the selected sample data. Furthermore, in order to control the quality of the amplified data, a generative pre-training language model GPT2 is taken to score the data, which discards the amplified data with low confidence and keeps the amplified data with high confidence.

Update

As time goes by, new data will be transmitted to the Data Lake, which needs to be annotated again. It is necessary to put the varied data into the active learning module again for updating.

Once the updated annotation results are available, they are applied to update the MKG, which can again be constructive for future work related to the medical domain.

5 Evaluation

MKGB has been deployed to Beijing Tsinghua Changgung Hospital[1] to support MKG construction in knee osteoarthritis domain. These knee osteoarthritis data, involving 128,000 people and a total of 230,000 visits, include structured EMRs and unstructured medical images and texts.

Based on 200GB structured and unstructured data, we construct 768,523 edges and 832,152 nodes in MKG. In the construction process, 15,360 samples are annotated by doctors and the model annotates 48,640 samples, which saves 76% labor.

6 Conclusion and Future Work

In this paper, we propose a MKG construction platform based on Data Lake and active learning. The platform consists of two core modules, which are the efficient data management module based on Data Lake and the active learning module with the addition of DITL. The data management method based on Data Lake is used to manage the complex large numbers of medical data, and then the data is reliably annotated by the active learning method of DITL, which provides a solid foundation for building a reliable MKG. In the future, we intend to optimize robustness of data management to adapt to more complex and huge amounts of medical data. For active learning, we intend to use additional extended knowledge to further improve the diversity and rationality of data selection strategies.

Acknowledgements. This work was supported by National Key R&D Program of China (2020AAA0109603), and Institute of Precision Medicine, Tsinghua University.

---

[1] http://www.btch.edu.cn/.

References

1. Zhang, Y., et al.: HKGB: an inclusive, extensible, intelligent, semi-auto-constructed knowledge graph framework for healthcare with clinicians' expertise incorporated. Inf. Process. Manage. **57**(6), 102324 (2020)
2. Huang, Z., Yang, J., van Harmelen, F., Hu, Q.: Constructing knowledge graphs of depression. In: Siuly, S., et al. (eds.) HIS 2017. LNCS, vol. 10594, pp. 149–161. Springer, Cham (2017). https://doi.org/10.1007/978-3-319-69182-4_16
3. Mitchell, J., Naddaf, R., Davenport, S.: A medical microcomputer database management system. Methods Inf. Med. **24**(2), 73–78 (1985)
4. Mohamad, B., Orazio, L., Gruenwald, L.: Towards a hybrid row-column database for a cloud-based medical data management system. In: Cloud-I, pp. 1–4 (2012)
5. Sebaa, A., et al.: Medical big data warehouse: architecture and system design, a case study: improving healthcare resources distribution. J. Med. Syst. **42**, 59 (2018)
6. Garani, G., Adam, G.K.: A semantic trajectory data warehouse for improving nursing productivity. Health Inf. Sci. Syst. **8**(1), 1–13 (2020). https://doi.org/10.1007/s13755-020-001 17-5
7. Hanisch, D., et al.: ProMiner: rule-based protein and gene entity recognition. BMC. Bioinform. **6**(1), S14 (2005)
8. Settles, B.: Biomedical named entity recognition using conditional random fields and rich feature sets. In: ACL, pp. 104–107 (2004)
9. Zeng G., Zhang C., Bo X., et al: CRFS-based Chinese named entity recognition with improved tag set. In: CSIE, pp. 519–522 (2009)
10. Huang Z., Wei X., Kai Y.: Bidirectional LSTM-CRF models for sequence tagging. Comput. Sci. (2015)
11. Konyushkova, K., Sznitman, R., Fua, P.: Geometry in active learning for binary and multi-class image segmentation. Comput. Vis. Image Underst. **182**, 1–16 (2019)
12. Smailagic, A., et al.: O-MedAL online active deep learning for medical image analysis. Wiley. Interdiscip. Rev. Data. Mining. Knowl. Discov. **10**(4), e1353 (2020)
13. Sheng, M., et al.: AHIAP: an agile medical named entity recognition and relation extraction framework based on active learning. In: Huang, Z., Siuly, S., Wang, H., Zhou, R., Zhang, Y. (eds.) HIS 2020. LNCS, vol. 12435, pp. 68–75. Springer, Cham (2020). https://doi.org/10.1007/978-3-030-61951-0_7
14. Carvallo, A., Parra, D., Lobel, H., Soto, A.: Automatic document screening of medical literature using word and text embeddings in an active learning setting. Scientometrics **125**(3), 3047–3084 (2020). https://doi.org/10.1007/s11192-020-03648-6
15. Li, X., Liu, H., Zhao, X., Zhang, G., Xing, C.: Automatic approach for constructing a knowledge graph of knee osteoarthritis in Chinese. Health Inf. Sci. Syst. **8**(1), 1–8 (2020). https://doi.org/10.1007/s13755-020-0102-4
16. Chen, I., et al.: Robustly extracting medical knowledge from EHRs: a case study of learning a health knowledge graph. In: PSB, pp. 19–30 (2019)
17. Dixon, J.: Pentaho, Hadoop, and data lakes (2015). https://jamesdixon.woedpress.com/2010/10/14pentaho-hadoop-and-data-lakes/. Accessed 15 June 2021
18. Mesterhazy, J., Olson, G., Datta, S.: High performance on-demand de-identification of a petabyte-scale medical imaging data lake (2020). arXiv preprint: https://arxiv.org/abs/2008.01827
19. Bozena, M., Marek, S., Dariusz, M.: Soft and declarative fishing of information in big data lake. IEEE Trans. Fuzzy Syst. **26**(5), 2732–2747 (2018)
20. Alhgaish, A., et al.: Preserve quality medical drug data toward meaningful data lake by cluster. Int. J. Recent Technol. Eng. **8**(3), 270–277 (2019)

21. Kachaoui, J., Larioui, J., Belangour, A.: Towards an ontology proposal model in data lake for real-time COVID-19 cases prevention. Int. J. Online Biomed. Eng. **16**(9), 123–136 (2020)

22. Nath, V., et al.: Diminishing uncertainty within the training pool: active learning for medical image segmentation (2021). arXiv preprint arXiv: https://arxiv.org/abs/2101.02323

23. Zhang, R., Yu, Y., Zhang, C.: SeqMix: augmenting active sequence labeling via sequence mixup. In: EMNLP, pp. 8566–8579 (2020)

HMDFF: A Heterogeneous Medical Data Fusion Framework Supporting Multimodal Query

Peng Ren[1], Weihang Lin[2(✉)], Ye Liang[2], Ruoyu Wang[3], Xingyue Liu[3], Baifu Zuo[4], Tan Chen[4], Xin Li[5], Ming Sheng[1], and Yong Zhang[1]

[1] BNRist, DCST, RIIT, Tsinghua University, Beijing 100084, China
`{renpeng,shengming,zhangyong05}@tsinghua.edu.cn`
[2] Beijing Foreign Studies University, Beijing 100089, China
`liangye@bfsu.edu.cn`
[3] Beihang University, Beijing 102206, China
`18377446@buaa.edu.cn`
[4] Henan University, Kaifeng 475004, China
`1912080073@henu.edu.cn`
[5] Beijing Tsinghua Changguang Hospital, School of Clinical Medicine, Tsinghua University, Beijing 102218, China
`Horsebackdancing@sina.com`

Abstract. As we move forwards to Healthcare Industry 4.0 era, more and more high accuracy and technological devices are applied into medical field, for the better services in health domain. However, the traditional storage methods of scaled data limit the application of data analysis. Besides, electronic medical data (EMR) and electronic health data (EHR), unstructured data including MRIs, CT scans, X-ray and PET scans are the fastest growing part of medical data. Due to different regulations between structured and unstructured data, and among various unstructured imaging data, though the traditional data warehouses can solve the problems of scalability and data fragmentation, the cost of solution is high and it is not real-time. The multimodal data are separated and this ineffective data storage is insufficient to enable further efficient hybrid query.

Therefore, to solve the fragmentation of multimodal data storage and enable hybrid query for further data analytics services, this paper proposes a high-efficiency heterogenous medical data fusion framework (HMDFF) for multimodal and heterogeneous data in medical field based on data lake. This framework aims to fuse the fragmented medical data and provide users with effective management methods and user-friendly interfaces to perform hybrid query.

Keywords: Heterogenous medical data · Data fusion framework · Multimodal query

1 Introduction

Tremendous amounts of multimodal and heterogeneous medical data are generated every day from medical smart devices and healthcare events. Besides, data generated from the

© Springer Nature Switzerland AG 2021
S. Siuly et al. (Eds.): HIS 2021, LNCS 13079, pp. 254–266, 2021.
https://doi.org/10.1007/978-3-030-90885-0_23

mentioned devices grow in large amount and complexity. The medical data types are very complicated and diverse [1]. The collected high dimensional data require matching methods to interpret and further organize and analyze in knowledge graph to obtain more valuable information, where data fusion, analytics technologies, and knowledge graph construction in medical field is employed [2]. These multimodal and heterogeneous medical data includes structured data, such as electronic medical records (EMRs) and electronic health records (EHRs), and unstructured imaging data, such as MRIs, CT scans, X-ray and PET scans etc. According to healthcare study, the imaging data generated in modern hospital environments are up to hundreds of terabytes [3].

With the variety and diversity of plenty of medical data, researches on data-driven decision-making approaches have long been conducted. In traditional computer-aided medical expert systems, decision making is assisted by employing feature-level fusion or rule-based reasoning [4]. These computer-aided diagnosis systems focus on semantic perception and entity association mining with the big medical data collection. Artificial intelligence techniques are also implemented in recent studies [5–7, 14], including deep neural networks for feature extractions for the purpose of data fusion [5, 7]. There are also frameworks proposed based on ML or DL for extraction of complementary information for multimodal data, extracting text features and image features for assistance of decision making [6, 7, 15, 16]. Due to the data fragmentation, the concept of "panoramic interactive decision-making" and relevant mechanisms were also proposed to overcome the problem due to regional and departmental multi-source, cross-border and multimodal medical data [4].

However, among all of these mentioned frameworks, mechanisms or systems, the fusion of multimodal data lacks the consideration on using a unified format for multimodal and cross-border data storage. Moreover, though with researches on panoramic decision-making, state-of-the-art techniques didn't enable any user-friendly hybrid queries based on the fused data. The analytics and utilization based on data fusion is insufficient to provide hybrid queries in medical scenarios.

Contributions. In this paper, we propose a framework based on data lake aiming to solve the current problem in multimodal query based on data fusion in medical field. The data lake is designed to accomplish the tasks of multimodal data fusion as a unified format with the high-calculability platform spark. On the top of the data lake, multimodal queries are performed with interfaces. We address our contributions as follows:

1. We implement the fusion of heterogeneous data based on Data Lake. Different formats of structured and unstructured data are transformed into one unified format for persistence.
2. We propose dynamic index management strategy on unstructured data. The generation of index to manage the high-dimensional feature vectors is in accordance with the characteristic of the unstructured data.

In the following sections, we will provide the details of HMDFF. Section 2 discusses related work. Section 3 introduces the overall architecture of HMDFF. Section 4 presents our designs and implementations of multimodal and heterogeneous data fusion. Section 5 presents our dynamic index management strategy on unstructured medical data. Section 6 presents our implementations and medical scenarios of the interfaces. Section 7 concludes the paper.

2 Related Work

In the aspect of storage, we aim to fuse the multimodal and heterogenous medical data. In traditional researches, structured data are usually stored in a relational database. As for unstructured data, there are researches on them to extract the feature information using machine learning tools for data analysis [5–7, 14]. Different algorithms are proposed for efficient embedding generation.

There are also researches about unstructured data storage systems. Zhu et al. [8] proposed a storage system, CTDGM, especially for unstructured data and merging strategy but only concerned the small-sized unstructured data in the way of storing them in a consecutive location for operation and index efficiency. Sun et al. [9] proposed INSMA, a system for medical field, transforming data from different patient monitor into a big text file including the monitoring results. An intelligent system is also proposed for patients' similar text information retrieval by information from template, topic, and latent semantic indexes [10]. None of these researches have focused on the fusion of multimodal data. The storage strategy was very limited and types of unstructured data doesn't include medical images.

Hybrid query is developed based on multimodal data storage. A hybrid query method concerning textual information retrieval is proposed [11], using both statistical approach based on term frequency and semantic approach with embedding information from WordNet and domain ontology. And a similar hybrid query framework is also introduced [12], utilizing original lexical resources and word embedding information concerning question answering problem. Though such frameworks are proposed, researches are very lacking in hybrid query area. Moreover, considering the diversity of medical data, existing researches are not adequate to meet the complicated medical scenarios.

In the aspect of embedding and index, every embedding model or index construction method has its own advantage. Embeddings from different models can represent different aspects of information from unstructured data. For example, AU-aware Deep Networks (AUDN) designed by Liu et al. [13] is constructed for facial expression recognition. And with later findings and research on expression datasets including CK +, MMI and SFEW, the model can provide competitive and even Better results. Besides, different index construction method has different efficiency. But there is lack of researches to do some management work for these embedding models and index construction methods in application scenarios. In many experiments, they only use single method to solve problems.

We address the challenges as follows:

1. There are a large number of data sources with rich and diverse structures but lacking of feasible method for data fusion and storage, which limit the application of further heterogenous data analysis. How can we fuse the multimodal medical data for persistence?

2. The amount of unstructured data is accumulating rapidly at present. However, in many query methods, unstructured data is usually in exception due to the limitation of the traditional tools. How can we efficiently and sufficiently manage the unstructured data?

In comparison, HMDFF has two advantages. In the layer of data storage, we fuse the multimodal and heterogenous data in medical field, which further enables our hybrid query on the fusion table. What's more, we further propose a dynamic strategy to manage embeddings and indexes for unstructured data.

3 System Design

HMDFF is built on top of the data lake based on Apache Spark. It consists of three modules: data lake at the base for reliable and permanent data storage, dynamic index management layer for efficient unstructured data management and hybrid query layer for multimodal and heterogeneous data analytics. HMDFF utilizes the functions of data lake for multimodal data fusion and develops dynamic index management strategies, based on which hybrid fusion query is performed. In this section, we present key system designs that enable the realization of multimodal and heterogeneous data fusion, index management and hybrid query processing.

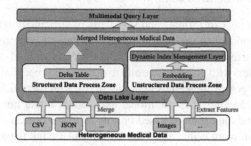

Fig. 1. HMDFF architecture overview

3.1 Architecture Overview

The architecture of HMDFF is presented in Fig. 1, which is mainly composed of three types of layers: data lake layer, dynamic index management layer, and multimodal query layer. Data lake Layer accept, parse and merge multimodal data, transforming data of different formats into delta tables. Index management layer constructs indexes on unstructured data dynamically according to users' request or data characteristics. With the results of data fusion and dynamic index, hybrid query is then performed on the transformed multimodal data. HMDFF adopts a typical read/write decoupling approach. Hence, write operation (i.e., INSERT, DELETE and UPDATE) about data is only performed in the data lake layer while read operation (i.e., SELECT) is performed in multimodal query layer.

Moreover, all of the mentioned operations are integrated into API interfaces, enabling users to operate as they wish based on some simple code sentences.

Data lake at the base uses Spark to implement the fusion of multimodal data, reframing variety of data into DataFrame including CSV, JSON, SQL file etc. As for the unstructured data, feature vector will be extracted first based on the pre-trained deep learning models. With the embedding of the unstructured data, indexes for the high-dimensional vector will be generated from the dynamic index management layer. The feature vectors with the indexes can be transformed into columns of DataFrame as well, realizing the fusion of multimodal data. Based on the two layers above, multimodal query layer is able to do fusion query after the generation of DataFrame for multimodal data. In this layer, we propose the RESTFUL interface using SQL dialects for the convenience of searching.

4 Multimodal Data Fusion and Management

The variety of source data formats makes it necessary to fuse the data before the efficient query. The fusion relies heavily on the data lake based on Spark. In this section, we introduce how to implement the fusion process on the structured and unstructured data respectively.

4.1 The Fusion of Structured Data

There are a large number of formats and standards of structured data in order to meet different practical demands in various situation. For example, various standards contain SQL, NoSQL etc.; in terms of file formats, CSV, JSON, XML and others are included. Among all of these data with diversity, we aim to use a unified concept for representation.

We regard that each of these files contains items with identified key and attached features. For data searching, it is traditional and common that query is processed on separated datasets and data sources based on join or union operation, which can lower the efficiency. The problem is that all of the stored data are not regarded as a whole.

In HMDFF, we use a different way of considering these multi-source data. Each data file is considered as a set containing different elements. Inside the sets, elements are represented as tree graphs (see Fig. 2). Every tree is an identified item and nodes are features or keys.

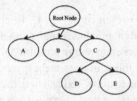

Fig. 2. Element tree graph

The fusion of multi-source data is represented as the union of different sets. Supposed that we have set A and set B, the target set S of the fusion can be represented as:

$$S = A \cup B \tag{1}$$

Then, the problem of fusing two sets can be further decomposed as the merge of various tree graphs representing elements.

To merge elements, we first distinguish two elements by comparing their keys. The algorithm of fusion can be expressed as follows. Because a key can be either on root node or leaf node, we have to trace back to root node initially for further subtree comparison. Three kinds of situation are included: if keys and all the subtrees are identical, the two trees are the same and only one is reserved; if keys are the same while subtrees are slightly different, they are partly the same and needs further fusion; if keys are different, then both elements are retained.

```
Algorithm 1:  Fusion of two trees
Input:   Tree T1, Tree T2, Target set S
Output: Target set S
1.    If    T1.key1 == T2.key2
2.          #Trace back to Root node
3.          If  T1.root node.all subtrees==T2.root   node.all subtrees
4.                T1==T2
5.          Else
6.                T1 = T1 + (T2 − T1 ∩ T2)
7.          S = S + {T1}
8.    Else
9.          S = S + {T1} + {T2}
10.   return S
```

4.2 The Fusion of Unstructured Data

Besides structured data, unstructured data is a very important component in HMDFF. To further develop the concepts in Sect. 4.1, unstructured data are regarded as one of the subtrees in the tree-presented element (See Fig. 3), which means we view unstructured data as one of the features of the elements.

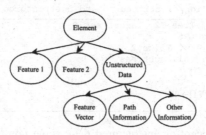

Fig. 3. Element tree graph including unstructured data

Unstructured data node is a concept node that contain the relevant information including feature vector node for representation and similarity calculation, path information node for tracing back to file, and some other underlying information nodes.

In healthcare unstructured data like images, types of images vary differently according to healthcare equipment including CT, MRI etc. The type differences lead to different features. For example, feature of gray scale in an X-ray image is more important than in a line-consisting electrocardiogram in which features of edges will be emphasized. Besides, in a specific medical image, features are usually more than one. It is difficult to cover all aspects of information within only one embedding vector. For example, background information, edges information and gray scale information of an MRI image work together to assist a doctor's decision. But using only one vector generated from a single model may lead to loss of key information. To solve the mentioned problem, we propose to use multi-version feature vectors generated from different embedding models to represent unstructured data in order to cover all of the information in an image for meeting the doctors' practical requests accordingly.

Therefore, feature vector node can be further demonstrated as Fig. 4. Multi-version embedding nodes are attached to the feature vector node. The attached leaf nodes demonstrate information including embedding model name and extracted vector itself.

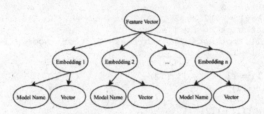

Fig. 4. Multi-version feature vector

When we consider the fusion of unstructured data, it is worthy to note that it doesn't indicate the fusion of different sources of unstructured data but the fusion of structured and unstructured data. The algorithm of the fusion of multimodal data including unstructured data is described in Algorithm 2.

Algorithm 2: Fusion of structured and unstructured data trees

---

Input: Tree T1, Tree T2, Target set S
Output: Target set S
1.   **If**   T1.key1 == T2.key2
2.   T1=T1+T2.all subtrees
3.   S = S + {T1}
4.   **Else**
5.   S = S + {T1} + {T2}
6.   **return** S

To illustrate the concept of unstructured data, some non-terminal concept nodes are introduced like feature vector node. In the actual process of storage after fusion, an element tree could be over-complicated and space-consuming when all of the embedding information (model names and feature vectors) are stored under one single root node. Hence, we regulate that an element root node will only contain one embedding model information along with the consistent feature vector. So, there will only be one embedding model in a fusion target set. Elements with different embedding information will be gathered and stored in another target set. The actual storage structure of an element consists of different features from structured data and nodes from unstructured data including model name, vector, path information and other information. The depth of the element tree is two.

4.3 Implementation

Based on the tree graph representation of elements and sets fusion, we further use our Data Lake to realize the theories on SparkSQL platform, utilizing the assistance of cluster computing, advantages of data structures and computing capability.

In SparkSQL, three kinds of data structures are offered, which are RDD, DataSet and DataFrame and they are immutable distributed collection of data. In comparison, RDD represents low-transformation and control of original datasets. The essence of DataFrame is RDD[ROW]. It organizes data into named columns with more APIs for data manipulation, providing detailed structural information. DataFrame is on a higher level of abstraction and RDD is more suitable for data with loose structure. Considering the data fusion and implementation of tree graph we are dealing with, the characteristics of DataFrame and the relevant APIs can provide us with convenience during data fusion and further query.

The attached structure information of the data can be parsed by DataFrame as schema. In essence, the schema information of the DataFrame can be expressed as a tree graph (See Fig. 5). Therefore, a tree graph can also be represented by a DataFrame. It means that each element represented by the tree graph in the set can be put into the DataFrame as a data row. Each node represents a feature column in a DataFrame. Moreover, feature vectors are extracted, where unstructured images are transformed into structured arrays and unstructured data can also be stored by DataFrame. Hence, a DataFrame containing all data rows can represent a data set containing all of the elements. According to this, the problem of merging different sets has become a problem of DataFrame fusion.

```
root
 |-- age: long (nullable = true)
 |-- myScore: array (nullable = true)
 |    |-- element: struct (containsNull = true)
 |    |    |-- score1: long (nullable = true)
 |    |    |-- score2: long (nullable = true)
 |-- name: string (nullable = true)
```

Fig. 5. DataFrame schema

The fusion is implemented by merge function in Spark, which enable us to utilize the calculation capability of this high-performing platform. There are three key equations in fusion algorithm that need to be further illustrated on data lake.

The Merge task of Data Lake can be divided into two scans. The first scan is an inner join based on the comparison of the key. When the keys are identical, two data rows will be taken out and perform inner join, which is equivalent to T1.allsubtrees == T2.allsubtrees in Algorithm 1; then outer join is performed in the second scan phase between the selected files, which accomplishes $T1 = T1 + (T2 - T1 \cap T2)$. Finally, the data rows will be added to the output DataFrame, which corresponds to TargetS = S + {T1} + {T2}.

Considering the two join phases above, merge is a combined optimized execution plan of join in essence. Therefore, based on the computing power of Spark, Spark queries can be optimized automatically, which provide the fusion process with great convenience and efficiency. Moreover, when executing join on Spark, the SparkSQL platform can automatically generate an optimized implementation plan based on the input file size. The implementation plan includes sort merge join, shuffle hash join and broadcast hash join, thereby improving the efficiency of join. In data lake, the mentioned advantages are utilized in our implementation of applied interfaces.

In the interface, various formats of data (including CSV, JSON, SQL) can be turned into a unified format as DataFrame. Besides, information from unstructured data after feature extraction are stored in JSON files and can be transformed into DataFrame. To complete the fusion process, we input the following parameters: file paths of delta table and json file, the primary key of delta table and the primary key of json file. Our Data Lake will then transform the separated files into a merged delta table containing heterogeneous data for further possible read operation and backtracking operation. When any query is required, the merged delta table will be directly read and searched with the user's SQL request. To record more embedding models, more delta tables will be created and stored for further use.

5   Index Management of Unstructured Data

Considering the characteristic of high dimension of feature vectors from different embedding models, it can be very inefficient if we directly use the vectors for similarity calculation. At the same time, it is time-consuming and not convenient for the management of such vectors. Hence, we propose methods of dynamic index management of unstructured data, using indexes to help improve the efficiency. According to different situation, three methods are proposed to meet different demands.

5.1   General Method

The general method is targeted to meet general requirements with general datasets. In this method, we use mono-index to construct the order of one particular feature that can best describe the overview of the images (See Fig. 6).

In the fusion delta table, indexes are generated according to user's actual requirements based on the feature vector columns. The way to generate indexes can be chosen by users. This method can be very simple and efficient in the situation that dataset is small and general.

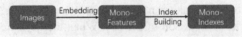

Fig. 6. General method

5.2 Data-Driven Method

However, the performance of general method may be affected when the unstructured data are accumulated in a very large amount. We then introduce a data-driven strategy to manage all of the indexes.

The embeddings of images in HMDFF are multi-version as is mentioned in Sect. 4 and multi-level indexes are constructed accordingly. These multi-version features are ranked in a specific order: features that represent the overall information of the image construct the first-level index; features representing more detailed information construct the second-level index. Other features are also constructed under this logic.

Supposed a practical healthcare scenario with the need for analysis of an electro-cardiogram. Features can include background, foreground, grayscale, pixels, edges etc. During the analysis, these feature genres can be ranked according to doctors' orders. So, the process of managing the indexes can be shown as Fig. 7:

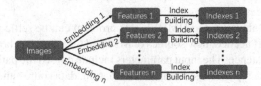

Fig. 7. Data-driven method of index management

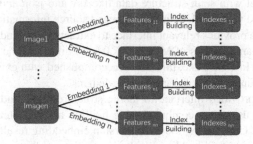

Fig. 8. Request-driven method of index management

5.3 Request-Driven Method

Besides multi-version embeddings of one image, there are also different types of images from various healthcare equipment with abundant information. Organization of unstructured data is more perplex and the diversity of image types like CRI, X-rays and CTs requires more human knowledge from doctors.

Supposed a healthcare scenario that a patient's medical record contains CRI, X-ray and CT at the same time. Three types of images can be ranked from high to low according to doctors' instructions to improve hybrid query. This method can be dynamic and changeable along with the actual situation in order to build efficient indexes. The process of request-driven methods bases itself on data-driven method in Sect. 5.2 (See Fig. 8).

6 Hybrid Query in Medical Field

6.1 Hybrid Query

In some medical scenarios, it is inevitable to use these heterogeneous data including EMRs, CTs, MRIs, X-rays etc. To accurately retrieve patients' records using heterogeneous data, healthcare multimodal query is executed based on both similarity constraints of feature vectors generated from medical scans and value conditions of structured data.

We can suppose a medical hybrid query scenario that a doctor needs to retrieve similar past cases for references when diagnosing a new patient, noted as A, over 60 years old with MRI and CT scans. In this typical situation, we need to search for the target records and retrieve the images according to A's scan results. So, the situation can be decomposed into two problems: first, filter condition on structured data about age which should be over 60 years old; second, filter condition on unstructured images including MRI scans and CT scans. Feature vectors of A's scans are query vectors and the scenario requires to find similar images in database.

Based on the Data Lake and HMDFF, this problem can be settled according to following steps: first, if needed, new sources of MRI and CT scans can be uploaded into our Data Lake for persistence. The input parameters include upload file path, destination path for persistence, data type, data structured information, data source and data description. The interface will return the first 10 lines of the data uploaded if successful but failure information if unsuccessful. The interface can manage data persistence in the data lake system and can deal with semi-structure data like csv and json and unstructured data like text, images and videos. Meta information and source information are also stored.

Next, Data Lake provides relevant interface to extract corresponding feature vectors according to the characteristics of MRI and CT and build dynamic indexes according to doctors' request. In Data Lake, this step is accomplished with existing techniques in Python and under supervision of doctors' knowledge.

Third, we use provided interface to merge structured data and unstructured data which can provide us with a combined table holding all the heterogeneous medical data as in Sect. 4.3. Considering the multi-version embedding results, one table would only contain one kind of embedding results in avoidance of information and storage redundance. Therefore, when there is more than one embedding result to consider, there will be several tables created with the dynamic index results.

Then, we are able to realize hybrid query on these tables in the form of SQL dialect. The results returned are hierarchical according to different priorities because of pre-set in dynamic index construction. In this interface, user can directly use SQL dialect to search on the target delta table with data type and path input. The output is returned in the form of json string.

With the mentioned results returned, several record items under the filter of age and suitable similarity between query feature vectors of MRI and CT and stored feature vectors from other patients. Doctors can further examine these comprehensive computing outcomes to diagnose and judge further for patients' treatment. At the same time, the path info recorded along with the feature vectors of these scan images can also help doctors to retrieve back to original scan images beyond getting merely the feature vectors.

6.2 Application

HMDFF has been applied to XXX hospital to implement heterogeneous data fusion and multimodal query in knee osteoarthritis domain. Compared to the traditional data system of XXX hospital, HMDFF implements knee osteoarthritis data fusion which was previously impossible and has very high query efficiency. The knee osteoarthritis data consists of 156.2 GB of structured data and 1.8 TB of unstructured data which mainly contains patients' X-ray scans. Oracle RDBMS processes unstructured data as Oracle LOB. It uses blob to transform scans into binary files with Base64 code and then stores them into clob type of database, based on which traditional indexes are constructed. In comparison, HMDFF utilizes embedding for compression of X-ray scans in order to construct dynamic indexes with more adaptable strategies. The experiment results of performance comparison between multimodal queries of HMDFF and queries based on Oracle RDBMS show that the fusion-based hybrid queries outperform the Oracle-based queries by 60% to 70%.

7 Conclusion

We present a framework called HMDFF based on Data Lake, implementing heterogeneous medical data fusion, index management and multimodal query. Based on the calculation capability and optimized execution plan of SparkSQL, we implement data fusion for structured and unstructured data and transform them into a merged file for further query. To represent all aspects of unstructured data, we introduce multi-version embedding with deep learning models. Dynamic index management strategies are also introduced for efficient high-dimensional feature management. Based on the fusion results, we implement multimodal query with interface for searching requirements involving both structured and unstructured data in SQL dialect.

Acknowledgements. This work was supported by Institute of Precision Medicine, Tsinghua University.

References

1. Li, T.: Enabling precision medicine by integrating multi-modal biomedical data. Georgia Institute of Technology, Atlanta, GA, USA (2021)
2. Zhang, Y., et al.: HKGB: an inclusive, extensible, intelligent, semi-auto-constructed knowledge graph framework for healthcare with clinicians' expertise incorporated. Inf. Process. Manage. **57**(6), 102324 (2020)
3. Mesterhazy, J., Olson, G., Datta, S.: High performance on-demand de-identification of a petabyte-scale medical imaging data lake. CoRR abs/ 2008.01827 (2020)
4. Qiong, C., Hao, W., Zhenmin, L., Xiao, L.: A survey on multimodal data-driven smart healthcare systems: approaches and applications. IEEE Access **7**, 133583–133599 (2019)
5. Jing, G., Peng, L., Zhikui, C., Jianing, Z.: A survey on deep learning for multimodal data fusion. Neural Comput. **32**(5), 829–864 (2020)
6. Dara, S., Tumma, P.: Feature extraction by using deep learning: a Survey. In: ICECA, pp. 1795–1801 (2018)

7. Huipeng, C., Niaoqing, H., Zhe, C., Lun, Z., Yu, Z.: A deep convolutional neural network based fusion method of two-direction vibration signal data for health state identification of planetary gearboxes. Measurement **146**, 268–278 (2019)

8. Dongjie Z., Haiwen D., Yundong S., Zhaoshuo T.: CTDGM: a data grouping model based on cache transaction for unstructured data storage systems. CoRR abs/2009.14414 (2020)

9. Yingcheng, S., Fei, G., Farhad, K., Jacono, F.J., Michael, D., Loparo, K.A.: INSMA: an integrated system for multimodal data acquisition and analysis in the intensive care unit. J. Biomed. Inf. **106**, 103434 (2020)

10. Saha, S.K., Prakash, A., Majumder, M.: Similar query was answered earlier: processing of patient authored text for retrieving relevant contents from health discussion forum. Health Inf. Sci. Syst. **7**(1), 1–9 (2019). https://doi.org/10.1007/s13755-019-0067-3

11. Hiba, A., Mossa, G., Ibrahim, A.: Al-Baltah: a hybrid semantic query expansion approach for Arabic information retrieval. J. Big Data **7**, 39 (2020)

12. Massimo, E., Emanuele, D., Aniello, M., Giuseppe, D., Hamido, F.: Hybrid query expansion using lexical resources and word embeddings for sentence retrieval in question answering. Inf. Sci. **514**, 88–105 (2020)

13. Mengyi, L., Shaoxin, L., Shiguang, S., Xilin, C.: AU-aware deep networks for facial expression recognition. In: FG, pp. 1–6 (2013)

14. Xu, Y., Mo, T., Feng, Q., Zhong, P., Lai, M., Chang, E.I.: Deep learning of feature representation with multiple instance learning for medical image analysis. In: ICASSP, pp. 1626–1630 (2014)

15. Liang, H., Sun, X., Sun, Y., Gao, Y.: Text feature extraction based on deep learning: a review. EURASIP J. Wirel. Commun. Netw. **2017**(1), 1–12 (2017). https://doi.org/10.1186/s13638-017-0993-1

16. Sitaula, C., Aryal, S.: Fusion of whole and part features for the classification of histopathological image of breast tissue. Health Inf. Sci. Syst. **8**(1), 1–12 (2020). https://doi.org/10.1007/s13755-020-00131-7

Author Index

Printed in the United States
by Baker & Taylor Publisher Services